Developing Holistic Care for Long-term Conditions

Developing Holistic Care for Long-term Conditions focuses on how to help people with long-term health conditions cope more effectively. It brings together physical and mental health, offering a holistic approach for students and practitioners in a variety of care settings.

Comprising four parts, this text introduces the policy and background to caring for people with chronic illness as well as the psychosocial impact of long-term conditions. Essential skills for practice are explored including holistic assessment, symptom control and the promotion of effective partnership between client and carer in supporting coping, recovery and end-of-life care. There is an emphasis on maximising individual health potential and resilience, with the role of nutrition, exercise, complementary therapy and spirituality considered. The focus is on client-centred care which addresses the whole person, mind and body. The extensive final part presents examples of key health issues where UK national guidelines have been published, including:

- long-term neurological conditions
- diabetes
- mental health
- cancer
- coronary heart disease
- older people.

This evidence-based book takes note of the relevant National Service Frameworks and offers an informative and pragmatic guide for all those learning about caring for the chronically ill, as well as providing a useful reference work for qualified nurses and allied health professionals.

Carl Margereson is Senior Lecturer and Programme Leader in the Faculty of Health and Human Sciences at Thames Valley University, UK.

Steve Trenoweth is Senior Lecturer in Mental Health in the Faculty of Health and Human Sciences at Thames Valley University, UK.

Developing Holistic Care for Long-term Conditions

Edited by Carl Margereson and
Steve Trenoweth

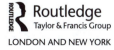

Routledge
Taylor & Francis Group

LONDON AND NEW YORK

First published 2010
by Routledge
2 Park Square, Milton Park, Abingdon, Oxon OX14 4RN

Simultaneously published in the USA and Canada
by Routledge
270 Madison Ave, New York, NY 10016

Routledge is an imprint of the Taylor & Francis Group, an informa business

Typeset in Baskerville by Wearset Ltd, Boldon, Tyne and Wear
Printed and bound in Great Britain by TJ International Ltd, Padstow, Cornwall

British Library Cataloguing in Publication Data
A catalogue record for this book is available from the British Library

Library of Congress Cataloging in Publication Data
Developing holistic care for long-term conditions/edited by Carl Margereson
and Steve Trenoweth.
p. ; cm.
Includes bibliographical references.
1. Chronic diseases–Alternative treatment. 2. Holistic medicine. 3. Holistic
nursing. I. Margereson, Carl. II. Trenoweth, Steve.
[DNLM: 1. Chronic Disease–Great Britain. 2. Evidence-Based Practice–Great
Britain. 3. Holistic Health–Great Britain. WT 500 D4885 2009]
RC108.D48 2009
616'.044–dc22   2009016674

ISBN10: 0-415-46080-8 (hbk)
ISBN10: 0-415-46081-6 (pbk)
ISBN10: 0-203-86736-X (ebk)

ISBN13: 978-0-415-46080-4 (hbk)
ISBN13: 978-0-415-46081-1 (pbk)
ISBN13: 978-0-203-86736-5 (ebk)

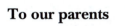

To our parents

Contents

Illustrations

Figures

Tables

Boxes

Contributors

Wasiim Allymamod BSc RN is a Staff Nurse at the West London Mental Health NHS Trust.

Tim Anstiss MB MEd DOccMed MFSEM is Principal Lecturer in Behavioural Medicine and Applied Positive Psychology in the Faculty of Health and Human Sciences at Thames Valley University.

Zoë Berry BSc(Hons) RN DN is a Lead Nurse Practitioner at the Orchard Practice, Hillingdon Primary Care Trust.

Paul Bromley PhD FESC is Lecturer in Clinical Physiology and Consultant Clinical Scientist (Cardiology) in the Department of Biological Sciences at the University of Essex.

Reverend Fr. Alan Brown MBA BSc(Hons) RGN RMN RNT AdvCert Theology is Bishop's Adviser for Hospital Chaplaincy at the Diocese of Bradford and former Senior Lecturer in the School of Healthcare at the University of Leeds.

Katie Burke MSc BSc RGN is a Lecturer Practitioner at the Royal Brompton and Harefield NHS Trust, London.

Deebs Canning MA RN PGDipN (Pall Care) PGDip (Teaching and Learning) is Lecturer at the St Joseph's Hospice/City University, London.

Shoela Detsios is Senior Lecturer in the Centre for Complementary Healthcare and Integrated Medicine at Thames Valley University.

Tim Duffy PhD BSc PGDip (Alcohol Studies) CQSW is Director of Distance Learning in the School of Health, Nursing and Midwifery at the University of the West of Scotland, Paisley.

Smita Hanciles MSc BSc is an Independent Nutritionist.

Janet Holt PhD MPhil BA(Hons) FHEA RN RM is Senior Lecturer and Head of Academic Unit as well as First Contact and Acute Care in the School of Healthcare at the University of Leeds.

Simon Jones MSc MA (Video) MA (Film) BA Hons PgCert (Teach) is Senior Lecturer (Research) in the Richard Wells Research Centre at Thames Valley University.

Breeda McManus BSc RN is Renal Consultant Nurse at Barts and The London NHS Trust.

Carl Margereson MSc BSc(Hons) DipN(Lond) CertEd RN(G) RN(M) is Senior Lecturer and Programme Leader in the Faculty of Health and Human Sciences at Thames Valley University.

Colin Martin PhD BSc RN YCAP CPsychol CSci AFBPsS is Chair in Mental Health in the School of Health, Nursing and Midwifery at the University of the West of Scotland, Paisley.

Robert Pratt CBE FRCN is Professor and Director of the Richard Wells Research Centre, Joanna Briggs Institute Collaborating Centre in the Faculty of Health and Human Sciences at Thames Valley University.

Samantha Prigmore MSc BSc(Hons) RGN is Respiratory Nurse Consultant in Chest Medicine at the St George's Healthcare Trust, London.

Jillian Riley MSc BA(Hons) RN RM is Head of Postgraduate Education (Nursing) at the Royal Brompton and Harefield NHS Trust, London.

Nicola Robinson PhD BSc(Hons) LicAc MFPHM FHEA FBAcC is Professor of Complementary Medicine and Head of the Centre for Complementary Healthcare and Integrated Medicine at Thames Valley University.

Helen Robson BSc DPSN RGN RMN RM is Lecturer in the Faculty of Health and Human Sciences at Thames Valley University.

Clair Sadler MSc, BSc, RGN, OncCert, DipCoun is Programme Leader at the School of Cancer Nursing and Rehabilitation, Royal Marsden Hospital, London.

Irrah Sibindi MA BA(Hons) RN(G) RN(M) is Senior Lecturer in the Faculty of Health and Human Sciences at Thames Valley University.

Jacqueline Sin MSc BSc(Hons) BN BGS PGCE CPN RMN RN(Psy) is the Education and Practice Lead in Psychosocial Interventions at the Berkshire Healthcare NHS Foundation Trust and Thames Valley University.

Sue Thomas BA(Hons) RN RM DN CPT is Long-term Conditions Adviser at the Nursing Department of the Royal College of Nursing.

Steve Trenoweth PhD MSc BSc(Hons) PGDipEA RMN FHEA is Senior Lecturer in Mental Health in the Faculty of Health and Human Sciences at Thames Valley University.

Swapna Williamson PhD MMEd MSc BSc LLB BA RNRM is Senior Lecturer in the Faculty of Health and Human Sciences at Thames Valley University.

Michele Wood BA(Hons) BSc DNMed is an Independent Nutritional Therapist.

Jacquie Woodcock MSc BEd RGN OncCert is Programme Leader at the School of Cancer Nursing and Rehabilitation, Royal Marsden Hospital, London.

Jan Worledge DipCOT is an Independent Occupational Therapist.

Introduction

Steve Trenoweth and Carl Margereson

> A human being is part of a whole, called by us the Universe, a part limited in time and space. He experiences himself, his thoughts and feelings, as something separated from the rest – a kind of optical delusion of his consciousness. This delusion is a kind of prison for us, restricting us to our personal desires and to affection for a few persons nearest us. Our task must be to free ourselves from this prison by widening our circles of compassion to embrace all living creatures and the whole of nature in its beauty.
>
> Albert Einstein

Modern healthcare is remarkable. Every day, dedicated, highly trained health professionals provide medical care and treatment and assist people to overcome the devastating effects of long-term illness. What is more, the biomedical model really delivers. There have been many remarkable achievements in the various fields of healthcare and the development of new and effective treatments continues apace, especially in pharmacotherapy. New medications offer relief to millions of people with long-term conditions ranging from chronic and enduring schizophrenia to HIV; new surgical interventions offer treatment with greater efficiency and in less time; and ever more specialist services are able to offer bespoke expert advice. As a result, medical interventions and treatments have increased survival rates, and overall life expectancy continues to rise.

This may seem to be an odd starting point for a book on *holism* but, as is apparent, our approach to this book is not anti-medical. Nor is our stance in any way anti-science. Many of the authors of the chapters are clinicians who are not only embedded in clinical 'reality' but actively draw upon empirical research to inform their discussion. Without question, medical science has been enormously successful in treating illness and disease and there is much to celebrate. However, much of the success of medical care and treatment, of course, comes from advances in understanding the germ theory of diseases and from isolating, caring for and treating *parts* of the body. Such developments have been accompanied by (and have perhaps even been necessitated by) an emphasis on reductionism, rationality, scientific objectivity and a persistence of Cartesian separation of the mind and the body. It has become clear that the medical model has become limited in its ability to account for, and respond to, the totality of the lived experience of the individual, and as such is inadequate in improving the overall sense of health and well-being of people. For example, medical explanations of disease processes continue to be accounted for by linear models and simplified unicausality at a time when the modern world has increased the complexity of lives. Traditional communities have been replaced by modern societies, and the erosion of family and social networks and a concomitant sense of isolation have become implicated in the development of psychological distress.

With growing expertise in medical areas has come increasing and inevitable specialisms, which has tended to also bring with it a disparate set of assumptions and ideologies about health and illness among healthcare practitioners, demarcated along professional lines. Expert healthcare practitioners may often find themselves 'living out their existence next door to each other but in altogether different subjective worlds' (Kelly 1955/1991, 56). Individuals and carers, likewise, may feel excluded from this increasing technological world and as such are in danger of being mere passive bystanders in their own care, or the care of their loved ones.

There is, therefore, an increasing awareness of gaps in the provision of modern medicine, and in the knowledge needed to participate in one's own care. People with long-term mental health problems, for example, often have poor access to specialist health services where diagnostic overshadowing may lead to a misinterpretation of physical symptoms as psychiatric phenomena. Further, many patients feel that modern medical services lack responsiveness to the totality of their healthcare-related needs, particularly mental health service users and those with functional health-related issues. Medical sociologists, such as Ivan Illich (1975), have argued that an exclusive interpretation of ill-health in purely medical terms attributes blame for an individual's illness or disease to factors located within the lifestyle choices they have made, rather than as a consequence of social and environmental factors brought about by industrialised societies. Furthermore, there is increasing evidence that social, psychological, emotional and even psychiatric factors are implicated in the aetiology and trajectory of physical illnesses. There is also much evidence that well-delivered holistic care where people feel connected with and involved in their own treatment have better clinical outcomes (Hassed 2004).

What is holism?

Holism is by no means a new concept but holism in a modern healthcare context seems to focus our attention on something that the Western world has lost – the care and treatment of the *whole person* (Shorter 2005) – for an holistic approach to life is an important concept within Islamic and Eastern religions (Rassool 2000). This has also been an essential component of the worldview of many ancient cultures, such as Australian Aborigines, Native Americans, Greeks and Chinese (Owen and Holmes 1993; Patterson 1998).

In the West, throughout the twentieth century there have been many who have recognised the potential value of holism, either directly or indirectly. For example, Jan Smuts, whose 1926 book *Holism and Evolution* encompassed the notion of wholeness being 'an inherent character of the universe', is often credited with giving us our modern conception of *holism*. Furthermore, the 'individual psychology' of Alfred Adler stressed the importance of understanding the individual as being embedded within the larger wholes of society, from interpersonal relationships to the social groups to which he belongs and ultimately to the larger whole of mankind, while in 1955, the psychologist George Kelly, in *The Psychology of Personal*

Constructs, recognised the interconnetedness of feelings, thoughts and behaviour. In 1977, George Engel sought a 'bio-psycho-social' model as a means of integrating the mind and body while recognising the social context of illness. Ludwig von Berta- lanffy, who was to have an influence on Engel, recognised the complexity of biologi- cal and social systems, and, more recently, James Lovelock in *Homage to Gaia* (2001) viewed the Earth as a complex, single and interconnected organism.

The term *holism* is used at times synonymously with the 'New Age' spiritual move- ment – which is not the focus of this book. The definition of holism that underpins this book is an approach and ideology which embraces all aspects of a person's func- tioning in an attempt to meet the healthcare needs and expectations. This encom- passes their physical, psychological, emotional and social aspects of self and the personal meaning that is attached to their experiences of health and illness. Such lived aspects are seen to be systemically interrelated and integrated, and contribute to the connectedness and wholeness of one's lived experience in healthcare terms. Furthermore, a holistic model of illness assumes multi-factorial aetiology and an array of influences on the trajectory, course and experience of health and illness. As such, optimal health outcomes require an integrated and holistic approach. Above all, 'holism is an aspiration, a direction' (Fulder 2005, 775) requiring attentiveness, skill and empathic understanding by those who seek to help the person in need.

Dualism is alive and well

However, we *should* be cautious about holism – the claims of holism can be over- stated and mired in fuzzy thinking and a poor evidence base. There is indeed much work to be done to demonstrate the effectiveness of this approach and there are many who remain unconvinced about the usefulness of the approach, arguing that holism is unaffordable and untenable given the increasing focus on quick 'fixes' to mind and body. If the holistic argument is to be won, and attempts to develop integ- rated and holistic care come to fruition, there is a need to demonstrate its relevance and value (real and potential) to service users and modern healthcare practitioners from differing disciplinary backgrounds. This book represents not an attempt to demedicalise modern healthcare, and a surrendering of the benefits that medical care has brought about, but an endeavour to suggest a symbiosis between various clinical approaches and ideologies while reconciling objective and subjective health- care 'realities'. In a world experiencing rapid change and an increasingly complex modern healthcare context which seeks to empower patients and service users, we may argue that such an approach is not only desirable but inevitable and essential.

References

Barker, P. (2003) The Tidal Model: Psychiatric Colonisation, Recovery and the Paradigm Shift in Mental Health Care. *Journal of Psychiatric and Mental Health Nursing*, 12, 96–102.

Engel, G. (1977) The Need for a New Medical Model: A Challenge for Biomedicine. *Science*, 196, 129–136.

Flaming, D. (2001) Duelling Dualisms: A Response to Thorne's 'People and Their Parts: Deconstructing the Debates Theorising Nursing's Clients'. *Nursing Philosophy*, 2, 263–265.

Fulder, S. (2005) Remembering the Holistic View. *Journal of Alternative and Complementary Med- icine*, 11(5), 775–776.

Hassed, C. (2004) Bringing Holism into Mainstream Biomedical Education. *Journal of Alternative and Complementary Medicine*, 10(2), 405–407.

Illich, I. (1975) *Medical Nemesis*. London: Calder & Boyars.

Kelly, G. (1955/1991) *The Psychology of Personal Constructs. Volume 1: Theory and Personality*. London: Routledge.

Kunitz, S. (2002) Holism and the Idea of General Susceptibility to Disease. *International Journal of Epidemiology*, 31, 722–729.

Lovelock, J. (2001) *Homage to Gaia: The Life of an Independent Scientist*. Oxford: Oxford University Press.

Owen, M. and Holmes, C. (1993) Holism in the Discourse of Nursing. *Journal of Advanced Nursing*, 18, 1688–1695.

Patterson, E. (1998) The Philosophy and Physics of Holistic Health Care: Spiritual Healing as a Workable Interpretation. *Journal of Advanced Nursing*, 17, 287–293.

Rassool, G.H. (2000) The Crescent and Islam: Healing, Nursing and the Spiritual Dimension. Some Considerations Towards an Understanding of the Islamic Perspectives on Caring. *Journal of Advanced Nursing*, 32(6), 1476–1454.

Shealy, C. (2003) Holism in Evolution. *Journal of Alternative and Complementary Medicine*, 9(3), 333–334.

Part I

Overview of holistic care

Introduction

Part I introduces a life course approach and psychosocial models of health to explain not only the aetiology of disorders but the many factors possibly contributing to recovery, chronic illness adjustment and death. Changing demographics and improved life expectancy with increasing numbers of older people often with co-morbid physical and mental health problems are explored. These developments are considered within the context of ongoing societal changes where lifestyle choices will increasingly challenge our ideas of community and caring.

For those living with an ongoing physical or mental health problem or indeed both, adjustment is necessary. For many people such adjustment is not always easy. Optimising symptom control alone will not increase the effectiveness of coping. In Chapter 2, Carl Margereson shows that we ignore people's thoughts, attitudes, feelings and behaviours regarding their health at our peril not least owing to the negative impact that psychological and social issues may have on the trajectory of the chronic illness. The principles of psychoneuroimmunology are introduced to demonstrate to readers the link between chronic stress and ill-health while focusing in particular on uncertainty, loss, changing identities, self-efficacy and disability.

In Chapter 3, policy initiatives driving the health and social care service changes regarding long-term conditions are explored along with initiatives designed to develop a more integrated and systematic approach to chronic illness. Models of care delivery drawing on international experiences are considered including

Wagner's Chronic Illness Model and Kaiser Permanente. Policy, however, does not take shape in a vacuum and cannot be carried out by health and social care agencies alone, and questions about user movements and increased expectations and caring in the future are also raised.

The care and treatment of people with chronic ill-health raises a number of ethical dilemmas. Chapter 4 explores such issues and considers the notion of autonomy and legal and ethical frameworks, and the resultant difficulties which may be encountered not least in the area of consent and choice. Janet Holt reflects on the withdrawal of treatment as well as overt/covert rationing of care in chronic illness and the crucial role of shared decision-making in all these areas. Advanced directives and power of attorney are also considered.

1 Epidemiology and aetiology of long-term conditions

Carl Margereson and Steve Trenoweth

Introduction

The terms 'long-term condition', 'long-standing disorder', 'chronic illness' and 'chronic disease' all refer to those health problems that are prolonged, do not resolve spontaneously, and are rarely completely cured (Dowrick *et al.* 2005). According to the Department of Health, in the United Kingdom (with a population of 61 million), approximately 17.5 million people have a long-term condition. Chronic illness is a significant health issue not least owing to the rising numbers of people with long-term health problems and the spiralling financial impact. World-wide, the prevalence of all the leading chronic diseases is increasing (World Health Organisation 2005) and although this book focuses mainly on the UK experience it is important to remember that numbers are greater in developing countries and are projected to rise substantially over the next two decades and beyond. Unfortunately, it appears that poorer countries are inheriting the problems of more affluent nations including diets rich in calories and fats, sedentary behaviour, increasing exposure to urban stresses, and the harmful consequences of tobacco, alcohol, drug use, accidents, suicide and violence (Holroyd and Creer 1986).

Life expectancy

Life expectancy in the UK has been increasing steadily and currently stands at 77.2 years for men and 81.5 years for women (ONS 2008) – the highest since records began. A number of factors have led to increased life expectancy including reduced infant mortality, obvious advances in medical knowledge, treatment, interventions and the development of skilled healthcare practitioners. Improved public health in the UK has also made a major contribution to life expectancy and there have, of course, been improvements in housing, sanitation and nutrition, with a decline in absolute poverty.

There is a price to be paid, however, for such longevity as it may bring with it a potential for an increased prevalence of age-related chronic disease. With increased longevity the primary causes of death and disability are conditions such as degenerative health problems (e.g. dementia), cardiovascular disease (heart disease and stroke), cancer and chronic respiratory disease, all affecting the older person more than the young. In 2005 the General Household Survey pronounced cardiovascular disease as the most commonly reported long-standing illness after musculoskeletal conditions (ONS 2005). However, while there is an increased likelihood and prevalence of such health problems, it must not be assumed that older people are all experiencing major chronic health problems or activity limitations (Kronenfeld 2006).

Co-morbidity

As medicine developed as a profession it was believed that the 'mind' had very little influence over the 'body', and over the years this dominant view has had a significant effect on healthcare delivery. One consequence is that there is often a tendency to consider physical health and mental health quite separately as a clear line of demarcation tends to exist between medical and psychiatric health services. Yet people with severe mental ill-health can also experience 'co-morbid' physical health problems, and having a severe and ongoing physical illness can significantly increase the likelihood of developing psychiatric problems (Cooke *et al.* 2007). Clients with long-term conditions may have very complex needs, but health services are often one-dimensional in their outlook (that is, they concentrate on either the medical or psychiatric but not both).

The reductive simplification of clients' problems can mean that significant aspects of their *whole* person (their psychological, social, emotional, biological or spiritual worlds) may be overlooked and, as a consequence, the holistic healthcare needs of clients may not be met effectively. It has been argued that such an artificial division between mental and physical illness is not only archaic and deeply misleading but incompatible with contemporary understanding of disease (Kendall 2001). The following section will help to show how important it is to consider both the mental health and physical health of clients with long-term conditions.

Prevalence of co-morbid mental and physical ill-health

About one in six adults aged 16 to 74 have mental health problems such as depression, anxiety or phobias while five in 1000 people were assessed in a single year as probably having schizophrenia and bipolar disorders (ONS 2001). Serious mental illness affects up to 3 per cent of the population in the United Kingdom and it is estimated that approximately 450 million people worldwide have a mental health problem (World Health Organisation 2001). However, there are many more people with long-term chronic and disabling conditions who experience mental distress which is not diagnosed, recognised or treated.

For example, the presentation of depression in the UK population has increased dramatically over recent decades and this has been accompanied by a decrease in the age of onset, with more cases being reported in children, adolescents and young adults (Mental Health Foundation 2006). Although the World Health Organisation (WHO) has highlighted depression as the second most common and economically costly long-term condition that will affect non-medically ill people globally over the next decades, depression is likely to be unrecognised and under-treated, particularly in primary care (Ballenger *et al.* 2001).

With the focus often on physical decline and physical health issues in the older person, together with an assumption that cognitive decline is inevitable, there is often a lack of awareness about the mental health of older people (DoH/CSIP 2005). This may result in mental health problems not being identified or referred to specialist mental health practitioners. However, 40 per cent of older people attending a GP and 50 per cent who are general hospital in-patients have a co-morbid mental health problem (most commonly depression, dementia or acute confusion). In care homes it is estimated that 60 to 70 per cent of residents have some form of dementia and 40 per cent have depression, and in the general community depression affects 15 per cent of older people with 5 per cent of those over 65 years affected by dementia (Department of Health/CSIP 2005). Out of 100,000 older people there will be 60 with ongoing mental illness such as chronic schizophrenia or relapsing mood disorder. Older women have twice the levels of depression as men and higher levels of anxiety and, sadly, women over the age of 55 account for over one-third of female suicides (Samaritans 2008).

Unfortunately, when compared with the general population, people with serious diagnosed mental health problems and learning disabilities have increased rates of physical illness and their overall physical health is poor (Harris and Barraclough 1998; Phelan *et al.* 2001; Robson *et al.* 2008). The Disability Rights Commission (DRC 2006) has recently drawn attention to the physical health inequalities experienced by people with mental health problems and those with learning disabilities. Many physical disorders including heart disease, diabetes and chronic respiratory disease are more likely to occur at a younger age in people with serious mental health problems, and who once diagnosed are more likely to die within five years compared with the general population (Harris and Barraclough 1998; DRC 2006). Sudden death caused by cardiac disease is three times as likely in patients with schizophrenia compared to the general population (Casey *et al.* 2004; Jindal *et al.* 2005) and there is an increased prevalence of chronic obstructive pulmonary disease (chronic bronchitis and emphysema) in people with serious mental disorders (Himelhoch *et al.* 2004). It is unacceptable that, on average, people with schizophrenia can expect to live ten years less than someone without a mental health problem (Mentality/NIMHE 2004) and, while it is true that suicide and accidental death contributes to this, mortality due to poor physical health is common (Jones *et al.* 2004)

When we consider people with physical health problems, a similar picture emerges in terms of co-morbidity, with mood disturbance and emotional difficulties common. For many individuals, mood changes are mild and do not affect coping ability. For others, severe mood disturbance may result in significant adjustment difficulties with increased disability and psychiatric co-morbidity. The Royal College of Physicians and Royal College of Psychiatrists reported in 1995 that at least 25 per cent of medical hospital patients have problems with adjustment and a further 15 to 18 per cent have anxiety and depression (RCP 1995). They also concluded that health providers in general medical care settings were often unable to carry out basic psychological assessments to detect problem areas.

There has been a great deal of research which has identified circumstances where physical illness is complicated by mental health issues. Depressed patients, for example, are twice as likely as non-depressed patients to have a major cardiac event within the first 12 months (Carney *et al.* 1988), and they are significantly more likely to die in the years following the diagnosis (Barefoot *et al.* 1996). Heart failure affects approximately 707,000 people over the age of 45 in the UK (Allender *et al.* 2008) and is the most frequent cause of hospitalisation. Major depression is present in 17 to 37 per cent of patients with heart failure and minor depression in 16 to 22 per cent (Freedland *et al.* 2003). Depression in patients with heart failure increases further their risk in terms of ongoing physical health and death (Jiang *et al.* 2001). In those with end-stage renal disease depression is identified as the most common psychiatric illness but its prevalence varies widely in different studies and populations (Kimmel 2001).

Chronic respiratory illness is common in the UK and when all these disorders are considered together, deaths from respiratory problems are greater than those due to heart disease. There is an increased prevalence of depression in patients with COPD (Yohannes *et al.* 2003), and in asthma, rates of psychiatric disorders, particularly anxiety and depression, have been shown to be up to six times more prevalent (16 to 52 per cent for anxiety, 14 to 41 per cent for depression), compared to rates observed in the general population (Netjeck *et al.* 2001; Lavoie *et al.* 2006). Psychosocial factors (that is, factors related to psychological phenomena and the social environment) can lead to disease changes in the body (Hemingway and Marmot 1999), and in people with asthma are known to contribute to poor control of symptoms, more accident and emergency admissions and increased risk of death (British Thoracic Society and Scottish Intercollegiate Guidelines Network 2008).

Stroke is a catastrophic event and depression is considered to occur in at least a quarter of patients in the first year (Hackett *et al.* 2005). In those with Parkinson's disease depression is one of the most common psychiatric disturbances reported and is often unrecognised (Aarsland *et al.* 1999), even though prevalence is thought to be around 40 to 45 per cent in both sexes. Depression is the most common mental disorder in multiple sclerosis and, with a lifetime prevalence of about 25 to 50 per cent (Minden and Schiffer 1990) is about three times higher than the rate in the general population.

Aetiology and risk factors for long-term conditions

Epidemiologists are not only involved in identifying how many people have long-term disorders but are also interested in why they develop them in the first place. Although a number of disease risk factors have been identified in research terms these are often statistical associations (or correlations) rather than definitive scientific 'cause and effect' proof. This might mean that an identified risk factor (such as lack of exercise) may be a cause *or* a consequence of a long-term condition (for example, coronary heart disease). Furthermore, risk factors are simply that – an indication that a phenomenon is associated with an increased *likelihood* but it is not a *certainty* that someone will develop a particular health-related problem as a consequence. For example, a significant number of heavy smokers will go on to develop chronic lung disease, but some will not, and not everyone who has high cholesterol, high blood pressure and smokes will develop cardiovascular disease, but many will. Even where there is a genetic predisposition for a disease this may manifest in some but not in others. The language of aetiology in long-term conditions is often one of probabilities and possibilities.

There is much that is not yet understood regarding the aetiology of health problems and perhaps the search for a single or simple cause (or causes) is too reductive to account for the complexity of long-term conditions. Instead of looking at biological risk factors in isolation, many epidemiologists are now looking at what happens during each life stage we pass through, from conception to old age, and the many complex factors we are exposed to during our lifetime which may contribute to the development of later ill-health.

Many support the view that we are exposed to risk the very moment we are conceived and as we grow in the uterus. These so-called 'early life' theories argue that the foetus is 'programmed' to develop adult disease later in life (Barker 1995) and there is evidence to support this. Good antenatal health is important for both intellectual development and adult health. Yet there are countless adverse factors that could increase the risk to both mother and foetus by causing complex biological changes, possibly resulting in both physical and mental health problems. However, poor health in adulthood cannot simply be due to problems during pregnancy alone. Indeed, epidemiologists have puzzled over this, and risk factors that we are exposed to during different stages of our life have become an important area of research. Scientists refer to this as a 'life-course' approach and recognise that there are many complex biopsychosocial factors involved. Although physical and social exposures are indeed considered important in foetal development, it is also argued that the long-term effects of physical and social exposures during childhood, adolescence, young adulthood and later adulthood should also be considered (Ben-Shlomo and Kuh 2002). The influence of childhood experiences on adult health should not be underestimated, with studies showing a strong association with childhood socioeconomic position in a number of areas (e.g. obesity, depression, health behaviours) independent of adult socioeconomic position (Kuh and Shlomo 2004).

It is in the area of heart disease that most research regarding risk factors has tended to focus and it is now accepted that high blood pressure, high cholesterol and smoking are independent risk factors for the development of cardiovascular disease. Since these early epidemiological studies, additional risk factors including dietary and activity factors have emerged and some of these will be considered in later chapters. But although we need to be aware of risk factors in order to reduce individual risk, we cannot consider this in isolation, and psychosocial factors and socioeconomic status appear to affect risk accumulation over the lifespan.

Professor Michael Marmot, a well-known epidemiologist, led a research project studying male civil servants known as the Whitehall Study (Marmot *et al.* 1978). The British Civil Service was chosen because workers are clearly separated into different grades with administrators at the top and messengers at the bottom. Marmot was interested in exploring the differences in health risk between high-status and low-status workers and demonstrated that death rates were higher in the lower grades, particularly for coronary heart disease. Contributing to this increased risk were factors such as obesity, smoking, high blood pressure, low physical activity and shorter height. Although much of this came as no real surprise, further statistical analysis revealed that these risk factors alone could not explain why there was greater cardiovascular disease mortality in the lower grades.

In a follow-up study (Whitehall II) both men and women were included, and the researchers were surprised to find that in the lower grades both sexes had poorer health compared to higher grade workers, but this was restricted not only to cardiovascular disease but also to some cancers, chronic lung disease, gastrointestinal problems, depression, suicide, sickness absence, back pain and self-reported feelings of ill-health (Marmot *et al.* 1991). What emerged was that not only was social position important but also complex psychosocial and behavioural pathways. Although the Whitehall II study initially investigated the relationships between work, stress and health, other areas are now considered significant. Differences between social groups may be related not only to the organisation of work and the work climate, but also to social influences beyond the work setting, influences from early life, and health behaviours which are largely socially determined. Social inequalities in health are an interesting area of study for epidemiologists, particularly how adult health and disease are influenced by socially patterned exposure during life. A major finding is that risks to health from poor socioeconomic circumstances accumulate over the life course (Graham 2002; Kuh *et al.* 2004).

In the United Kingdom, for research purposes the population is stratified according to occupation, and such social grouping provides information regarding the economic resources individuals have at their disposal. Social class based on occupational grouping can affect health in many different ways including work-related factors, housing, education and social standing and relationships. Exposure to physical hazards and stressful life conditions is more likely in the residential and occupational environments of manual socioeconomic groups (Bartley and Blane 1997). Low income throughout adult life can lead to poorer physical and mental health and is a strong predictor of mortality (Lynch *et al.* 1997). The constant stress experienced by individuals who are socially disadvantaged can be detrimental to their health.

Psychosocial aspects of health and illness

The development of long-term health problems may be due to differences in individual resilience. Resilience may be defined as the latent resources that can be activated in times of stress to aid in returning to a previous state following stress or trauma (Bergeman and Wallace 1999). How resilient a person is will be determined by both individual characteristics (based in part at least on a genetic predisposition) but also, and crucially, on social, cultural and environmental factors.

How we feel about ourselves and the situations in which we find ourselves has a significant impact on our health status. We know, for example, that those individuals who perceive life events as stressful have been found to have more health problems (Adler and Mathews 1994). Psychologists over the years have identified various components of our personality which are known to influence our physical and mental health. These are relevant not only when considering the possible reasons why people get sick in the first place, but in how they can influence coping ability in those living with a long-term health problem. It is during childhood and adolescence that some of these psychological attributes develop and which help to confer advantage with regard to positive health experiences in later life.

Certainly, how we perceive and respond to our environment can directly affect our health status, and our emotions are significant in this respect. For example, aspects of our personality have been found to have a negative effect on health with 'anger/hostility' associated with chronic over-stimulation of the sympathetic nervous system (Keefe *et al.* 1986). During rest, our parasympathetic nervous system normally dominates but with sustained sympathetic arousal as a result of negative emotions can result in increased heart rate and blood pressure causing adverse effects. The key role that self-confidence has on our health has been studied extensively. The psychologist Albert Bandura (Bandura 1977) suggests that belief in our own ability to succeed, which he refers to as our sense of 'self-efficacy', can play a major role in how we approach goals, tasks and challenges. A strong sense of efficacy enhances human accomplishment and personal well-being in many ways. Therefore, where there is pessimism and a sense of hopelessness, individuals may feel that they are unable to control events in their life. Consequently the accompanying negative emotions and subsequent behaviour can impact negatively on health.

Negative emotions outlined in the previous paragraph and anxiety and depression can also bring about biological changes in the body, demonstrating further that the mind and body are most definitely linked. The complex interplay of the mind (psyche), neurohormonal activation and immune system is a major focus in psycho-neuroimmunology, and studies have demonstrated many negative health outcomes as a result of chronic stress. The stress response is activated when there is additional demand placed upon us, particularly when this is sustained over a period of time. This physiological stress response involves complex neurohormonal pathways which can affect the immune system, increasing vulnerability in terms of poorer health.

Such chronic negative emotional states are associated with the release of inflammatory markers. Cytokines, for example, are molecules released by many different cell types, which by and large have a useful regulatory role in the body. Some cytokines released during chronic stress (e.g. interleukin 6) are linked to the inflammatory changes in cardiac disease and can increase the production of C-reactive protein, an important risk factor for myocardial infarction (Papanicolaou *et al.* 1998; Appels *et al.* 2000; Kiechl *et al.* 2001; Kiecolt-Glaser *et al.* 2003; Rozanski *et al.* 2005). Nor is it only cardiac disease where these cytokines have been found to have a more sinister role. Inflammatory changes linked to cytokines have also been identified in osteoporosis, arthritis, type 2 diabetes and some cancers (Ershler and Keller 2000). Kiecolt-Glaser *et al.* (2002) have also identified a relationship between chronic stressors, psychiatric syndromes/symptoms and altered immune function.

As well as the importance of individual characteristics influencing resilience, also important for the promotion of mental and physical well-being is the social environment. How individuals in communities feel in terms of participation and emotional well-being may be a critical factor in determining health (Kawachi *et al.* 1997; Cooper *et al.* 1999). Factors such as low social support as well as intense, individualised competitiveness, alcohol use and high social conflict in families/communities where individuals cannot escape from each other can have a detrimental impact on health (Gilbert 2006).

'Social capital' is an important concept in social epidemiology and stems from the social relationships within society, referring to social organisation and integration, including the quantity and quality of formal and informal social interactions, civic participation, norms of reciprocity and trust in others (De Silva *et al.* 2005). It is the perceived social support which is seen as a significant factor in 'buffering' the impact of chronic stress experienced by individuals. Positive social encounters can assist in the development of those individual characteristics outlined above including positive attitudes, values, self-esteem, self-efficacy, social and cognitive skills, and coping behaviours generally. As such, the aetiology of long-term conditions may well have roots in an individual's psychological world and social environment, and it follows, therefore, that the care and treatment of such clients requires a holistic and multi-factorial response.

Conclusion

Life expectancy in the UK continues to increase due to a range of factors. However, a consequence of increased longevity is a concomitant increase in chronic illness, and it is currently estimated that 17.5 million people have a long-term condition. However, health services are often clearly demarcated, for example, along medical and psychiatric lines, which can mean that significant aspects of a *whole* person (their psychological, social, emotional, medical or spiritual worlds) may be over-looked. As a consequence, the needs of people with co-morbid conditions may not be met effectively. Moreover, the aetiology of long-term conditions is complex and may not only be a reflection of pathophysiological changes within the body, but may also be rooted in an individual's psychological world and social environment over the life stages. It follows, therefore, that the care and treatment of such clients requires a holistic and multi-factorial response in assessing needs and assisting people to cope with long-term conditions. Such themes are explored throughout this book.

References

Aarsland, D., Larsen, J.P., Lim, N.G. *et al.* (1999) Range of Neuropsychiatric Disturbances in Patients with Parkinson's Disease. *Journal of Neurology, Neurosurgery and Psychiatry*, 67, 492–496.

Adler, N. and Mathews, K. (1994) Health Psychology: Why Do Some People Get Sick and Some Stay Well? *Annual Review of Psychology*, 45, 229–259.

Allender, S., Peto, V. and Scarborough, P. (2008) Coronary Heart Disease Statistics. *British Heart Foundation*. Online. Available at: www.heartstats.org/homepage.asp (accessed 23 February 2009).

Appels, A., Bar, F.W., Bruggeman, C. *et al.* (2000) Inflammation, Depressive Symptomatology and Coronary Artery Disease. *Psychosomatic Medicine*, 61, 378–386.

Ballenger, J.C., Davidson, J.R.T., Lecrubier, T. *et al.* (2001) Consensus Statement on Transcultural Issues in Depression and Anxiety from the International Consensus Group on Depression and Anxiety. *Journal of Clinical Psychiatry*, 62, 47–55.

Bandura, A. (1977) Toward a Unifying Theory of Behavioral Change. *Psychological Review*, 84, 191–215.

Barefoot, J.C., Helms, M.J., Mark, D.B. *et al.* (1996) Depression and Long-term Mortality Risk in Patients with Coronary Artery Disease. *American Journal of Cardiology*, 78, 613–617.

Barker, D.J.P. (1995) Fetal Origins of Coronary Heart Disease. *British Medical Journal*, 311, 171–174.

Bartley, M. and Blane, D. (1997) Health and the Life Course; Why Safety Nets Matter. *British Medical Journal*, 314, 1194–1196.

Ben-Shlomo, Y. and Kuh, D. (2002) A Life Course Approach to Chronic Disease Epidemiology: Conceptual Models, Empirical Challenges and Interdisciplinary Perspectives. *International Journal of Epidemiology*, 31, 285–293.

Bergeman, C.S. and Wallace, K.A. (1999) Resiliency in Later Life. In: Whitman, T.L., Merluzzi, T.V. and White, R.D. (eds) *Life Span Perspectives on Health and Illness* (pp. 207–225). London: Lawrence Erlbaum Associates.

British Thoracic Society and Scottish Intercollegiate Guidelines Network (2008) *British Guideline on the Management of Asthma*. *British Thoracic Society*. Online. Available at: www.brit-thoracic.org.uk/ClinicalInformation/Asthma/AsthmaGuidelines/tabid/83/Default.aspx (accessed 23 February 2009).

Carney, R.M., Rich, M.W., Freedland, K.E. *et al.* (1988) Depressive Disorder Predicts Cardiac Events in Patients with Coronary Artery Disease. *Psychosomatic Medicine*, 50, 627–633.

Casey, D.E., Haupt, D.W., Newcomer, J.W. *et al.* (2004) Antipsychotic Induced Weight Gain and Metabolic Abnormalities: Implications for Increased Mortality in Patients with Schizophrenia. *Journal of Clinical Psychiatry*, 65(7), 257–269.

Cooke, D., Newman, S., Sacker, A. *et al.* (2007) The Impact of Physical Illnesses and Non-psychotic Psychiatric Morbidity: Data from the Household Survey of Psychiatric Morbidity in Great Britain. *British Journal of Health Psychology*, 12, 463–471.

Cooper, H., Arber, S., Fee, L. *et al.* (1999) *The Influence of Social Support and Social Capital on Health.* London: Health Education Authority.

De Silva, M.J., McKenzie, K., Harpham, T. *et al.* (2005) Social Capital and Mental Illness: A Systematic Review. *Journal of Epidemiology and Community Health*, 59, 619–627.

Department of Health/Care Services Improvement Partnership (DoH/CSIP) (2005) *Everybody's Business.* Online. Available at: http://kc.csip.org.uk/upload/everybodysbusiness.pdf (accessed 20 February 2009).

Disability Rights Commission (DRC) (2006) *Equal Treatment: Closing the Gap.* Online. Available at: www.drc.gov.uk/library/health_investigation.aspx (accessed 15 January 2009).

Dowrick, C., Dixon-Woods, M., Holman, H. *et al.* (2005) What is Chronic Illness? *Chronic Illness*, 1, 1–6.

Ershler, W. and Keller, E. (2000) Age-associated Increased Interleukin-6 Gene Expression, Late Life Diseases and Frailty. *Annual Review of Medicine*, 51, 245–270.

Freedland, K.E., Rich, M.W., Skala, J.A. *et al.* (2003) Prevalence of Depression in Hospitalised Patients with Congestive Heart Failure. *Psychosomatic Medicine*, 65, 119–128.

Gilbert, P. (2006) Evolution and Depression: Issues and Implications. *Psychological Medicine*, 36, 287–297.

Graham, H. (2002) Building an Inter Disciplinary Science of Health Inequalities: The Example of Lifecourse Research. *Social Science Medicine*, 55, 2005–2016.

Hackett, M.L., Yapa, C., Parag, V. *et al.* (2005) Frequency of Depression after Stroke: A Systematic Review of Observational Studies. *Stroke*, 36, 1330–1340.

Harris, E.C. and Barraclough, B. (1998) Excess Mortality of Mental Disorder. *British Journal of Psychiatry*, 173, 11–53.

Hemingway, H. and Marmot, M. (1999) Evidence Based Cardiology: Psychosocial Factors in the Aetiology and Prognosis of Coronary Heart Disease: Systematic Review of Prospective Cohort Studies. *British Medical Journal*, 318, 1460–1467.

Himelhoch, S., Lehman, A., Kreyenbuhl, J. *et al.* (2004) Prevalence of Chronic Obstructive Pulmonary Disease Among Those with Serious Mental Illness. *American Journal of Psychiatry*, 161, 2317–2319.

Holroyd, K.A. and Creer, T.L. (1986) *Self Management of Chronic Disease; A Handbook of Clinical Interventions and Research.* Orlando: Academic Press.

Jiang, W., Alexander, J., Christopher, E. *et al.* (2001) Effect of Depression on Mortality and Morbidity in Patients with Congestive Heart Failure. *Archives of Internal Medicine*, 161, 1849–1856.

Jindal, R., Mackenzie, E.M., Baker, G.B. *et al.* (2005) Cardiac Risk and Schizophrenia. *Journal of Psychiatry Neuroscience*, 30(6), 393–395.

Jones, D.R., Macias, C., Barreira, P.J. *et al.* (2004) Prevalence, Severity and Co-occurrence of Chronic Physical Health Problems of Persons with Serious Mental Illness. *Psychiatric Services*, 55, 1250–1257.

Kawachi, I., Kennedy, B. and Lochner, K. (1997) Social Capital, Income Inequality and Mortality. *American Journal of Public Health*, 87, 491–498.

Keefe, F.J., Castell, P.J. and Blumenthal, J.A. (1986) Angina Pectoris in Type A and Type B Cardiac Patients. *Pain*, 27, 211–218.

Kendall, R.E. (2001) The Distinction between Mental and Physical Illness. *British Journal of Psychiatry*, 178, 490–493.

Kiechl, S., Egger, G., Mayr, M. *et al.* (2001) Chronic Infections and the Risk of Carotid Atherosclerosis: Prospective Results from a Large Population Study. *Circulation*, 103, 1064–1070.

Kiecolt-Glaser, J.K., McGuire, L., Robles, T.F. *et al.* (2002) Psychoneuroimmunology and Psychosomatic Medicine: Back to the Future. *Psychosomatic Medicine*, 64, 15–28.

Kiecolt-Glaser, J.K., Preacher, K.J., MacCallum, R.C. *et al.* (2003) Chronic Stress and Age-related Increases in the Proinflammatory Cytokine IL-6. *Proceedings of the National Academy of Sciences U.S.A.*, 100, 9090–9095.

Kimmel, P.L. (2001) Psychosocial Factors in Dialysis Patients. *Kidney International*, 59, 1599–1613.

Kronenfeld, J.J. (2006) Changing Conceptions of Health and Life Course Concepts. *Health*. 10, 501–517.

Kuh, D. and Shlomo, Y. (2004) Socioeconomic Pathways between Childhood and Adult Health. In: Kuh, D. and Shlomo, Y. (eds) *A Life Course Approach to Chronic Disease Epidemiology*. Oxford: Oxford University Press.

Lavoie, K.L., Bacon, S.L., Barone, S. *et al.* (2006) What is Worse for Asthma Control and Quality of Life: Depressive Disorders, Anxiety Disorders, or Both? *Chest*, 130, 1039–1047.

Lynch, J.W., Kaplan, G.A. and Shema, S.J. (1997) Cumulative Impact of Sustained Economic Hardship on Physical, Cognitive, Psychological and Social Functioning. *New England Journal of Medicine*, 337, 1889–1895.

Marmot, M.G., Davey Smith, G., Stansfield, S. *et al.* (1991) Health Inequalities Among British Civil Servants: The Whitehall II Study. *Lancet*, 337, 1387–1393.

Marmot, M.G., Rose, G., Shipley, M. *et al.* (1978) Employment Grade and Coronary Heart Disease in British Civil Servants. *Journal of Epidemiology and Community Health*, 32, 244–249.

Mental Health Foundation (2006) *Feeding Minds: The Impact of Food on Mental Health*. Online. Available at: www.mentalhealth.org.uk/campaigns/food-and-mental-health/ (accessed 10 November 2008).

Mentality/NIMHE (2004) *Healthy Body and Mind: Promoting Healthy Living for People who Experience Mental Distress*. Online. Available at: www.neyh.csip.org.uk/silo/files/hbhmprimary-care.pdf (accessed 24 February 2009).

Minden, S.L. and Schiffer, R.B. (1990) Affective Disorders in Multiple Sclerosis. Review and Recommendations for Clinical Research. *Archives of Neurology*, 54, 531–533.

Netjeck, V., Brown, E., Khan, D. *et al.* (2001) Prevalence of Mood Disorders and Relationship to Asthma Severity in Patients at an Inner-city Asthma Clinic. *Annals of Allergy, Asthma and Immunology*, 87, 129–133.

Office for National Statistics (ONS) (2001) *Psychiatric Morbidity among Adults Living in Private Households, 2000*. Online. Available at: www.statistics.gov.uk/statbase/Product.asp?vlnk=8258&More=N (accessed 18 December 2008).

Office for National Statistics (ONS) (2005) *General Household Survey 2005*. Online. Available at: www.statistics.gov.uk/StatBase/Product.asp?vlnk=5756 (accessed 16 December 2008).

Office for National Statistics (ONS) (2008) *Life Expectancy. September 2008*. Online. Available at: www.statistics.gov.uk/cci/nugget.asp?id=168 (accessed 23 February 2009).

Papanicolaou, D.A., Wilder, R.L., Manolagas, S.C. *et al.* (1998) The Pathophysiologic Roles of Interleukin-6 in Human Disease. *Annals of Internal Medicine*, 128, 127–137.

Phelan, M., Stradins, L. and Morrison, S. (2001) Physical Health of People with Severe Mental Illness. *BMJ*, 322, 443–444.

Robson, H., Trenoweth, S. and Margereson, C. (2008) Co-morbidity in Physical and Mental Ill Health. In: Lynch, J. and Trenoweth, S. (eds) *Contemporary Issues in Mental Health Nursing*. Chichester: John Wiley & Sons.

Royal College of Physicians and Royal College of Psychiatrists (RCP) (1995) *Psychological Care of Medical Patients: Recognition and Service Provision. A Joint Working Party Report*. London: RCP.

Rozanski, A., Blumenthal, J.A., Davidson, K.W. *et al.* (2005) The Epidemiology, Pathophysiology and Management of Psychosocial Risk Factors in Cardiac Practice: The Emerging Field of Behavioral Cardiology. *Journal of the American College of Cardiology*, 45, 637–651.

Samaritans (2008) *Information Resource Pack 2008*. Online. Available at: www.samaritans.org/PDF/SamaritansInfoResourcePack2008.pdf (accessed 24 February 2009).

World Health Organisation (2001) *The World Health Report 2001 – Mental Health: New Understanding, New Hope.* Geneva: WHO.

World Health Organisation (2005) *Preventing Chronic Disease: A Vital Investment.* Geneva: WHO.

Yohannes, A.M., Baldwin, R.C., Connolly, M. *et al.* (2003) Prevalence of Sub-threshold Depression in Elderly Patients with Chronic Obstructive Pulmonary Disease. *International Journal of Geriatric Psychiatry,* 18, 412–416.

2 Trajectory and impact of long-term conditions

Carl Margereson

Introduction

The term *trajectory* has been utilised for a number of years by researchers interested in the complexities of long-term conditions, and was used by Glaser and Strauss (1968) in a seminal study which explored the experiences of dying patients in hospital. Listening to the patients' own stories enabled Glaser and Strauss to gain new insights into the trajectory or 'path travelled' by each individual, and in doing so were able to identify similar stages experienced. The Chronic Illness Trajectory Framework was developed later to assist in anticipating possible phases likely to be experienced by patients so that more holistic care might be delivered (Corbin and Strauss 1992) (see Table 2.1). The trajectory begins more often than not with physiological change/impairment; there then follow various phases representing the cumulative effects of disabling illness, including physical symptoms and the impact of the illness on the individual's social world, possibly challenging perceptions of self-identity (Burton 2000).

Trajectory framework

Use of a trajectory framework (Table 2.1) is not to suggest that there are clearly identified stages that can always be easily predicted and therefore anticipated. Long-term and chronic illnesses are, of course, unpredictable and complex, necessitating the individual to make adjustments, and involves fluctuations and movement back and forth as they grapple with the strong reactions to the loss of life as it was (Paterson 2001; Kralik 2002). Although these experiences will vary widely from one person to another, some understanding of the potential difficulties possibly encountered is important. While medicine of course has a role to play, treatments alone will not be enough to address the highly complex behavioural, cognitive, physical, emotional and psychological processes involved in the progression of long-term health problems (Marks *et al.* 2005).

Although the chronic illness trajectory can be useful when applied to physical health disorders, it does not provide a satisfactory explanatory framework where there are mental health problems. The terms 'long-term conditions' and 'chronic illness', for instance, may not be considered appropriate for individuals with mental health problems, where the emphasis is very much on rehabilitation, personal growth, support and recovery (NIMHE 2005). In one study, a model was developed which reflected the personal experiences of people with schizophrenia and other

Table 2.1 Chronic illness trajectory framework

- Pre-trajectory – before signs and symptoms/possible risk factors present
- Trajectory – signs and symptoms
- Crisis – life-threatening
- Acute – intermediate care/hospitalisation
- Stable – recovery/rehabilitation
- Unstable – ongoing difficulties
- Downward – deterioration
- Dying – palliation

Source: Corbin and Strauss (1992).

serious mental illness (Andreson *et al.* 2003). The five stages of this framework, viewed as more compatible with the idea of psychological recovery, may be seen in Table 2.2. The 'moratorium' stage is characterised by denial, confusion, hopelessness, identity confusion and withdrawal. There follows 'awareness' with hope of a better life and the possibility of recovery. 'Preparation' involves taking stock of the intact self, and of one's values, strengths and weaknesses. The hard work of recovery takes place in the 'rebuilding' phase where the individual begins to forge a positive identity and becomes more responsible for managing the illness and taking control. Finally there is 'growth', and although there may not be total freedom from symptoms, resilience is increased and the individual knows how to manage the illness, remains positive and starts to look to the future.

In a more recent study the recovery model was viewed as a continuum, where at times individual resilience is compromised (Geanellos 2005). Geanellos developed a model to facilitate appropriate intervention, based on her findings that individuals with mental illness can be anywhere on a 'resilience continuum' and can therefore be assisted to move along it. Understanding of how resilience can be compromised is important and four phases are identified (Table 2.3). The concept of resilience, however, where 'self' is compromised, is relevant to individuals with either mental or physical health problems and this idea will be explored later.

There are many different physical and mental health disorders which can result in ongoing problems, not only for the individual but also for family members. Sometimes the onset will be slow and diagnosis may be delayed, often resulting in uncertainty with varying degrees of distress. For some there is slow deterioration over a relatively long period, and for others deterioration is more rapid with the illness trajectory punctuated by frequent relapses and acute or chronic exacerbations. Chronicity may occasionally begin suddenly, for example, following a stroke, or some traumatic event resulting in perhaps paralysis or limb injury, or when abnormalities are discovered unexpectedly during routine health screening. What is certain is that

Table 2.2 Five-stage recovery framework

1 Moratorium
2 Awareness
3 Preparation
4 Rebuilding
5 Growth

Source: Andreson *et al.* (2003) Reproduced with permission.

Table 2.3 Adversity as opportunity: living with schizophrenia and developing a resilient self

Theme 1	Fragmentation – compromised resilience and the vulnerable self
Theme 2	Disintegration – broken resilience and the submerged self
Theme 3	Reintegration – recovered resilience and the re-established self
Theme 4	Reconstruction – renewed resilience and the recast self

Source: Geanellos (2005). Reproduced with permission.

following diagnosis, in an attempt to achieve a degree of 'normality' in their lives, individuals must learn that a great deal of hard and heavy work is needed for defining the self, coping and carrying on (May 2006).

Living with either physical or mental health problems, or indeed both, is done so within a specific cultural setting and this is important to remember when trying to understand the experiences of individuals. In a chapter such as this it is impossible to explore fully the experiences of all groups coping with ongoing health difficulties. The trajectory will be affected by a range of complex factors, not least the type of disorder as well as the life stage during which symptoms arise, diagnosis is made and ongoing difficulties are experienced. What emerges from research, however, is that there are common themes occurring, reflecting similar difficulties across many groups with different long-term conditions. This chapter will therefore focus on these common themes across different groups, and in Part IV, where each chapter explores a specific client group, specific psychosocial aspects will be considered.

The sick role

Talcott Parsons, a sociologist, was interested in how society responded to the 'deviance' of being sick and described the 'sick role' as a state where there is temporary exemption from role responsibilities (Parsons 1951). Most readers will have taken on the 'sick role' at some point, and even those who have been fortunate to have had nothing more than a bad cold can probably remember the 'benefits' that being unwell brought. It was probably totally acceptable to take time out from the many stresses that day-to-day life may bring. Perhaps this involved time off from work or college, and perhaps a partner or friend helped with domestic chores where there was little energy to perform them. There may also have been additional benefits such as welcomed visitors, flowers, chocolates and other rewards. Indeed, Parsons noted that in Western culture there is a general belief that the sick have a right to be cared for, but have an obligation to want to become well, and must seek and cooperate with health professionals. In other words, the timeframe in which it is acceptable to inhabit the sick role, be cared for and recover is relatively short, and a speedy return to 'health' is desirable and indeed expected.

What has just been described is the sick role relating to acute ill-health where the timeframe is often short. Yet Parsons' observations offer insight not only into the sick role inhabited by those with acute health problems, but help us to understand why those with ongoing health problems may experience a number of difficulties, especially from others who may have expectations regarding the timeframe of their recovery. However, chronic health problems are very different to acute health problems in a number of ways. They are long term, unpredictable, irreversible, characterised by remissions and relapses, and often result in negative consequences such as physical suffering, loss, worry, grief and disability (Lundman and Jansson 2007). Furthermore, the temporary role exemption referred to earlier may not apply to long-term conditions, as role changes and associated difficulties may be ongoing and indeed permanent. With the idea that those who are ill are obligated to get well as soon as possible, there may be tension where the sick role becomes permanent and further difficulties may be encountered by individuals where others judge them negatively and apportion blame. Those with mental health problems, for example, may be perceived to display unacceptable social behaviour and medical disorders seen to be the consequence of unhealthy lifestyles, and these misattributions may result in less tolerance within communities and society. There may also be tension regarding the obligation to cooperate with health professionals, particularly where partnership and collaboration is not fostered. Professional carers sometimes fail to acknowledge that individuals with long-term health problems have a wealth of knowledge and experiences which they bring to any health encounter.

The sick role does not always necessitate a visit to the doctor's surgery, but when this is necessary there may be yet an additional benefit. For example, there may be validation of the illness by the doctor in terms of a medical certificate, or a prescription of medicine which is proof to others that we are truly sick! The legitimisation of the 'sick role' by a doctor is particularly important and powerful in cultures with a strong work ethic, and where there is a positive and functionalist view that professions contribute to the overall well-being of society (Barber 1963). Those individuals who are not working and seen not to be contributing to society can soon experience the disapproval of others. Until the 'sick role' has been officially validated by a diagnostic label, individuals may find themselves in a prolonged pre-diagnosis period with ongoing diagnostic tests and endless referrals to specialists. This can be a stressful time when there are attempts to make sense of deteriorating health and can result in further distress and uncertainty.

At each stage along the trajectory there are many factors which, either independently or more often than not together, will influence the ability of the individual with ongoing health problems to adjust. But perhaps we should start on a positive note and remember that there is also a significant number of people with long-term conditions who adjust perfectly well. There are many who, despite major disability, manage to live life with purpose and maintain a positive attitude and outlook. Although some may view ongoing health problems in terms of loss and threat, others may redefine this time more positively, seeing it as an opportunity for re-evaluation and modification of future goals and ambitions.

There may also be a genetic predisposition towards better physical and mental health and conversely poorer health. Personality characteristics, the physical and social environment and individual behaviour are all important in contributing to increased resilience and coping. In the elderly, for example, successful ageing is associated with zest, resolution and fortitude, happiness, relationships between desired and achieved goals, self-concept, morale, mood and overall well-being (Bowling and Dieppe 2005). In this section we will focus on the impact of ongoing health problems and the coping attempts made.

Symptoms

The first area of difficulty that people with ongoing health problems must struggle with usually involves the biological or pathological aspects of the disorder. Symptoms may be difficult to control, resulting in a great deal of distress, and in physical disorders may be wide-ranging and include pain, breathlessness, fatigue, nausea, vomiting, to name but a few. While these may be as a direct result of the disease process, such symptoms may also develop due to the side-effects of medication or other treatments. Multiple symptoms may occur, resulting in distress, and skilled symptom assessment and management are vital aspects of care if quality of life is to be improved (see Chapter 5) (Fu *et al.* 2007). In individuals suffering from leukaemia, for example, experiences of pain, gastrointestinal problems and infections have been reported, with fatigue, breathlessness and sleep disturbance the most severe (Perrson and Hallberg 2004). Fatigue or low energy, often underestimated or not acknowledged at all, can have a further impact on both physical and mental health (Breitbart *et al.* 1998).

Where there are mental health problems, symptoms can include lack of energy and motivation, attention impairment, depression, anxiety and false sensory perceptions such as hallucinations, delusions and paranoid states (Glynn 1998). In schizophrenia symptoms such as emotional withdrawal, motor retardation, uncooperativeness, somatic concern, hostility, suspiciousness, hallucinations, guilt feelings, tension, anxiety and depressive mood have all been found to have a negative impact on coping ability (Bengtsson-Tops and Hansson 2001). However, there are times when physical health problems may be more important than psychiatric symptoms in limiting role function (Dixon *et al.* 2001).

Maximising symptom control should be conducted wherever possible and health professionals need to work closely together with clients to ensure that this is achieved. In an attempt to alleviate symptoms it may be necessary to alter normal lifestyle routines to accommodate complex treatment regimens. Physical factors such as fatigue and medical illness, together with psychological factors, can reduce vitality, defined as a positive state associated with a sense of enthusiasm and energy (Kubzansky *et al.* 2001; Rozanski and Kubzansky 2005). Where there is difficulty in coping with high levels of anxiety and stress, the presentation and interpretation of symptoms may be complex. Individuals may present with medically unexplained symptoms which may include chronic neck and low back pain, stomach pain and headaches, as well as mental health complaints such as sleeping disorders, nervousness, anxiety and depression, unrelated to the primary disorder (Ringsberg and Krantz 2006) (see Chapter 15).

The relationship between physical symptoms and coping is not straightforward, and psychological and psychosocial factors are likely to be far more important than symptoms in terms of the individual's quality of life. Symptoms which are not well controlled may affect the ability to self-care and it may no longer be possible to carry out the activities of living independently. Dependency on others as disability increases can undermine perceptions of control, and can result in much frustration and feelings of helplessness and powerlessness, further reinforcing the sick role.

Experiencing loss

Loss as a result of ongoing health problems is experienced by many and may result in unresolved grief, anxiety and depression. There can be many losses over the course of the chronic illness trajectory including loss of physical health, employment, independence, hope, stamina, social relations, sexual function, intimacy, role fulfilment, and leisure pursuits that were previously enjoyed. However, loss may be experienced for not only what has been but what could have been. There may be grieving for the loss of personal control and spontaneity in life as well as loss of dignity. In individuals with multiple sclerosis, for example, there was a feeling of loss of identity and not being the person they used to be, with some longing for their earlier healthy life (Isaksson *et al.* 2007).

Cumulative losses may result in chronic sorrow where there is pervasive sadness which is permanent, periodically intense and progressive in nature (Burke *et al.* 1992). Intensity in the feelings of loss may occur at specific points along the trajectory, as when there is a crisis possibly requiring hospitalisation or residential care, or when there is a significant negative life event such as bereavement, divorce or redundancy. Loss of 'self' has been viewed as a fundamental form of suffering in those with ongoing health problems (Charmaz 1983) where there is a crumbling away of the former self-image without the development of an equally valued new one. According to Charmaz there are four major consequences of this which contribute to this negative self-evaluation: leading a restricted life, experiencing social isolation, being discredited and burdening others.

Self-esteem

At times we compare the view we have of ourselves with that of what we feel 'we should be', and these self-evaluations are often based on media images of what is seen as perfect and desirable. Such comparisons are difficult enough in good health, but for those with health problems can be a major source of anxiety and distress. Negative stereotypes exist in the community about those who are chronically ill or have a disability (Telford *et al.* 2006) and those with ongoing health problems are only too aware that they are often judged accordingly.

Self-esteem refers to the positive regard we have for ourselves and the beliefs we hold about our place in the world, and these feelings are powerful, inner influences which help to guide, steer and nurture us through life (Mann *et al.* 2004). Additional terms such as self-concept, self-worth, self-image and self-perception have all been of interest to researchers, and it is clear that positive images of self can contribute significantly not only to how well we cope with life, but also to how much personal control we perceive ourselves to have. Positive self-esteem contributes to increased resilience in life and is a prerequisite for mental, emotional and social health (Macdonald 1994) which, of course, will also contribute to improved physical health. Impacting negatively on self-esteem can be distortions of body image whether these are real or imagined. Difficulties with body image have been identified in a number of groups, and may arise as a direct result of the disorder itself, or perhaps as a result of treatment leading to low self-esteem, depression, relationship difficulties, loneliness and even suicidal thoughts (Sprangers *et al.* 1995; Vironen *et al.* 2006) (see Chapter 15). Healthcare treatment plans which are perceived as threatening to self-concept can result in emotionally centred responses, and body image can continue to be a significant influence on health behaviour beyond adolescence (Thomas 2007).

Sexuality and how we see ourselves as sexual beings is also very much part of our self-identity and is linked to self-esteem. Expressing sexuality is an important activity of living but difficulties with intimacy may be experienced by many with ongoing health problems. Neither increasing age nor disability diminishes the need to be valued as a vital, sexually attractive person. Men and women, though suffering similar forms of impairment, experience their meanings and consequences in ways that relate to wider constructions of masculinity and femininity (Twigg 2006). Although sexuality is often considered an important health concern in women with chronic illness and needs to be acknowledged (Kralik 2002), ideas about gender are changing and being challenged all the time. Yet issues around sexuality need to be acknowledged in those with chronic ill-health whatever the gender or sexual orientation. In men with prostate cancer, problems with urinating, loss of urinary control, sexual dysfunction, hormonal alterations and fatigue are major problems, and the presence of an indwelling catheter can have particular consequences for sexual expression (Chapple and Ziebland 2002). For men, changes in self-image from being a strong man, successful in work to becoming a weaker sick man can lead to fears of being discounted and emasculated (Elmberger *et al.* 2002; Schacht and Ewing 1998).

Social stigma

Embarrassment and shame may be devastating for those with long-term health problems, particularly where there are visible signs of 'being different'. This can result in feelings of being stigmatised. Stigma occurs when people are defined in terms of a distinguishing characteristic or mark, and as a consequence are often devalued (Dinos *et al.* 2004; Johnson *et al.* 2007). Individuals thus perceived are labelled in a negative way, suggesting that they are less desirable (Goffman 1963). Although visible signs set the individual apart as different, thereby subjecting him/her to negative stereotypes and possible discrimination, problems can arise through the invisibility of disability where others may be less sensitive to their needs. In the absence of visible signs individuals are generally subjected to the expectations placed upon healthy individuals (Stephenson and Murphy 1986; Fraser *et al.* 2006) and this can result in further frustration and distress. Thus people with long-term health issues, such as those with mental health problems, are particularly vulnerable to being stigmatised, discriminated, marginalised and disadvantaged. Negative labelling is particularly likely where the person is held responsible for the disease and where the disease leads to serious disability, disfigurement, lack of control or disruption of social interactions (Albrecht *et al.* 1982). In a study of women who had contracted HIV infection in heterosexual and monogamous relationships, for example, it was often assumed that they had become infected owing to promiscuity, intravenous drug use or prostitution (Sandelowski *et al.* 2004).

Negative encounters with relatives, friends, local community, media and even health professionals can all reinforce feelings of being stigmatised. Perceived stigma can have a major psychological impact, not least on self-esteem (Link *et al.* 2001) and confidence, and can adversely affect communication and relationships. The individual may socially withdraw to avoid anxiety and distress, thus becoming even more isolated. Stigma management refers to the hard work involved in trying to reduce stigmatisation and enhance normalisation (Joachim and Acorn 2000). Devaluing of individuals may be due not only to health problems but also because of being elderly in cultures where ageing is viewed negatively. There may also be serious consequences where younger people with diabetes and asthma, in an attempt to be no different from their healthy and 'normal' friends, stop taking their medication or adopt unhealthy lifestyle patterns, such as drinking excessive amounts of alcohol or smoking. In people living with chronic respiratory disease, a sense of stigmatisation may be felt as a direct result of using supplemental oxygen around other people and this may lead to feelings of embarrassment and social isolation (Earnest 2002). Although there are some disorders that are more likely to result in stigma, it is possible for an individual to feel stigmatised no matter what the disorder is, and such feelings need to be explored sensitively.

Social networks and support

An area which can have a profound impact on those with long-term health problems relates to the fracturing of networks and ultimately support. We have a profound need for social connection, and a lack of positive relationships or social isolation leads to stress, disease and premature death (Berkman and Syme 1979; Cacioppo and Hawkley 2003). Loneliness may also be a significant problem for those with ongoing physical and/or mental health disorders and is a challenge not only for all involved in health and social care but for society generally. As Geanellos (2005, 11) suggests:

> When people suffer alone, cannot express their fears and pain, struggle to appear normal, go without needed aid and are marginalized in relationships with others and society, the vulnerable self moves toward disintegration.

Social support may be classified as being instrumental (helping with tasks), financial, informational, appraisal (help in evaluating a situation) and emotional (an affective restorative function) (Rozanski *et al.* 2005). Yet for some, there may be no human contact for weeks on end. Even where practical assistance is available (for example, through social care agencies) this may still not offer the emotional support which gives individuals a sense that they 'belong' and are therefore esteemed and valued. For those not able to work there may be limited opportunities for contact outside the home, which can impact not only on financial remuneration but on perceived self-worth (Lauder *et al.* 2004).

A number of factors may be responsible for reduced social interaction. Where there is increasing disability due to physical symptoms, mobility may be severely restricted. Relatives may not be able to give the support needed for various reasons, or there may be interference with the ability to participate as before in various social interactions. Social engagement and inclusiveness in local communities contributes significantly to physical and mental health. Being involved in activities that many of us take for granted (e.g. shopping, meeting friends) is essential for those with ongoing health problems. For people with mental health problems there may be exclusion and segregation in the form of distancing, where groups in society maintain boundaries separating themselves from what they perceive as frightening behaviour (Kelly *et al.* 2001; Granerud and Severinsson 2003). As individuals with mental health problems experience increasing difficulty with everyday activities and in forging positive interpersonal relationships, social isolation may increase further. In people with schizophrenia, involvement in social activities may also play a part in helping to manage symptoms such as hallucinations (Kelly *et al.* 2001).

Although supportive personal relationships are associated with better coping and immune function, close personal relationships that are chronically abrasive or stressful may provoke depression and other negative emotions, as well as contributing to increased health risk (Kiecolt-Glaser *et al.* 2002a). It must not be assumed, therefore, that members of an individual's close social network, such as their spouse, are best placed to provide the support needed. Those who are unable or reluctant to provide support may actually contribute to increased stress and distress. It is also important to remember that where an individual has an ongoing health problem, the dynamics of family relationships can change dramatically, particularly where there are role losses and changes. Gender may be a significant factor here where role change possibly impacts on being perhaps a husband/wife, mother/father, with enforced role change resulting in feelings of uselessness contributing to increased family tension and conflict.

There are many individuals, both adults and children, caring for a loved one, yet the contribution made to health and social care is not fully recognised. Care agencies often assume that where there is a close family member or friend, care will be given willingly and without difficulty. The impact on carers can be profound and in partners who are carers, females report a higher burden than do male partners (Baanders and Heijmans 2007). The care-giving burden is often perceived in terms of feelings of a heavy responsibility; an uncertainty about care needs; constant worries; restraints in social life; and feelings that only they are relied on for their care (Scholte op Reimer *et al.* 1998). Gender differences are seen here, and traditionally women have been more likely to take on the responsibility for caring. In an effort to maintain normality in the home, carers may experience an uphill struggle where they are often aware of their limitations in attempting to balance caring duties given the challenging circumstances that present, and at times often feeling like an outsider in their partner's life (Eriksson and Svedlund 2005).

Carers may also experience loss and feelings of guilt, and together with the inevitable stress involved in caring for a loved one, it is no surprise that they too are at increased risk of developing health problems. It has been demonstrated that men and women who provide care to a spouse with a stroke or dementia are at increased risk for a whole range of health problems, including infections, hypertension and heart disease (Kiecolt-Glaser *et al.* 1991; Grant *et al.* 2002; Vitaliano *et al.* 2002).

Perceived social support of individuals with long-term health problems and their carers is an important factor in coping, and society is faced with an enormous challenge. The concept of community is changing all the time and by 2020 a significant proportion of households will consist of people living alone, so society will need to decide how our older members and the most vulnerable are best supported, or the burden of care will continue to be shouldered by informal carers (if available) and the health and social sectors (if financially sustainable) (Margereson 2006).

Coping and adjustment

Given the psychosocial impact of long-term health problems, individuals must learn to cope with the inevitable changes imposed by their declining health status. Much has been written about coping, which may be viewed as the cognitive and behavioural efforts directed towards successful adaptation to stressful situations (Lazarus and Folkman 1984). What this means is that appropriate psychological and behavioural strategies must be developed in order to manage the complex demands which inevitably challenge on a daily basis. A great deal of energy may be used by individuals in trying to maintain a sense of 'normality' not only to avoid embarrassment but in a desperate attempt to get on with their lives. Strategies must be learned so that there are the physical, emotional and psychological resources to cope with each day (see Chapter 8). In a study of individuals with chronic breathlessness, strategies were adopted through trial and error, and involved pacing activities and learning how to conserve energy and adapt daily tasks such as sitting down to complete tasks in the kitchen, washing and dressing, as well as sometimes using tricks to hide their problems from others (Barnett 2004).

Behavioural responses include the many self-care skills that are required to control symptoms and treat the underlying disorder. Many behavioural responses made by individuals to cope with ongoing health problems may be observed by healthcare workers and these can be either health promoting or indeed health damaging. Lifestyle behaviours such as smoking, poor diet, lack of exercise and excessive alcohol intake may increase further individual health risk. Other behavioural responses may involve poor use of healthcare facilities and non-concordance with treatment and care plans generally. Anger, verbal abuse, withdrawal, excessive dependence, immature behaviour and denial may all be observed, and it is important that these behaviours are understood, since no matter how inappropriate they may sometimes seem, they reflect the individual's attempts to cope, although perhaps not very successfully (see Chapter 6).

It is important to recognise the individual differences in coping and adjustment, and there is a need to consider the impact of individual thoughts and beliefs, for what 'we think' is closely linked to our behavioural and emotional responses (see Chapter 8). Whether or not an individual perceives his or her personal situation as stressful, for example, will depend on their own interpretation. Such interpretation is influenced by physical, psychological and socioeconomic factors, and cultural background is particularly significant (McCabe and Priebe 2004). Earlier we referred to symptoms which are experienced by most people with long-term health problems, and whether these are intermittent or continuous. Symptoms can also sometimes be ambiguous and the precise aetiology of the illness can be elusive. When ill we have our own personal theories about what is wrong, what the cause is, as well as what the treatment and outcome should be. Sometimes such 'mini-theories' can be helpful but sometimes they can result in action which is at best unhelpful or at worst negatively impact on the trajectory of the illness.

These personal 'mini-theories' are referred to as 'illness representations' and describe how the illness is 'pictured and stored' in the mind (Leventhal and Diefenbach 1991; Brownlee *et al.* 2000; Insel *et al.* 2005). If adaptation to long-term health problems is to be effective and individuals are able to engage in adaptive tasks it is important that appropriate illness representations are developed (Scharloo *et al.* 2000). Care workers need to work collaboratively in this process and must listen carefully to the client's narrative in order to gain some understanding of their unique illness representations (see Chapter 8). Difference in interpretation between client and health professional may result in practice which is not culturally sensitive and may contribute to inappropriate help-seeking and self-care behaviours, non-concordance and ineffective coping (Bhui and Bhugra 2002; Bhui *et al.* 2003). Illness representations, along with social support, have been shown to have a positive impact on a range of disorders, and effective interventions will help individuals change inappropriate illness perceptions and improve health outcome (Petrie *et al.* 2007).

The power of 'perceived control'

One mechanism whereby active coping might influence health is through the control we believe we have over stressful events. The impact of ongoing health problems may be so overwhelming that individuals may believe that there is nothing that can be done to influence events. Martin Seligman explored the concept of 'learned helplessness', a state occurring when people are bombarded with unsolvable problems, becoming helpless, passive, slower to learn, anxious and sad (Seligman 1975). Conversely, optimism has been shown to be linked with superior emotional well-being in people with chronic and acute health problems (Bedi and Brown 2005) (see Chapter 7). Resilience is another central pillar which can support an individual's perceived sense of control and relates to all those resources both internal and external that can be activated in times of stress, allowing us to face challenges and make appropriate adjustments (Bergeman and Wallace 1999).

Although many with long-term disorders are self-caring, there is a small yet significant group of individuals with complex health and social care needs who do not feel in control and lack confidence, and this can contribute to frequent hospitalisation. Although these feelings may have developed partly due to the nature of the disorder and also as a result of individual personality traits, healthcare workers can also disempower individuals, resulting in loss of confidence. Individuals, particularly the elderly, who find themselves in a care setting may find their personal integrity threatened, where not only their health but their dignity and autonomy are diminished (Jacelon 2004). Removing choice and control, and not involving individuals in decision-making about their own care, can quickly lead to feelings of helplessness and increased dependency. In those with mild to moderate mental health problems there are often feelings of powerlessness and of being lost in a system that is more responsive to severe and acute episodes of illness (Campbell *et al.* 2007).

Being in control, also referred to as 'self-efficacy', is associated with better health outcomes, and refers to the confidence one feels about being able to carry out behaviours which can lead to an improvement in one's own health (Bandura 1977, 1996). Where self-efficacy is high and the individual has confidence in their ability, this has been shown to influence motivation levels, mood, and enables them to cope more effectively with their symptom management and other health-promoting aspects (Lorig *et al.* 1993; Marks *et al.* 2005). Although an individual may be more than capable of carrying out a self-care task, if self-efficacy is low then performance of the task may not be successful.

Making sense of what is happening to us and what is going on in our lives is an important factor in perceived control. This has been referred to as a 'sense of coherence' (SOC) and three components have been identified: comprehensibility, manageability and meaningfulness, all contributing to increased confidence and self-efficacy (Antonovsky 1987, 1993; Wolff and Ratner 1999). Where there are long-term health problems with poor coping ability, 'sense of coherence' may be weak, and any additional demands may therefore be viewed as uncontrollable and threatening, increasing further personal conflict and tension. In addition, negative emotions (both anxiety and depression), anger-suppression coping style and cynical hostility are associated with a weak sense of coherence (Hart *et al.* 2006). Sense of coherence may be further weakened by inadequate physical, emotional, social, financial and community resources which can all affect individual resistance and the ability to 'bounce back'.

Chronic stress

Depression and social isolation is a reality for many individuals with long-term health difficulties and their carers. Where there are problems with resilience and coping, ongoing stress, anxiety and depression can have a negative impact on immune function with periods of worsening physical health (Kiecolt-Glaser *et al.* 2002b, 2003; Tosevski and Milovancevic 2006). This is a good example of how potentially powerful the mind–body connection is, where negative thoughts and emotions can activate complex neurohormonal pathways as part of the stress response. Most of us experience occasional stress, but while brief increases in stress hormones may offer benefit, longer term increases are associated with immunological problems. This increased risk of poorer heath as a result of stress has been observed over a range of different medical disorders. Stress management interventions may need to be considered for some individuals with ongoing health problems who are experiencing adjustment difficulties.

Conclusion

There are many issues which can impact both positively and negatively on the trajectory of long-term conditions. A number of explanatory frameworks have been generated in an attempt to offer new insights into the experiences of those with ongoing health problems. Inevitably, many will experience ongoing loss and this will necessitate ongoing efforts to cope with the changes imposed by their deteriorating health. Healthcare workers need to be sensitive to the devastating impact that chronic ill-health can have on day-to-day life. Although symptom management is crucial, it is psychosocial factors that are likely to be the most important in terms of effective coping. Time needs to be taken to listen to the client's story, since each individual has a unique biography and narrative which needs to be heard and understood. Confidence in terms of self-efficacy should not be underestimated, and strategies need to be identified which facilitate personal control and maintain human dignity. Most people with long-term conditions are in the community, either living alone or in some kind of residential care with relatively few in acute care facilities, so the fostering of self-care ability where appropriate is important. Effective coping will be influenced by a range of intrapersonal and environmental factors which have been introduced in this chapter. We should remember that we ignore how people think about themselves and their illness at our peril, and we need to understand the processes driving the behaviours and emotions of those for whom we care.

References

Albrecht, G., Walker, V. and Levy, J. (1982) Social Distance from the Stigmatised: A Test of Two Theories. *Social Science Medicine*, 16, 1319–1327.

Andreson, R., Oades, L. and Caputi, P. (2003) The Experience of Recovery from Schizophrenia: Toward an Empirically Validated Stage Model. *Australian and New Zealand Journal of Psychiatry*, 37(5), 586–594.

Antonovsky, A. (1987) *Unraveling the Mystery of Health: How People Manage Stress and Stay Well.* San Francisco: Jossey-Bass.

Antonovsky, A. (1993) The Structure and Properties of the Sense of Coherence Scale. *Social Science and Medicine*, 36, 725–733.

Baanders, A.N. and Heijmans, M.J.W.M. (2007) The Impact of Chronic Diseases: The Partner's Perspective. *Family and Community Health*, 30, 305–317.

Bandura, A. (1977) Toward a Unifying Theory of Behavioral Change. *Psychological Review*, 84, 191–215.

Bandura, A. (1996) *Social Foundations of Thought and Action: A Social Cognitive Theory.* Englewood Cliffs: Prentice Hall.

Barber, B. (1963) Some Problems in the Sociology of Profession. *Daedalus*, 92, 4.

Barnett, M. (2004) Supported Discharge for Patients with COPD. *Nursing Standard*, 18, 33–37.

Bedi, G. and Brown, S.L. (2005) Optimism, Coping Style and Emotional Well-being in Cardiac Patients. *British Journal of Health Psychology*, 10, 57–70.

Bengtsson-Tops, A. and Hansson, L. (2001) The Validity of Antonovsky's Sense of Coherence Measure in a Sample of Schizophrenic Patients Living in the Community. *Journal of Advanced Nursing*, 33, 432–438.

Bergeman, C.S. and Wallace, K.A. (1999) Resiliency in Later Life. In: Whitman, T.L., Merluzzi, T.V. and White, R.D. (eds) *Life Span Perspectives on Health and Illness* (pp. 207–225). London: Lawrence Erlbaum Associates.

Berkman, L.F. and Syme, S.L. (1979) Social Networks, Host Resistance and Mortality: A Nine Year Follow Up Study of Alameda County Residents. *American Journal of Epidemiology*, 109, 186–204.

Bhui, K. and Bhugra, D. (2002) Explanatory Models for Mental Distress: Implications for Clinical Practice and Research. *British Journal of Psychiatry*, 181, 6–7.

Bhui, K., Stansfield, S., Hull, S. *et al.* (2003) Ethnic Variations in Pathways to and Use of Specialist Mental Health Services in the UK. Systematic Review. *British Journal of Psychiatry*, 182, 105–116.

Bowling, A. and Dieppe, P. (2005) What is Successful Ageing and Who Should Define It? *BMJ*, 331, 1548–1551.

Breitbart, W., McDonald, M.V., Rosenfeld, B. *et al.* (1998) Fatigue in Ambulatory AIDS Patients. *Journal of Pain Symptom Management*, 15, 159–167.

Brownlee, S., Leventhal, H. and Leventhal, E. (2000) Regulation, Self Regulation and the Construction of the Self in the Maintenance of Physical Health. In: Boekaerts, M., Pintrich, P. and Zeidner, M. (eds) *Handbook of Self Regulation* (pp. 369–416). San Diego, CA: Academic Press.

Burke, M.L., Hainsworth, M.A., Eakes, G. *et al.* (1992) Current Knowledge and Research on Chronic Sorrow: A Foundation of Inquiry. *Death Studies*, 16, 231–245.

Burton, C.R. (2000) Re-thinking Stroke Rehabilitation: The Corbin and Strauss Chronic Illness Trajectory Framework. *Journal of Advanced Nursing*, 32, 595–602.

Cacioppo, J.T. and Hawkley, L.C. (2003) Social Isolation and Health, with an Emphasis on Underlying Mechanisms. *Perspectives in Biological Medicine*, 46, S39–S52.

Campbell, S., Gately, C. and Gask, L. (2007) Identifying the Patient Perspective of the Quality of Mental Healthcare for Common Chronic Problems: A Qualitative Study. *Chronic Illness*, 3, 46–65.

Chapple, A. and Ziebland, S. (2002) Prostate Cancer: Embodied Experience and Perceptions of Masculinity. *Sociology of Health and Illness*, 24, 820–841.

Charmaz, K. (1983) Loss of Self: A Fundamental Form of Suffering in the Chronically Ill. *Sociology of Health and Illness*, 5, 168–197.

Corbin, J.M. and Strauss, A. (1992) A Nursing Model for Chronic Illness Management Based Upon the Trajectory Framework. In: Woog, P. (ed.) *The Chronic Illness Trajectory Framework* (pp. 9–28). New York: Springer.

Dinos, S., Stevens, S., Serfaty, M. *et al.* (2004) Stigma: The Feelings and Experiences of 46 People with Mental Illness: Qualitative Study. *British Journal of Psychiatry*, 184, 176–181.

Dixon, L., Goldberg, R., Lehman, A. *et al.* (2001) The Impact of Health Status on Work, Symptoms, and Functional Outcomes in Severe Mental Illness. *Journal of Nervous and Mental Disease*, 189, 17–23.

Earnest, M.A. (2002) Explaining Adherence to Supplemental Oxygen Therapy: The Patient's Perspective. *Journal of General International Medicine*, 17, 749–755.

Elmberger, E.R., Bolund, C.P. and Lutzen, K.P. (2002) Men With Cancer: Changes in Attempts to Master the Self-image as a Man and as a Parent. *Cancer Nursing*, 25, 477–485.

Eriksson, M. and Svedlund, M. (2005) 'The Intruder': Spouses' Narratives About Life with a Chronically Ill Partner. *Journal of Clinical Nursing*, 15, 324–333.

Fraser, D.D.M., Kee, C.C.P. and Minick, P.P.R. (2006) Living with Chronic Obstructive Pulmonary Disease: Insiders' Perspectives. *Journal of Advanced Nursing*, 55, 550–558.

Fu, M.R., McDaniel, R.W. and Rhodes, V.A. (2007) Measuring Symptom Occurrence and Symptom Distress: Development of the Symptom Experience Index. *Journal of Advanced Nursing*, 59, 623–634.

Geanellos, R. (2005) Adversity as Opportunity: Living with Schizophrenia and Developing a Resilient Self. *International Journal of Mental Health Nursing*, 14, 7–15.

Glaser, B. and Strauss, A. (1968) *Awareness of Dying*. Chicago, IL: Aldine.

Glynn, S. (1998) Handbook of Social Functioning in Schizophrenia. In: Mueser, K. and Tarrier, N. (eds) *Psychopathology and Social Functioning in Schizophrenia* (pp. 66–78). Boston, MA: Allyn & Bacon.

Goffman, E. (1963) *Stigma*. Englewood Cliffs, NJ: Prentice Hall.

Granerud, A. and Severinsson, E. (2003) The New Neighbour: Experiences of Living Next Door to People Suffering from Long-Term Mental Illness. *International Journal of Mental Health Nursing*, 12, 3–10.

Grant, I., Adler, K.A., Patterson, T.L. *et al.* (2002) Health Consequences of Alzheimer's Caregiving Transitions: Effects of Placement and Bereavement. *Psychosomatic Medicine*, 64(3), 477–486.

Hart, K., Wilson, T.L. and Hittner, J.B. (2006) A Psychosocial Resilience Model to Account for Medical Well-being in Relation to Sense of Coherence. *Journal of Health Psychology*, 11, 857–862.

Insel, K.C., Meek, P.M. and Leventhal, H. (2005) Differences in Illness Representation among Pulmonary Patients and their Providers. *Journal of Health Psychology*, 10, 147–162.

Isaksson, A.K., Gunnarsson, L.G. and Ahlstrom, G. (2007) The Presence and Meaning of Chronic Sorrow in Patients with Multiple Sclerosis. *Journal of Clinical Nursing*, 16(11c), 315–324.

Jacelon, C.S. (2004) Managing Personal Integrity: The Process of Hospitalization for Elders. *Journal of Advanced Nursing*, 46, 549–557.

Joachim, G. and Acorn, S. (2000) Stigma of Visible and Invisible Chronic Conditions. *Journal of Advanced Nursing*, 32, 243–248.

Johnson, J.L., Campbell, A.C., Bowers, M. *et al.* (2007) Understanding the Social Consequences of Chronic Obstructive Pulmonary Disease: The Effects of Stigma and Gender. *Proceedings of the American Thoracic Society*, 4, 680–682.

Johnstone, M.J. (2001) Stigma, Social Justice and the Rights of the Mentally Ill: Challenging the Status Quo. *Australian and New Zealand Journal of Mental Health Nursing*, 10, 200–209.

Kelly, S., McKenna, H., Parahoo, K. *et al.* (2001) The Relationship between Involvement in Activities and Quality of Life for People with Severe and Enduring Mental Illness. *Journal of Psychiatric and Mental Health Nursing*, 8, 139–146.

Kiecolt-Glaser, J.K., Dura, J.R., Speicher, C.E. *et al.* (1991) Spousal Caregivers of Dementia Victims: Longitudinal Changes in Immunity and Health. *Psychosomatic Medicine*, 53(4), 345–362.

Kiecolt-Glaser, J.K., McGuire, L., Robles, T.F. *et al.* (2002a) Emotions, Morbidity and Mortality: New Perspectives from Psychoneuroimmunology. *Annual Review of Psychology*, 53, 83–107.

Kiecolt-Glaser, J.K., McGuire, L. and Robles, T.F. *et al.* (2002b) Psychoneuroimmunology and Psychosomatic Medicine: Back to the Future. *Psychosomatic Medicine*, 64(1), 15–28.

Kiecolt-Glaser, J.K., Preacher, K.J., MacCallum, R.C. *et al.* (2003) Chronic Stress and Age-related Increases in the Proinflammatory Cytokine IL-6. *Proceedings of the National Academy of Sciences U.S.A.*, 100, 9090–9095.

Kralik, D. (2002) The Quest for Ordinariness: Transition Experienced by Midlife Women Living with Chronic Illness. *Journal of Advanced Nursing*, 39, 146–154.

Kubzansky, L.D., Sparrow, D., Vokonas, P. *et al.* (2001) Is the Glass Half Empty or Half Full? A Prospective Study of Optimism and Coronary Heart Disease in the Normative Aging Study. *Psychosomatic Medicine*, 63, 910–916.

Lauder, W., Sharkey, S. and Mummery, K. (2004) A Community Survey of Loneliness. *Journal of Advanced Nursing*, 46, 88–94.

Lazarus, R. and Folkman, S. (1984) *Psychological Stress and the Coping Process*. New York: Springer.

Leventhal, H. and Diefenbach, M. (1991) The Active Side of Illness Cognition. In: Skelton, J.A. and Croyle, R.T. (eds) *Mental Representation in Health and Illness* (pp. 247–272). New York: Springer-Verlag.

Link, B.G., Struening, E.S., Neese-Todd, M.A. *et al.* (2001) The Consequences of Stigma for the Self Esteem of People with Mental Illness. *Psychiatric Services*, 52, 1621–1626.

Lorig, K., Mazonson, P.D. and Holman, H. (1993) Evidence Suggesting that Health Education for Self Management in Patients with Chronic Arthritis Has Sustained Health Benefits While Reducing Health Care Costs. *Arthritis and Rheumatism*, 36, 439–446.

Lundman, B.P. and Jansson, L.M. (2007) The Meaning of Living with A Long-term Disease. To Revalue and Be Revalued. *Journal of Clinical Nursing*, 16, 109–115.

Macdonald, G. (1994) Self Esteem and the Promotion of Mental Health. In: Trent, D. and Reed, C. (eds) *Promotion of Mental Health* (pp. 19–20). Aldershot: Avebury.

Mann, M., Hosman, C.M.H., Schaalma, H.P. *et al.* (2004) Self Esteem in a Broad-Spectrum Approach for Mental Health Promotion. *Health Education Research*, 19, 357–372.

Margereson, C.B. (2006) Challenges in Caring for People with Long Term Conditions. *British Journal of Cardiac Nursing*, 1, 6.

Marks, R., Allegrante, J.P. and Lorig, K. (2005) A Review and Synthesis of Research Evidence for Self-Efficacy-Enhancing Interventions for Reducing Chronic Disability: Implications for Health Education Practice (Part I). *Health Promotion Practice*, 6, 37–43.

May, C. (2006) The Hard Work of Being Ill. *Chronic Illness*, 2, 161–162.

McCabe, R. and Priebe, S. (2004) Explanatory Models of Illness in Schizophrenia: Comparison of Four Ethnic Groups. *British Journal of Psychiatry*, 185, 25–30.

National Institute for Mental Health In England (NIMHE) (2005) *NIMHE Guiding Statement on Recovery*. Online. Available HTTP: www.psychminded.co.uk/news/news2005/feb05/nimherecovstatement.pdf (accessed 5 March 2009).

Parsons, T. (1951) *The Social System*. New York: Free Press.

Paterson, B.L. (2001) The Shifting Perspectives Model of Chronic Illness. *Journal of Nursing Scholarship*, 33, 21–26.

Perrson, L. and Hallberg, I.R. (2004) Lived Experience of Survivors of Leukemia or Malignant Lymphoma. *Cancer Nursing*, 27, 303–313.

Petrie, K.J., Jago, L.A. and Devcich, D.A. (2007) The Role of Illness Perceptions in Patients with Medical Conditions. *Current Opinion in Psychiatry*, 20, 163–167.

Ringsberg, K.C. and Krantz, G.K. (2006) Coping with Patients with Medically Unexplained Symptoms. *Journal of Health Psychology*, 11, 107–116.

Rozanski, A. and Kubzansky, L.D. (2005) Psychologic Functioning and Physical Health: A Paradigm of Flexibility. *Psychosomatic Medicine*, 67, 47–53.

Rozanski, A., Blumenthal, J.A., Davidson, K.W. *et al.* (2005) The Epidemiology, Pathophysiology and Management of Psychosocial Risk Factors in Cardiac Practice: The Emerging Field of Behavioural Cardiology. *Journal of the American College of Cardiology*, 45, 637–651.

Sandelowski, M., Lambe, C. and Barroso, J. (2004) Stigma in HIV-positive Women. *Journal of Nursing Scholarship*, 36, 122–128.

Schacht, S. and Ewing, D. (1998) *Feminism and Men: Reconstructing Gender Relations*. New York: New York University Press.

Scharloo, M., Kaptein, A.A., Weinman, J.A. *et al.* (2000) Physical and Psychological Correlates of Functioning in Patients with Chronic Obstructive Pulmonary Disease. *Journal of Asthma*, 37(1), 17–29.

Scholte op Reimer, W.J.M., de Haan, R.J. and Rijnders, P.T. (1998) The Burden of Caregiving in Partners of Long-term Stroke Survivors. *Stroke*, 29, 1605–1611.

Seligman, M.E.P. (1975) *Helplessness*. San Francisco, CA: Freeman.

Sprangers, M., Taal, B., Aaronson, N. *et al.* (1995) Quality of Life in Colorectal Cancer: Stoma vs Non-Stoma Patient. *Disease Colon Rectum*, 35, 361–369.

Stephenson, J.S. and Murphy, D. (1986) Existential Grief. The Special Case of the Chronically Ill and Disabled. *Death Studies*, 10, 133–145.

Telford, K., Kralik, D. and Koch, T. (2006) Acceptance and Denial: Implications for People Adapting to Chronic Illness: Literature Review. *Journal of Advanced Nursing*, 55, 457–464.

Thomas, C.M.R. (2007) The Influence of Self-concept on Adherence to Recommended Health Regimens in Adults with Heart Failure. *Journal of Cardiovascular Nursing*, 22, 405–416.

Tosevski, D.L. and Milovancevic, M.P. (2006) Stressful Life Events and Physical Health. *Current Opinion in Psychiatry*, 19, 184–189.

Twigg, J. (2006) *The Body in Health and Social Care*. New York: Palgrave-Macmillan.

Vironen, H., Kairaluoma, M., Aalo, A. *et al.* (2006) Impact of Functional Results on Quality of Life after Rectal Cancer Surgery. *Disease Colon Rectum*, 49, 568–578.

Vitaliano, P.P., Scanlan, J.M., Zhang, J. *et al.* (2002) A Path Model of Chronic Stress, the Metabolic Syndrome, and Coronary Heart Disease. *Psychosomatic Medicine*, 64, 418–435.

Wolff, A.C. and Ratner, P.A. (1999) Stress, Social Support, and Sense of Coherence. *Western Journal of Nursing Research*, 21, 182–197.

3 Going forward with long-term conditions

Towards a true health system

Tim Anstiss

Introduction

Long-term conditions are common, costly and becoming more prevalent. Health systems which developed to deal with acute episodes of ill-health are finding themselves poorly designed and poorly prepared for the current epidemics of chronic illness and long-term conditions. Many are engaged in radical transformation efforts to make themselves fit for purpose.

This chapter outlines the historical and current drivers behind this transformation effort, describes some of the policies put in place to push/pull the system forward, and makes some suggestions as to what a true health system might look like. The focus of the chapter is the UK National Health Service, but reference is made to issues and developments from elsewhere.

Socioeconomic context and drivers

The current and future cost of caring for people with long-term conditions is one of the key factors driving healthcare reform, along with concerns about the poor quality of care being delivered to so many voters and taxpayers. People are living longer with ongoing health problems and increasing numbers are living with more than one disorder.

In England, people with chronic illness account for 80 per cent of general practice consultations and the approximately 15 per cent of people with three or more problems account for almost 30 per cent of inpatient days (Wilson *et al.* 2005). In the UK treatment and care for people with long-term conditions accounts for almost 70 per cent of the primary care and acute budget, and chronic illness care may consume 75 per cent of the total cost of national healthcare expenditure in the US (Hoffman *et al.* 1996). Eighty-five per cent of deaths in the UK may be from chronic disease. Some studies suggest that long-term conditions can consume up to 7 per cent of a country's gross domestic product (Oxford Health Alliance Working Group 2005) – not just a result of the impact they have on health service costs (Jonsson 2002) but also due to their impact on decreased work productivity (Oxford Health Alliance Working Group 2005). The UK economy may lose £16 billion over the next ten years through premature deaths due to heart disease, stroke and diabetes.

And of course all these statistics are merely one way of representing the huge and growing burden of suffering, impairment, chronic pain, loneliness, fear and grief experienced by millions of individuals and families year upon year.

The policy and initiative response

For all the difference in the aetiology and pathophysiology of long-term conditions, chronic illnesses have several things in common, including the need for healthcare systems and health and social care professionals to activate, empower and support the person with the condition to ensure optimum outcomes.

The wider policy context

In the UK, the NHS reforms (DoH 2000, 2007a) must be considered part of a wider and ongoing reform of the public sector as a whole which aims to transfer more power to parents, pupils and patients and to enable public sector workers delivering services to respond in new and innovative ways. Perhaps the two main principals of public sector reform in the UK are:

- Putting people first by placing power in the hands of those who use public services.
- Personalising services and providing greater choice.

In the health and social care sector this is being done via a wide range of policies, initiatives and programmes, some of which are outlined in this chapter. A key aim is to provide people with personalised budgets and accurate information so that they can choose the specific care they most need, underpinned by an 'information revolution' to enable patients to share information and experiences on the performance of the services they receive.

Specific policies and initiatives

The UK Department of Health (DoH) is currently managing one of the largest organisational development projects the world has ever seen – attempting to transform one of the world's largest organisations into a semi-coordinated network of lean and nimble organisations delivering timely, effective, integrated and quality controlled care to people with and without long-term conditions. The aim is that people with long-term conditions pull what they value (treatment, care, advice, support, reassurance) from the system on an as-needed basis to increase their choice, health, well-being and sense of control, while the government 'pushes' screening and preventive services towards people backed by social marketing initiatives to try to change people's health behaviour so that they do not develop long-term conditions in the first place.

A vast array of semi-aligned policies, initiatives and programmes are pushing and pulling the UK health and social care system in the direction of a first-class service for people with long-term conditions, including the following.

Common Assessment Framework (CAF) for adults (DoH 2009a)

A commitment of the White Paper *Our Health, Our Care, Our Say* (DoH 2006a) was to develop a generic, common assessment framework for adults which would:

- improve outcomes for adults by ensuring a personalised and holistic assessment of need, focused on delivering individual outcomes;

- support improved joint working between health and social services;
- increase efficiency through better information sharing.

Common core principles to support self-care (DoH 2008a)

A document aiming to help all those who work in health and social care (e.g. commissioners, service providers, educators) make personalised services, enablement and early intervention to promote independence a reality. The government wants health and social care organisations to embed these principles in their organisational policies, agreements with other agencies, and their own culture and practices. Developed by Skills for Health and Skills for Care in partnership with people who use services, carers and other stakeholders, these principles are also making their way into skills and competency frameworks to shape training and professional development.

The Dignity in Care campaign

A programme aiming to eliminate tolerance of indignity in health and social care by raising awareness and inspiring people to take action. If patients and their carers were treated with more respect, health and well-being outcomes for people with long-term conditions would likely improve (see Chapter 19).

Direct payments and individual budgets (DoH 2007b; Samuel 2009)

A major strand of policy aiming to accelerate the transformation in social care. Direct payments and individual budgets will place more power in the hands of people with long-term conditions, giving them more choice and control, bringing together separate income streams and helping people secure more joined-up packages of support. Once people know the level of resources at their disposal, it can help them plan and control how their support needs are met.

Caring with Confidence Programme (Caring with Confidence 2009)

Previously referred to as the Expert Carers Programme (ECP), this is designed to support and train carers, helping them to develop new skills to manage the condition of the person they care for and to cope with their own health needs better on a day-to-day basis. Many carers suffer ill-health as a result of their caring activities, and if their health breaks down, so do the care arrangements. Helping them care for the person they care for, and themselves, more effectively and with less stress, makes good sense.

The Expert Patients Programme (EPP) (DoH 2007c)

This is run by the EPP Community Interest Company, a not-for-profit social enterprise (EPP CIC 2006). This relatively long-running programme provides training for people with chronic or long-term conditions, delivered by trained and accredited but lay tutors who are also living with a long-term health condition. The programme aims to give people the confidence to better manage their own health, while working collaboratively with health and social care professionals.

NHS Direct

Now multi-media, this telephone service was launched in 1998 and now gets over six million calls a year. The Internet service *NHS Direct Online* was launched in 1999 and gets over half a million hits a month, while the digital TV service *NHS Direct Interactive* covers 60 per cent of the population and has about one million page viewings a month, and the NHS Direct self-care guide delivered to 20 million homes.

Personalisation (DoH 2008b)

The personalisation of health and social care services is a shared ambition across government, and a common theme throughout health and social care policies. The intention is to put people first through a radical reform of public services, helping people to live their own lives as they wish: confident that services are of high quality, are safe and promote their individual needs for independence, well-being and dignity. The government sees personalisation as:

> the way in which services are tailored to the needs and preferences of citizens. The overall vision is that the state should empower citizens to shape their own lives and the services they receive.
>
> (HM Government 2007)

Personalised care planning

Personalised care planning is another main strand of policy, designed to address *'an individual's full range of needs, taking into account their health, personal, family, social, economic, educational, mental health, ethnic and cultural background and circumstances'* (DoH 2009b). To skilfully develop a personalised care plan, collaboratively with an individual, taking the above factors and others besides into consideration, is a very different task from assessing someone with an acute illness and deciding how best to treat them. This illustrates the nature of the change required by healthcare systems to meet the needs of people with long-term conditions.

Integrated care pilots (DoH 2009c)

This programme aims to test and evaluate new models of integrated care, models which aim to empower clinicians to work more closely with patients and other partners. Integration in this context may refer to partnerships, systems and models as well as organisations, and the pilots have been chosen for geographical spread as well as examples crossing boundaries across primary, community, secondary and social care. The insights which flow from this programme should be substantial, and this is a good example of how innovation and risk-taking can be stimulated in a sometimes slow-to-react public service.

Pharmacy in England (DoH 2008c)

A White Paper setting out the government's vision of the future role of pharmacists and pharmacy services, including the promotion and support of healthy living and healthy lifestyles, advice and support on self-care, offering services to people with minor ailments and supporting people living with long-term conditions with routine monitoring, vascular risk assessment and support in making the best use of their medicines. Another example of how the government wants to make local support available to help people with long-term conditions look after themselves better, and avoid complications of their condition.

Practice-based commissioning (DoH 2007d)

Practice-based commissioning aims to place decisions about which services should be commissioned for a patient closer to the patient, helping to deliver a more personalised service with more choice. Practice-based commissioning should be supported by PCTs to help them deliver 'world class commissioning', helping them in turn to commission services more responsive to the needs of local people identified, in part, via the personalised care planning process.

Supporting People with Long Term Conditions to Self Care: A Guide to Developing Local Strategies and Best Practice (DoH 2006b)

This document explains how health and social care services can support people with long-term conditions to self-care through an integrated package including information, self-monitoring devices, self-care skills education and training, and self-care support networks.

Year of care programme

A three-year project to test a commissioning, care planning and service delivery approach – initially around diabetes. This programme will produce practical guides, training programmes and insights for service improvement along the way, and like some of the other initiatives and pilots mentioned in this chapter, the results of this programme will inform future policy development in what people hope will be a cycle of continuous improvement.

Elements and models

The above policies, programmes and initiatives are designed to bring a better healthcare system into existence. Much is known about the elements or components of a healthcare system required to deliver superior outcomes for people with long-term conditions (Renders et al. 2001; Bodenheimer et al. 2002; Weingarten et al. 2002; Ouwens et al. 2005; Singh and Ham 2006) – indeed, there have even been reviews of systematic reviews! (Ouwens et al. 2005). One review (Singh 2005) found evidence to support the beneficial impact of a range of initiatives on patient and system outcomes including: the use of broad chronic care management models; involving people with long-term conditions in decision-making; greater reliance on primary care; providing accessible structured information; self-management education; and the use of nurse-led strategies.

Models are abstractions that help us understand how the world works and what causes what. They simplify things – leaving some things out, and focusing our attention on what the model developers consider to be the most important features and relationships. The following models were developed by different organisations for different purposes and one is not necessarily better than another.

The Kaiser Permanente triangle

A useful way of stratifying populations to inform service planning, service delivery and workforce development, the model divides the population into three levels (DoH 2005a) (Figure 3.1):

- *Level 3: People with complex needs requiring skilled case management.* Individuals in this group may be high-intensity users of unplanned secondary care, and the case management approach involves anticipating their future needs and coordinating and joining up health and social care services.
- *Level 2: People experiencing high risk of disease progression and complications requiring skilled disease/care management.* Individuals in this group may have a complex single need or multiple conditions and benefit from responsive, specialist services using multi-disciplinary teams and disease-specific protocols and pathways (such as the National Service Frameworks). Skilled disease management may deliver better health outcomes, slow disease progression, reduce the associated disability and ensure better management of any sudden deterioration. Good care management for this group involves identifying their needs early and responding promptly with the right care and support using systematic and tailored programmes for individual patients.
- *Level 1: The remainder of the population requiring help and support to care for themselves.*

The Chronic Care Model

The main elements of a system designed to improve care for people with long-term conditions is depicted in the Chronic Care Model (Figure 3.2). This empirically informed and extensively tested model was developed by Ed Wagner and the MacColl Institute (Wagner *et al.* 1999, 2001) and implementation of the model has led to favourable outcomes in a range of long-term conditions (Asch *et al.* 2005; Mangione-Smith *et al.* 2005; Vargas *et al.* 2007).

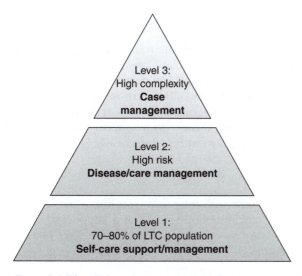

Figure 3.1 The Kaiser Permanente triangle (source: Department of Health (2005a). Reproduced with permission).

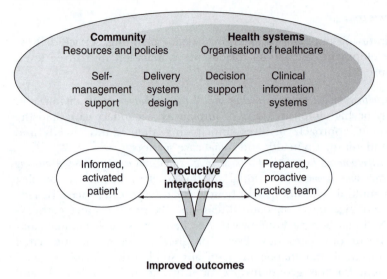

Figure 3.2 Chronic Care Model (source: Wagner (1998). Reproduced with permission).

The model emphasises a 'productive interaction' as the essential element of chronic illness care, an interaction in which the work of evidence-based chronic disease care is conducted in a systematic way with patient needs being met. The whole system is designed to help co-produce 'informed, activated patients'. These are patients who have goals and a plan to improve their health, along with the motivation, information, skills and confidence required to manage their illness well. A recent article by Anstiss (2009) shows how motivational interviewing can help healthcare systems deliver these essential elements of high-quality care for people with long-term conditions.

The NHS and Social Care Long Term Conditions Model (DoH 2005a)

The Chronic Care Model has been combined with the triangular population model of Kaiser Permanente to create the NHS and Social Care Long Term Conditions Model (Figure 3.3). The model builds on UK and international experience and is designed to help improve the health and quality of life of those with long-term conditions by providing personalised yet systematic ongoing support. It details the infrastructure available to support better care for those with long-term conditions as well as a delivery system designed to match support with patient needs.

Lean healthcare

Improving care and outcomes for people with long-term conditions may be seen as one big, lean transformation package, redesigning care and support around the patient/service user. When organisations decide to 'go lean' and deliver better services while driving up efficiency, many follow a five-step programme of:

1   Understanding what service users truly value (as opposed to what providers want to give them).

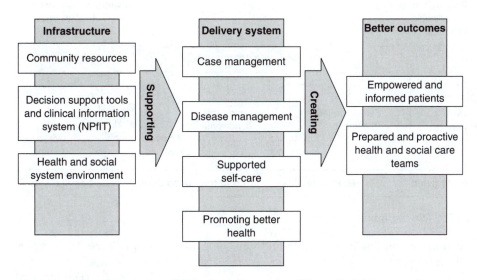

Figure 3.3 The NHS and Social Care Long Term Conditions Model (source: Department of Health (2005a). Reproduced with permission).

2   Understanding how this value flows to service users, and how and why it often does not (commonly using mapping tools).
3   Making this value flow to service users (by continuously identifying and eliminating causes of waste, delay and complexity, as well as by innovating).
4   Enabling service users to pull what they want and need from the system when, where and how they want it.
5   Striving for perfection in service delivery.

The desired end state of all the policies and initiatives described above could be considered 'lean consumption', in which the health and social care system gives people with long-term conditions exactly what they want, in exactly the right amount, at exactly the right time and place with minimum delay, waste and cost (Womack and Jones 2005).

Promoting and supporting self-care

Promoting self-care is a major strand of policy and a core element of chronic care models. Self-care has been defined as

> the activities individuals, families, and communities undertake with the intention of enhancing health, preventing disease, limiting illness, and restoring health.
> (Kickbush and Hatch 1983, 4)

and

> the actions people take for themselves, their children and their families to stay fit and maintain good physical and mental health; meet social and psychological needs; prevent illness or accidents; care for minor ailments and long-term

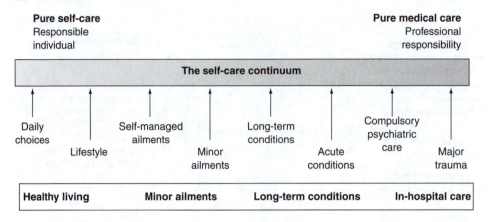

Figure 3.4 The continuum of care.

conditions; and maintain health and well-being after an acute illness or discharge
from hospital.

(DoH 2005b)

Self-care may be considered as existing towards one end of a care continuum
(Figure 3.4) with professional care at the other end. Wearing a safety belt can be
considered 100 per cent self-care, and abdominal aortic surgery 100 per cent professional care. Shared care lies between these ends of the spectrum (DoH 2005b).

A recent UK study suggested that most people treat their minor ailments themselves, that nearly two-thirds of people often monitor their acute illness following
discharge from hospital and that over 80 per cent of people with a long-term health
condition say they play an active role in caring for their condition themselves
(DoH/MORI Survey: DoH 2005c). People also seem interested in engaging in more
or better self-care, especially if support is provided. Over 75 per cent of people in
the survey said they would be far more confident about taking care of their own
health if they had guidance and support from an NHS professional. However, over
50 per cent of people who had seen a care professional in the previous six months
said they have rarely been encouraged to self-care and one-third said they have *never*
been encouraged by their professional to self-care.

In view of the importance of self-care in long-term conditions, the White Paper
Our Health, Our Care, Our Say (DoH 2006a) gave the approach a big boost by:

- stating that the Expert Patients Programme will increase capacity from 12,000
  course places to over 100,000 and investment in this initiative will be trebled;
- outlining plans to improve self-care through assistive technology, health checks,
  health trainers and NHS Direct;
- providing primary care providers with a much stronger focus on improving self-
  care through both the Quality and Outcomes Framework and on commissioning services that support self-care. Self-care is considered as one of the highest
  priorities for future changes to contractual arrangements;
- describing professional education to encourage support for individual empowerment and self-care with a clear self-care competency framework for staff and
  to work with the professional bodies to embed self-care in core curricula;

- stating that everyone with a long-term condition or long-term need for support, and their carers, would routinely receive self-care support through networks.

To help the health and social care system deliver better, more holistic care for people with long-term conditions, the UK government has set out seven principles it wishes to see embedded in local policies and agreements, as well as local culture and practice (DoH 2008a):

1 Ensuring individuals are able to make informed choices to manage their self-care needs.
2 Communicating effectively to enable individuals to assess their needs, and to develop and gain confidence to self-care.
3 Supporting and enabling individuals to access appropriate information to manage their self-care needs.
4 Supporting and enabling individuals to develop skills in self-care.
5 Supporting and enabling individuals to use technology to support self-care.
6 Advising individuals how to access support networks and to participate in the planning, development and evaluation of services.
7 Supporting and enabling risk management and risk taking to maximise independence and choice.

Two sector skills agencies (Skills for Care and Skills for Health) are piloting these principles in an attempt to embed them into people's daily working practice, while also embedding them in the National Occupational Standards and qualifications for health and social care.

Towards a true health service

Continuous improvements in the care we offer people with long-term conditions must progress in parallel and harmony with continuous improvements in the care we offer people with acute conditions. These improvements must in turn progress alongside improvements in primary prevention and of the social, economic and material environments in which we all live, move and have our being. Continuously reducing the stress and allostatic load experienced by the less well-off will help reduce the intergenerational transmission of poor health, well-being and life chances that blight our communities and will help us control the growth of future health and social costs (Case *et al.* 2005).

Delivering holistic care to people with long-term conditions may be considered a vital stepping stone along the path from a healthcare service focused on treating

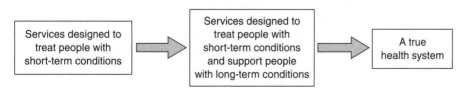

Figure 3.5 Stepping stones to a true health system.

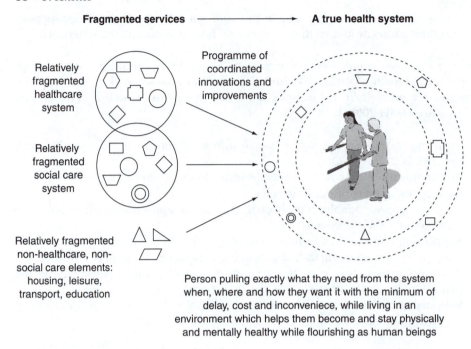

Figure 3.6 Evolving a true health system.

acute injury and illness to a true health system focused on keeping people healthy and helping them flourish (Figure 3.5).

But changes in health services alone will never be enough to create a true health system, a fact that has been recognised for decades, if not centuries:

> A real Health Service must surely concern itself with the way people live, with town and country planning, houses and open spaces, with diet, with playgrounds, gymnasia, baths and halls for active recreation, with workshops, kitchens, gardens and camps, with the education of every child in the care and use of his body, with employment and the restoration to the people of the right and opportunity to do satisfying creative work. The true 'health centre' can only be a place where the art of healthy living is taught and practised: it is a most ominous and lamentable misuse of words to apply the name to what is and should be called a 'medical centre'.
>
> (*Lancet* 1944, 443)

The emergence of a true health system out of today's somewhat fragmented, variable quality health and social care services (Figure 3.6) requires policy development, clinical leadership and public service of the highest order. But if we can work together to create a true health system, the rewards, like the challenges, are great – including having contributed to one of the world's outstanding feats of human cooperation.

References

Anstiss, T. (2009) Motivational Interviewing in Primary Care. *Journal of Clinical Psychology in Medical Settings*, 16(1) published online, 1 March 2009.

Asch, S., Baker, D., Keesey, J. *et al.* (2005) Does the Collaborative Model Improve Care for Chronic Heart Failure? *Medical Care*, 43, 667–675.

Bodenheimer, T., Wagner, E.H. and Grumbach, K. (2002) Improving Primary Care for Patients with Chronic Illness: The Chronic Care Model, Part 2. *JAMA*, 288, 1909–1914.

Caring with Confidence (2009) Online. Available at: www.caringwithconfidence.net/ (accessed 15 April 2009).

Case, A., Fertig, A. and Paxson, C. (2005) The Lasting Impact of Childhood Health and Circumstance. *Journal of Health Economics*, 24(2), 345–389.

Crocker, L. (1936) Pioneer Health Centre, Annual Report for 1936. PHC Papers, SA/PHC/PP/I. 107.

Department of Health (2000) *The NHS Plan: A Plan for Investment; A Plan for Reform.* London: Department of Health.

Department of Health (2005a) *Supporting People with Long Term Conditions: An NHS and Social Care Model to Support Local Innovation and Integration.* London: Department of Health.

Department of Health (2005b) *Self Care – A Real Choice.* London: Department of Health.

Department of Health (2005c) *Public Attitudes to Self Care: Baseline Survey.* London: Department of Health.

Department of Health (2006a) *Our Health, Our Care, Our Say: A New Direction for Community Services.* London: Department of Health.

Department of Health (2006b) *Supporting People with Long Term Conditions to Self Care: A Guide to Developing Local Strategies and Good Practice.* London: Department of Health.

Department of Health (2007a) *Our NHS Our Future: NHS Next Stage Review – Interim Report.* London: Department of Health.

Department of Health (2007b) *Putting People First: A Shared Vision and Commitment to the Transformation of Adult Social Care.* London: Department of Health.

Department of Health (2007c) The Expert Patients Programme. Online. Available at: www.dh.gov.uk/en/Aboutus/MinistersandDepartmentLeaders/ChiefMedicalOfficer/ProgressOnPolicy/ProgressBrowsableDocument/DH_4102757 (accessed 15 April 2009).

Department of Health (2007d) *World Class Commissioning: Vision.* London: Department of Health.

Department of Health (2008a) *Common Core Principles to Support Self Care: A Guide to Support Implementation.* London: Department of Health.

Department of Health (2008b) *Transforming Adult Social Care.* London: Department of Health.

Department of Health (2008c) *Pharmacy in England. Building on Strength – Delivering the Future.* London: Department of Health.

Department of Health (2009a) *Common Assessment Framework for Adults – A Consultation on Proposals to Improve Information Sharing Around Multi-disciplinary Assessment and Care Planning.* London: Department of Health.

Department of Health (2009b) *Supporting People with Long Term Conditions. Commissioning Personalised Care Planning. A Guide for Commissioners.* London: Department of Health.

Department of Health (2009c) Integrated Care Pilots. Online. Available at: www.dh.gov.uk/en/Healthcare/IntegratedCare/DH_091112 (accessed 14 April 2009).

Expert Patients Programme Community Interest Company (EPP CIC) (2006) Expert Patients Programme Update. Online. Available HTTP: www.expertpatients.co.uk/epp_update/eppupdate16.pdf (accessed 13 April 2009).

HM Government (2007) *Policy Review Building on Progress: Public Services.* Online. Available at: www.cabinetoffice.gov.uk/media/cabinetoffice/strategy/assets/building.pdf (accessed 15 April 2009).

Hoffman, C., Rice, D. and Sung, H.Y. (1996) Persons with Chronic Conditions. Their Prevalence and Costs. *JAMA*, 276, 1473–1479.

Jonsson, B. (2002) Revealing the Cost of Type II Diabetes in Europe. *Diabetologia*, 45, S5–12.

Kickbush, I. and Hatch, S. (1983) *Self Help and Health in Europe: New Approaches to Care*. Geneva: WHO.

Lancet (1944) *White Paper Reviewed*. VI. By an Urban Practitioner. *Lancet*, I, 443.

Mangione-Smith, R., Schonlau, M., Chan, K. *et al.* (2005) Measuring the Effectiveness of a Collaborative for Quality Improvement in Pediatric Asthma Care: Does Implementing the Chronic Care Model Improve Processes and Outcomes of Care? *Ambulatory Pediatrics*. 5, 75–82.

Ofman, J.J., Badamgarav, E., Henning, J.M. *et al.* (2004) Does Disease Management Improve Clinical and Economic Outcomes in Patients with Chronic Diseases? A Systematic Review. *American Journal of Medicine*, 117, 182–192.

Ouwens, M., Wollersheim, H., Hermens, R. *et al.* (2005) Integrated Care Programmes for Chronically Ill Patients: A Review of Systematic Reviews. *International Journal of Quality Health Care*, 17, 141–146.

Oxford Health Alliance Working Group (2005) *Economic Consequences of Chronic Diseases and the Economic Rationale for Public and Private Intervention*. Oxford: Oxford Health Alliance [draft report].

Renders, C.M., Valk, G.D., Griffin, S. *et al.* (2001) Interventions to Improve the Management of Diabetes Mellitus in Primary Care, Outpatient and Community Settings. *Cochrane Database Syst Rev*, 1: CD001481.

Samuel, M. (2009) Expert Guides. Direct Payments, Personal Budgets, and Individual Budgets. CommunityCare.co.uk. Online. Available at: www.communitycare.co.uk/Articles/2009/04/08/102669/direct-payments-personal-budgets-and-individual-budgets.html (accessed 15 April 2009).

Schonlau, M., Mangione-Smith, R., Chan, K.S. *et al.* (2005) Evaluation of a Quality Improvement Collaborative in Asthma Care: Does it Improve Processes and Outcomes of Care? *Annals of Family Medicine*, 3, 200–208.

Singh, D. (2005) *Transforming Chronic Care. Evidence about Improving Care for People with Long-term Conditions*. Birmingham: University of Birmingham, Surrey and Sussex PCT Alliance.

Singh, D. and Ham, C. (2006) *Improving Care for People with Long-term Conditions. A Review of UK and International Frameworks*. Birmingham: University of Birmingham, NHS Institute for Innovation and Improvement.

Skills for Care, Skills for Health (2008) Common Core Principles to Support Self Care: A Guide to Support Implementation.

Vargas, R., Mangione, C.M., Asch, S. *et al.* (2007) Can a Chronic Care Model Collaborative Reduce Heart Disease Risk in Patients with Diabetes? *General Internal Medicine*, 22, 215–222.

Wagner, E. (1998) Chronic Disease Management: What Will it Take to Improve Care for Chronic Illness? *Effective Clinical Practice*, 1, 2–4.

Wagner, E., Davis, C., Schaefer, J. *et al.* (1999) A Survey of Leading Chronic Disease Management Programs: Are they Consistent with the Literature? *Managed Care Quarterly*, 7, 56–66.

Wagner, E., Austin, B., Davis, C. *et al.* (2001) Improving Chronic Illness Care: Translating Evidence into Action. *Health Affairs*, 20, 64–78.

Weingarten, S.R., Henning, J.M., Badamgarav, E. *et al.* (2002) Interventions Used in Disease Management Programmes for Patients with Chronic Illness: Which Ones Work? Meta-analysis of Published Reports. *BMJ*, 325, 925.

Wilson, T., Buck, D. and Ham, C. (2005) Rising to the Challenge: Will the NHS Support People with Long-term Conditions? *BMJ*, 330, 657–661.

Womack, J. and Jones, D. (2005) *Lean Solutions*. New York: Simon & Schuster.

4 Legal and ethical issues

Janet Holt

Introduction

Ethical and legal issues are a common feature of contemporary healthcare, mainly because research and advances in technology, pharmaceuticals and treatment options allow people in some circumstances to be given effective and even curative treatment where in the past this was not available. Even when the condition cannot be eradicated, symptom management and palliative care can slow down the disease trajectory, improve the prognosis or allow someone to lead a relatively normal life while living with the condition. Individuals with long-term conditions can particularly benefit from such advances in medical science, but this in turn can give rise to a number of ethical dilemmas. Long-term treatment options can be costly, and in a publicly funded health service, difficult questions inevitably arise about how worthwhile such treatments are and how they are to be funded. Individuals with long-term conditions will have to make decisions about a range of treatment options over a period of time. While UK law presumes (unless proven otherwise) that a person has the capacity to make decisions, overt and subtle influences on service users made vulnerable because of their health status can affect their ability to make autonomous decisions. Perhaps the most complex and difficult decisions that service users, their carers, family and friends face are those at the end of life, when choices may need to be made about continuing or discontinuing treatment or even assisted dying.

This chapter will explore the concept of vulnerability within the context of ethics and law. The importance of the ethical principle of autonomy and its relationship to the legal requirements for informed consent and mental capacity will be examined with reference to the recent Mental Capacity Act 2005. The theory and practicalities of advance decisions will be considered and the difficulties in the allocation of resources to a group with multiple and lengthy health needs discussed. The chapter will close with an exploration of end-of-life decisions. Throughout the chapter, examples of ethical dilemmas will be used to illustrate the issues raised, and reference will be made to significant legal judgements where controversial cases were settled in law.

Vulnerability

Individuals with long-term conditions are usually considered to be vulnerable to a greater or lesser degree. In the context of health and social care this may mean that the person is not able to protect their own interests because of physical or mental ill-health, disability and cognitive impairment. Mechanic and Tanner (2007, 1220) describe vulnerability as susceptibility to harm but broaden the understanding of this by describing how the vulnerable state can emanate from 'developmental problems, personal incapacities, disadvantaged social status, inadequacy of personal networks and supports, degraded neighbourhoods and environments, and the complex interactions of these factors over the life course'. Levels of vulnerability therefore vary between individuals, and people may have phases in their lives where they are more vulnerable than others. To describe someone as vulnerable can be useful to ensure that due recognition is given to protecting their interests and rights. This is a key feature of the National Service Framework for Long-term Conditions which sets a target of improving health outcomes for vulnerable people most at risk of long-term conditions (DoH 2005).

However, the term should be used with caution as it can stereotype and lead to paternalistic behaviour. Paternalism as its name suggests resembles the care a parent may exercise over a child and means that decisions may be made for someone without expressly consulting them or even by overriding their express wishes (Fletcher *et al.* 1995). On the whole, paternalistic behaviour in healthcare is usually well meant and founded on a concern for a person's welfare. Suppose Jim, an older service user in a nursing home, has a degree of dementia and also hypertension. Despite the best efforts of the carers in the home, Jim refuses to take his prescribed medication for hypertension. The nurses are concerned about the detrimental affect this will have on his health state so conceal the medication in some food which Jim readily eats. The nurses are acting paternalistically towards Jim, but in their defence they could argue that they are doing so out of a genuine concern for his welfare. However, paternalistic relationships are dependent and imbalanced in favour of the care giver and the real danger is that the dominant voice then becomes that of the care giver rather than that of the service user. To act paternalistically, no matter how well meant, is contrary to one of the most important concepts in healthcare ethics: respecting autonomous decision-making.

Autonomy and moral decision-making

Autonomy is derived from the Greek *autos*, meaning self and *nomos* meaning rule, governance or law, and literally means self-rule (Beauchamp and Childress 2009). Hence, an autonomous person is one who is able to act independently, is not constrained by others and someone who is capable of meaningful choice. It is an important concept legally and morally in contemporary healthcare as well as being a pivotal issue in codes of conduct and/or practice for health professionals. To be meaningful, autonomy needs to be not simply acknowledged but respected. Just to recognise that a person is autonomous or capable of making rational autonomous choices is not enough. The person must also be respected as an autonomous agent; that is, someone with a right to hold views, make choices and to decide upon a course of action based on personal values and beliefs. As Beauchamp and Childress (2009, 103) point out, respecting autonomy means recognition of an individual's right to hold views, make choices and to act based on their personal values and beliefs. 'Such respect involves respectful action, not merely a respectful attitude.'

Nevertheless, recognising autonomous choices is not always immediately obvious, as even people who in normal circumstances are considered to be autonomous may have temporary constraints placed upon them that affect their freedom of choice and diminish their autonomy. An example of this is seen in the scenario with Jim discussed above. Jim has a degree of dementia and the nurses are faced with the moral dilemma of reconciling concern for Jim's welfare while respecting his autonomous choice to refuse the medication. The situation is further complicated if Jim's autonomy is diminished owing to the dementia.

Harris (1985) suggests that defects in the person's ability to control their desires or actions, in reasoning; in the information available and defects in the stability of the person's desires diminishes autonomy. A person with a long-term condition could experience one or more of these defects through the period of their illness. For example, suppose that Sarah, an 85-year-old, lives independently with support from members of her family. Her family members all work and have children of their own, and Sarah is acutely aware of how much time they spend helping her with personal and household tasks. Sarah perceives herself to be a burden on her family and decides to move into residential care so that she will be less reliant upon her family. For Sarah's choice to be considered autonomous, we would need to be convinced that she had decided upon this course of action based on her own personal beliefs, that she was not coerced by any members of her family into making the decision, that she is capable of rational thought, has correct and accurate information, and that there is some stability in the final decision she makes. If all of these criteria are met, then Sarah's decision may be considered to be autonomous even if her family do not agree with her. Perhaps Sarah's family willingly help her maintain her independence and never suggest that she is a burden to them, but Sarah perceives this to be the case and, in the absence of any clear indication that she is not capable of rational thought, it would be difficult to assess Sarah's decision as being anything other than fully autonomous.

Many decisions made by individuals are not controversial and there are few or no difficulties in recognising the decisions as autonomous. But as well as the temporary constraints discussed above, there are other situations where conflict can arise between the service user and the carers (professional or otherwise) involved in their care. The person may be competent to make an autonomous choice, but the decision they make is one that the carer does not agree with. While respecting someone's autonomy is an important moral principle, it is not the only issue that needs to be taken into consideration. Autonomy is not an absolute moral principle; that is, one that will take precedence in every case, as a person's autonomous choice can be legitimately constrained by the rights of others. For example, a service user may decide that their life is not worth living and ask their carer to assist them to die by providing them with appropriate medication to commit suicide. Even if the carer was convinced that the person had made a rational choice, it does not follow that in order to act ethically and respect the autonomous decision, the carer is morally obliged to accede to the person's request. The service user may have a rational self-chosen plan upon which they wish to act, but in doing so, they are asking the carer to act unlawfully. In this example the carer also has the right to make an autonomous decision on how to act. She may of course agree to the request, obtain the medication and accept the consequences of her actions, or she may choose not to do so. What is important here is that the course of action decided upon by the carer is based upon her own autonomous decision, not because she considers herself to be obliged to respect the autonomous decision of the service user and fulfil the request. Respecting autonomy is therefore a *prima facie* right; that is, one that must be fulfilled unless it conflicts with an equal or even stronger claim. In this example, the carer's obligation to act within the law would arguably be stronger than the service user's claim that they should have their autonomy respected (Holt 2002).

Autonomy and the law

Autonomy is the foundation of the law surrounding informed consent and for consent to be recognised as valid in law the person must fulfil three criteria, namely have capacity, be acting voluntarily and be broadly aware of what is being consented to (Pattinson 2006). The understanding of capacity in a legal sense has been made more explicit in the United Kingdom with the introduction of the Mental Capacity Act 2005 which came into force in April 2007. Section 1 of the Act states that:

> A person must be assumed to have capacity unless it is established that he lacks capacity.
>
> (Department of Constitutional Affairs 2007, 19)

The emphasis of this is important, as it establishes that everyone is presumed to have capacity unless it is proven that they do not. An individual therefore does not have to prove they have the capacity to make autonomous decisions, but can expect (given the caveats discussed above) to have his or her decisions respected in law unless they are proven to lack capacity. The focus of the Mental Capacity Act 2005 is on individuals who lack capacity and to put them at the centre of holistic decision-making processes and allow those with capacity to plan ahead should they lose the ability to make autonomous decisions in the future (Griffith 2008). This is of particular importance for individuals with long-term conditions such as dementia, brain injury, progressive neurological disorders or mental illness and who may at some point be unable to communicate their preferences regarding care and treatment. The Re C Test (based on the case of Re C Advice: refusal of treatment [1994] 1 WLR 290) is used to determine if an individual does have the necessary capacity to make autonomous choices. As capacity is presumed, this test is not carried out routinely, but an assessment is made only where there are doubts about the person's ability to make decisions. In Re C, a 68-year-old man with paranoid schizophrenia refused to have a below-the-knee amputation despite being told that he had a very poor chance of survival if he did not have the surgery. The judge found that C's mental illness did not prevent him from being capable of making the decision to refuse the amputation and a three-stage test emerged from this case as a test for capacity. The stages of the Re C Test are:

- Can the patient understand and retain the treatment information?
- Can he believe it?
- Can he weigh it sufficiently to make a choice?

> (Pattinson 2006, 134–135)

To return to the scenario with Jim, as well as the moral dilemma the nurses face, they must also act in accordance with professional guidance and the law. If a person is competent, then it is neither lawful nor professionally acceptable to administer covert medication even if the nurses believe it is in the individual's best interests. People who have capacity have a legal right to refuse any medication, treatment or procedures even if such a decision is considered to be unwise or irrational. If Jim's capacity was tested using the Re C Test, then unless it could be shown that his dementia caused impairment or disturbance to the functioning of his mind, the nurses would have to accept that although Jim's refusal of medication may be unwise, he cannot be treated as though he were unable to make the decision (Griffith and Tengnah 2008). This example shows the difficulties of reconciling moral, legal and professional decision-making in practice. The nurses may feel morally justified in giving Jim the medication covertly on the grounds that they have an obligation to maintain his health, yet if Jim is found to have capacity, legally and professionally they must not administer medication against his will.

If a person is found to lack capacity, then the Mental Capacity Act 2005 allows a third party to give proxy consent for the person based on what they consider to be in the service user's best interests. This is achieved either by the service user nominating someone to do this through a lasting power of attorney, or by the appointment of a deputy (Law Commission 2005). A person with a mental disorder (such as paranoid schizophrenia) may or may not lack capacity and some aspects of their care and treatment may be subject to the Mental Health Act 2007. However, it should be noted that the Mental Health Act 2007 only covers treatment of mental disorder and not other treatment decisions, and Re C (discussed above) is a clear example of this. Under the Mental Health Act, if necessary C could have been treated for his mental disorder without giving consent, but the powers of this Act did not extend to performing an amputation without his consent.

Advance decisions

One way that individuals may exercise their autonomy is through the preparation of a document known as an advance decision or living will. Living wills were proposed by an American lawyer Louise Kutner in 1969 and introduced in the UK by the Voluntary Euthanasia Society in the 1980s. Different terms are used such as advance directives, active declarations and living wills, and these tend to be used interchangeably, but the Mental Capacity Act 2005 uses the term 'advance decision'. Drawing up an advance decision gives individuals an opportunity to express their preferences to others, particularly health professionals, if at a later date they are unable to communicate them verbally. The advance decision therefore is:

> A decision to refuse specified treatment made in advance by a person who has capacity to do so. This decision will then apply at a future time when that person lacks capacity to consent to, or refuse, the specified treatment.
> (Department of Constitutional Affairs 2007, 280)

Prior to the Mental Capacity Act coming into force in 2007, there was no statute in the UK governing advance decisions, but their use was recognised in common law; that is, law made by the judges who adjudicate in different cases. The BMA also published a Code of Practice to guide health professionals in the use of advance statements in clinical practice (British Medical Association 1995). It is difficult to estimate how many advance decisions have been drawn up either prior or subsequent to the Mental Capacity Act 2005, and there is some evidence in the literature that although many people are unaware of living wills, once informed of the subject, they are interested to hear about them (Schiff *et al.* 2000).

The Mental Capacity Act 2005 gives legal effect to advance decisions if made by a person over 18 years with capacity and the emphasis is on refusal of treatment, although the person can change their mind at any time and cancel the advance decision. There are certain criteria that must be adhered to and the advance decision must specify what treatment the individual wishes to refuse. If the advance decision refuses life-sustaining treatment, there are three additional criteria:

1   It must be in writing (it may be written by someone else or recorded in the notes).
2   It must be signed and witnessed.
3   It must state clearly that the decision applies even if life is at risk.

(Department of Constitutional Affairs 2007)

It should be noted that advance decisions are only applicable to appropriate and lawful requests and cannot be used to request assisted suicide, euthanasia, or to ask doctors to act against their professional judgement.

The changes to the legal position on advance decisions recognise and respect a person's autonomy and can give an opportunity for dialogue with healthcare professionals about treatment options when drawing up the document. Furthermore, a written expression of the person's preferences serves to guide those making decisions when dilemmas arise and the person lacks capacity. There are also some shortcomings to consider in that there may be difficulty in predicting how a person may feel about their illness, debilitating symptoms or incapacity in the future, and judgements could be based upon misunderstanding. It is important for the person making the advance decision to be as specific as possible about what treatments they would like to refuse, as this will be open to interpretation by those faced with implementing treatment decisions and may be complicated by the clinical picture at the time. While the advance decision can be amended at any time, there is also always the possibility that new treatments may become available that, had the person been aware of them, they would have wanted to receive (Samuels 1996). Useful practical information on how to go about making an advance decision is available from the Directgov website: www.direct.gov.uk/en/Governmentcitizensandrights/Death/Preparation/DG_10029683.

Allocation of resources

Weale (1998) refers to the inconsistent triad of healthcare provision as a set of three propositions, any two of which are compatible but which together form a contradiction. In healthcare, the three propositions are comprehensive care, high-quality care and care available on the basis of need (rather than the ability to pay). Weale (1998) contends that we can have any two combinations of the propositions but not all three together, so care can be comprehensive and high quality but not necessarily provided on the basis of need, or we can have comprehensive care on the basis of need, but such care will not necessarily be high quality. The inconsistent triad neatly illustrates the problems in providing care and treatment to individuals with long-term conditions which by definition may be numerous and/or extend over a long period of time and thus are expensive. The problem is made more acute in a publicly funded health service where decisions have to be made between what sort of treatment individuals may want to have provided and the treatment the health service has the ability to provide. As Butler (1999) points out, in the National Health Service, the allocation of care does not rely on market forces and access to all aspects of healthcare is not determined by a person's ability to pay. Therefore, to bridge the gap between supply and demand, a variety of rationing strategies have been developed.

One of the most influential methods for this in current practice is by recourse to the objective and quantifiable system of evidence-based medicine or practice. Evidence can show which treatments are effective and thus the ones that should be publicly funded. Proponents of this view argue that to provide less effective treatments or those considered to be futile is a waste of public money and by definition unethical (Parker and Dickenson 2001). However, this view is based on the assumption that, first, such objective, quantifiable evidence exists and, second, that there is a shared understanding of what is ineffective or futile. Differences of opinion of what treatment may be considered futile are illustrated in the Leslie Burke case, a man with the degenerative brain disease Fredrich's ataxia who challenged the General Medical Council on their guidelines for withdrawal of treatment. Mr Burke knew that he would eventually need nutrition and hydration to be administered artificially, and was concerned that should he lose the ability to communicate, doctors might assess his quality of life as poor, the treatment futile, and subsequently withdraw nutrition and hydration from him. Mr Burke did not view the administration of nutrition or hydration as futile, and argued that withdrawing this would cause him mental and physical suffering, and be in violation of his human rights (Samanta and Samanta 2005). Mr Burke eventually lost his case on appeal in the House of Lords and the European Court of Human Rights which held that doctors should not be expected to continue treatment of a patient if, in their professional judgement, the treatment was futile (Buka 2008). At first sight, this case appears to centre on the status of advance decisions, but by defining the treatment Mr Burke requested be given to him as futile this makes certain assumptions about the value of Mr Burke's life. If administering treatment is futile, that is, pointless, useless or ineffective, then by definition Mr Burke's life is seen to be less valuable and therefore not worth saving.

The ethical principle at the heart of this problem is justice or fairness; that is, ensuring that individuals have 'fair, equitable and appropriate treatment in light of what is due or owed to persons' (Beauchamp and Childress 2009, 241). But, in the NHS, there are a number of competing factors to consider in funding a service, and decisions may be based on social criteria (e.g. age), clinical need, treating the first in line (e.g. with waiting lists) or by calculating the efficacy of treatments using the system of quality-adjusted life-years (QALYs). In response to criticisms of a so-called 'postcode lottery' of treatment, the UK government established the National Institute for Health and Clinical Excellence (NICE) to evaluate the cost-effectiveness of medicines and treatment, and to provide guidance on best practice. While this system does appear to be in keeping with Beauchamp and Childress's (2009) definition of justice, NICE guidelines and recommendations can only be based on the available evidence and are dependent on shared understandings of cost-effectiveness.

Generally speaking, NICE bases its recommendations on value for money which is undoubtedly beneficial to the NHS (and arguably taxpaying citizens) as a whole, but such decisions do not obviate the need to choose between people. A recent example of this concerned NICE's decision on the use of a medicine used to treat people with Alzheimer's disease. NICE concluded that the medicine could be prescribed for people in moderate stages of the disease, but not for those in the early or late stages, even though individuals with the disease considered it to be helpful in the early stages. A key issue in this example is the discrepancy in the outcome measures used to assess the effects of the medication and the way in which the symptoms of dementia are rated by people with Alzheimer's disease and those caring for them (Chalmers 2007). The properties that NICE considers to be important are simply different to those that individuals with Alzheimer's disease and/or their carers rate as being important. Hence, prescribing the medication using NICE guidelines is cost-effective to the public purse, but not necessarily effective in alleviating the symptoms of those with the condition. The importance of not squandering public resources should not be minimised, but allocating health resources is a complex issue and cannot be easily done in a fair and just manner. Inevitably, decisions do have to be made from which some individuals will benefit and some will lose out. Owing to potentially complex or lengthy healthcare needs, this will not always be to the advantage of individuals with long-term conditions.

Assisted dying

One of the most complex ethical dilemmas which people caring for individuals with long-term conditions face is when the service user decides that they would like to bring their life to an end but lack the ability to do so without assistance. This may take the form of assisting someone with their suicide or by carrying out acts of euthanasia; that is, deliberately taking measures to end the person's life. In the UK, suicide is not a criminal offence but helping another to do so is, and if found guilty the person may face imprisonment for up to 14 years (Pattinson 2006). A recent case that received much media attention was that of Diane Pretty, a woman with motor neurone disease who unsuccessfully sought leave from the courts for her husband to assist her suicide without fear of prosecution (House of Lords 2001). Mrs Pretty died in 1998 having finally lost her case in the European Court of Human Rights. In February 2003, an assisted suicide bill was introduced by Lord Joffe in the House of Lords, but was eventually blocked in May 2006 as peers backed an amendment to delay the bill (House of Lords 2005). Other terminally ill people including some from the UK have turned to the Swiss organisation Dignitas, a euthanasia group that claims to offer a dignified death to terminally ill people. Since it began in 1998, Dignitas claims to have helped about 85 British people end their lives with some of the cases being reported in the media. Doctors and patients' relatives have been questioned by British police over their role in the suicide, although no criminal charges or prosecutions have been brought to date (Minelli 2007).

While the literal definition of euthanasia is 'a good death' (from the Greek *eu*, good and *thanatos*, death), the term is more commonly used in contemporary society to refer to mercy killing. There are a range of definitions used to describe different forms of euthanasia with active euthanasia defined as a deliberate act bringing about the death of another (such as administering a poison), while passive euthanasia refers to withdrawing or withholding treatment and subsequently allowing the person to die. Other definitions that may be used depend upon consent with euthanasia performed at the individual's request described as voluntary, while euthanasia carried out without the request of the patient is involuntary. The term non-voluntary is used where the person lacks capacity to consent; for example, someone who is unconscious but who has not made their preferences known, or a baby.

In the UK, active euthanasia is unlawful, and consent of the patient, their health status, who carries out the act (be it a health professional or the person's friend or relative) and what their intentions are are all irrelevant, since active euthanasia is not differentiated from any other act of deliberate killing. If a person did carry out an act of active euthanasia, they would face a mandatory life sentence should they be found guilty. While it is rare for health professionals to be charged with murder, even on grounds of compassion, one exception was the case of Dr Cox. Lillian Boyes, a 70-year-old woman with rheumatoid arthritis, repeatedly asked her consultant Dr Cox to end her life as she was in intractable pain unrelieved by analgesia. Dr Cox administered a lethal dose of potassium chloride and she died a short time later. Dr Cox was subsequently charged and found guilty of attempted murder. The lesser charge (rather than murder) was brought, as Mrs Boyes had been cremated before the case was reported to the police, and the absence of forensic evidence coupled with her general health state would have made it extremely difficult to prove beyond all reasonable doubt that she had died directly as result of the injection of potassium chloride. Dr Cox was treated sympathetically by the court as he was given a 12-month suspended sentence, and by the GMC who allowed him to remain on the medical register subject to training and supervision (Pattinson 2006).

While assisted suicide and active euthanasia are not lawful, UK law does recognise the doctrine of double effect which may be summarised as being 'always wrong intentionally to do a bad act for the sake of good consequences that will ensue, but that it may be permissible to do a good act in the knowledge that bad consequences will ensue' (Glover 1977, 87). An example of this is when analgesia is administered to a service user (usually by a doctor) which shortens their life but where the primary motive is to relieve suffering and not to kill the patient (Grubb 2001). The courts have recognised in some circumstances that it may be legitimate to withhold treatment or administer large doses of opiates, even if the incidental effect hastens the person's death (McHale *et al.* 2006). Since 1957, there have been several examples where the distinction between active and passive euthanasia has been demonstrated in legal cases where the defence has relied upon the doctrine of double effect. Recently, the principle was reiterated when permission was sought from the courts to discontinue artificially feeding Tony Bland, a young man in a permanent vegetative state as a result of injuries sustained during the Hillsborough football disaster (*Airedale NHS Trust* v. *Bland 1993*). However, as discussed in the Leslie Burke case above, it cannot be assumed that the best course of action is always to discontinue artificial feeding.

Conclusion

Many of the ethical issues that people with long-term conditions and/or their carers face are not unique. Nonetheless, because such people may need access to medicines, treatment and care for protracted periods of time, they may be vulnerable to resource allocation decisions made on the basis of value for money. Ironically, this state of affairs has arisen precisely because they are a group of people likely to have benefited from research and development into the conditions, technological advances and new treatment options available to them. The principle of respect for autonomy is crucially important in healthcare ethics and law. While new legislation such as the Mental Capacity Act 2005 focuses on ensuring those who may lack capacity in the future can articulate their preferences, a service user's autonomy may be diminished in a range of circumstances. Furthermore, if there is doubt over a person's ability to make an autonomous decision, capacity needs to be formally assessed. Preferably, service users will be full participants in decisions about their treatment and care, with the expectation that their preferences will be respected even if their preferred course of action is deemed unwise. A useful way in which individuals with long-term conditions can make their preferences known is by use of advance directions, the legality of which has been made more explicit in the Mental Capacity Act 2005. This is particularly important when the service user has views about how they would like to be treated at the end of their life. End-of-life decisions are fraught with ethical dilemmas but rising to this challenge constitutes an important aspect of caring for people with long-term conditions and ensuring that, wherever possible, the principles of a good death may be put into practice.

References

Airedale NHS Trust v. *Bland* [1993] 2WLR316.

Beauchamp, T.L. and Childress, J.F. (2009) *Principles of Biomedical Ethics.* New York: Oxford University Press.

British Medical Association (1995) *Advance Statements about Medical Treatment.* London: BMA.

Buka, P. (2008) *Patients' Rights, Law and Ethics for Nurses.* London: Hodder Arnold.

Butler, J. (1999) *The Ethics of Health Care Rationing.* London: Cassell.

Chalmers, I. (2007) The Alzheimer's Society. Drug Firms and Public Trust. *British Medical Journal,* 335 (7616), 4000.

Department of Constitutional Affairs (2007) *Mental Capacity Act 2005. Code of Practice.* London: The Stationery Office.

Department of Health (2005) *The National Service Framework for Long-term Conditions.* London: Department of Health.

Fletcher, N., Holt, J., Brazier, M. *et al.* (1995) *Ethics, Law and Nursing.* Manchester: Manchester University Press.

Glover, J. (1977) *Causing Death and Saving Lives.* Harmondsworth: Penguin.

Griffith, R. (2008) Deprivation of Liberty Safeguards. *British Journal of Community Nursing,* 13 (11), 532–537.

Griffiths, R. and Tengnah, C. (2008) Mental Capacity Act 2005: Statutory Principles and Key Concepts. *British Journal of Community Nursing,* 13(5), 233–237.

Grubb, A. (2001) Euthanasia in England – A Law Lacking Compassion? *European Journal of Health Law,* 8(2), 89–93.

Harris, J. (1985) *The Value of Life.* London: Routledge.

Holt, J. (2002) In *Advancing Practice in Cancer and Palliative Care Nursing,* Ed. Clarke, D., Flanagan, J., Kendrick, K. Basingstoke: Macmillan.

House of Lords (2001) Vol. 2005. Online. Available at: www.publications.parliament.uk/pa/ld200102/ldjudgmt/jd011129/pretty-1.htm. (accessed 4 March 2009).

House of Lords (2005) Vol. 2006. Online. Available at: www.publications.parliament.uk/pa/ld200506/ldbills/036/06036.i.html. (accessed 4 March 2009).

Law Commission (2005) *Mental Capacity Act.* London: The Stationery Office.

McHale, J., Fox, M., Gunn, M. *et al.* (2006) *Healthcare Law; Text, Cases and Materials.* London: Sweet & Maxwell.

Mechanic, D. and Tanner, J. (2007) Vulnerable People, Groups and Populations. *Health Affairs*, 26 (5), 1220–1230.

Minelli, L.A. (2007) Vol. 2008. Online. Available at: www.dignitas.ch/WeitereTexte/FriendsAtTheEnd.pdf. (accessed 10 July 2008).

Parker, M. and Dickenson, D. (2001) *The Cambridge Medical Ethics Workbook.* Cambridge: Cambridge University Press.

Pattinson, S. (2006) *Medical Law and Ethics.* London: Sweet & Maxwell.

Samanta, A. and Samanta, J. (2005) End of Life Decisions. *British Medical Journal*, 331(7528), 1284–1285.

Samuels, A. (1996) The Advance Directive (Or Living Will). *Medical Science Law*, 36, 2–8.

Schiff, R., Rajkumar, C. and Bulpitt, C. (2000) Views of Elderly People on Living Wills. Interview Study. *British Medical Journal*, 320, 1640–1641.

Weale, A. (1998) Rationing Health Care. *British Medical Journal*, 316, 831–841.

Part II

Developing holistic care

Introduction

A crucial aspect of being able to develop and deliver holistic care is a thorough understanding of the needs and wishes of the person with a long-term condition. In Chapter 5 the authors discuss and illustrate how the reader can develop skills and knowledge in undertaking systematic, comprehensive and holistic assessments for the purposes of understanding a client's physical, psychological and social functioning. The reader is guided through the principles and practice of screening for a wide range of health and social care needs, and to consider the importance of not only assessing for healthcare deficits but also, and crucially, to be able to balance such deficits against the overall backdrop of the client's life, recognising the individual as a person with abilities, aspirations, strengths and goals.

Assisting clients to maximise control over their physical symptoms (such as pain, fatigue and breathlessness) and psychological experiences (such as affective disturbances, stress and anxiety, alterations to self-image and self-esteem) is an important part of the holistic care of people with chronic ill-health. In Chapter 6, guidance is offered on how to best assist clients to cope with, and adjust to, their conditions and how clients may be supported to communicate their needs, and to access services effectively to ensure that the right care is offered. Central to maximising the client's ability to develop their personal perceptions of self-efficacy is self-management, and links between the person's cognitive appraisals of their condition are considered, as is the importance of developing a sense of hope for their future and personal mastery and control over their symptoms. Related policy initiatives are also discussed, including the Expert Patient Programme (EPP).

Chapter 7 gives an overview of specific psychological and therapeutic strategies, both individual and in a group context, which can facilitate and support recovery across a wide range of conditions. Problem-solving therapies, brief therapies, cognitive behavioural interventions, psychoeducational programmes and motivational interviewing are highlighted in particular. This chapter assists the reader to become focused on factors which aim to promote the overall health and well-being of the person with a long-term condition – recognising the individual as a sentient individual with hopes and fears, which can impact on their perceptions of their recovery and overall quality of life. The authors offer advice regarding how to empower people to make meaningful choices, to enhance coping ability and to consider the impact of perceived positive social support in promoting recovery and preventing relapse and remission.

5 Frameworks for comprehensive and holistic assessment

Carl Margereson, Steve Trenoweth and Jan Worledge

Introduction

If all needs relating to ongoing health problems are to be met effectively, and if individuals are to be assisted with improving their overall quality of life, then comprehensive and holistic assessments are crucial. Such assessments will focus on both immediate and potential future needs and will consider the psychological, social, emotional, physical and spiritual dimensions of the whole person. This will require attentive listening to the individual's narrative of their illness so that their needs, views and wishes are at the centre of all decisions made. The overall aim of such assessments is to establish the type and range of support needed to maintain independent living and to improve psychological well-being and resilience, while maintaining and developing social networks and delaying deterioration in physical or mental health. The assessment of needs, and decision-making to address health issues, are never one-off activities but ongoing processes dictated by the changing needs of the person, their family and carers (DoH 2005a). This is by no means an easy task and will depend on a number of factors, not least the setting in which care is provided and the background and skill of the assessor. However, what is crucial is that assessments are sufficiently structured and detailed to afford an overview of the totality of the individual's needs, problems, wishes and, indeed, strengths.

The process of comprehensive and holistic assessments

In comprehensive and holistic assessments a systematic approach needs to be taken and skills acquired in order to collect and analyse health and social care information. This process should be collaborative, involving the person, their carer and family whenever appropriate and possible. It is vital that a complete and wide-ranging assessment is undertaken to enable a full understanding of each individual. If healthcare professionals focus too much on the specific areas relating to what they perceive to be the 'primary' problem(s), such as a particular medical diagnosis or social needs, the individual becomes 'splintered' and the bigger picture is lost. As such, other areas which may impact upon, or be related to, the perceived primary need may be unknown, ignored or go unmet. Chapter 8 provides details regarding how interviews may be undertaken to elicit sometimes personal and painful information relating to an individual's life and the clinical skills required in this endeavour. It is important, however, that such questions are framed by the use of active listening, the demonstration of empathy, skilled interpersonal skills and sensitivity.

Subjective assessments

A subjective assessment is one in which data are meaningful primarily to the individual and should begin by asking about the difficulties the person feels they have currently. Their responses should be recorded wherever possible in their own words. A credulous approach should be taken recognising the importance of the person's perception of symptoms and the possible cause of health problems. This may help to establish whether there are gaps in an individual's knowledge or understanding that need to be addressed later. If coping skills and self-management are to be developed, including self-monitoring skills, then individuals need to understand the underlying disorder and the medication prescribed (Margereson 2008). Where there is misunderstanding, this can contribute to non-concordance and have an impact on the trajectory and possible prognosis of the long-term condition.

Subjective assessments may also include 'psychosocial' aspects which recognise the importance of psychological (thoughts, feelings and behaviours), interpersonal and environmental factors on the client's overall well-being. Indeed, there is overwhelming evidence that subjective psychosocial factors can impact on the aetiology and trajectory of long-term conditions, and have a significant influence on clinical outcomes and satisfaction with treatment. Subjective assessments are so-called as data gathered are based on individual responses which can be influenced by a number of factors, not least memory. Nevertheless, the meaning that a client attributes to their lives is of central concern. Appropriate communication skills should be used to encourage the individual to 'tell their personal story'. In their encounters with health professionals, individuals present their problems as stories and this has led to a 'narrative-based approach' which helps in understanding their accounts (Launer 2002). For example, in 'motivational interviewing' – a client-centred counselling technique centring on health behaviour change (Miller and Rollnick 2002) – a useful approach which facilitates and structures the individual's sharing of their frame of reference is that of the 'typical day' strategy. Here, the client is asked to conversationally describe a usual or common day in their life, and to annotate how their health status or condition impacts upon this (Rollnick *et al.* 1999).

As such, data are likely to include information relating to their perception of their overall health and illness, and will include:

- their perception of, and meaning that is attributed to, the current presenting problem;
- the client's perception of their prior health-related experiences and the sense that they make of this;
- their beliefs surrounding the aetiology of the current problem;
- the impact that the present problem has on their social, vocational, sexual, spiritual, domestic and interpersonal life;
- the impact that the present problems have on their perceptions of 'self', for example, self-esteem, self-worth, body image and self-concept;
- what they feel might improve or make the condition worse;
- what skills and abilities they believe they have in being able to cope with their health-related problems.

Personal biography

There is clearly a need to capture factual information which provides a contemporary snapshot of the individual's life and such information is usually subject to local policy. It is important to realise that personal details captured should be relevant to the current health issue in question, and should be contemporaneous. This information is likely to include, for example: name; age; address; marital status and next of kin; children; name of primary carer; hobbies and interests; ethnicity; cultural and religious observances; employment status; and receipt of benefits.

Personal history

In attempting to understand holistic needs, the individual's personal history can be of major importance and significance. Sometimes, however, an individual with long-term health problems may have already had a comprehensive assessment of their physical and/or psychiatric 'needs' which may already be documented. Often, assessments can be duplicated with health and social care professionals seeking to collect the same or very similar information. Effective strategies might involve the single assessment process such as that described in the National Service Framework for Older People (DoH 2001) as well as the accessing of personal information by other means such as through previous notes and electronic records.

It is important that information is sought out if available. Much of this information is likely to be a matter of historical record – and time should not be wasted, or the client's patience tested, in asking for information when it could be easily obtained elsewhere. The importance of understanding the client's view of their personal history is that it helps the professional to develop an understanding which grounds the client in their own personal, biographical context. In this sense, the history assessment should be seen as the starting point of a subjective assessment (see below) rather than a 'mere' collection of prior health-related data.

The assessment of personal history should include details of:

- previous ill-health (medical and psychiatric if appropriate) with diagnosis if possible;
- risk (previous history of, for example, falls, hospitalisations, self-neglect, suicide attempts, alcohol, smoking and/or drug use) (see Lifestyle section, p. 77, for examples of assessment tools);
- previous medical/surgical history with dates;
- allergies and immunisation with dates;
- treatment information, such as prescribed medication and any equipment used;
- relevant family history, including medical conditions of parents, grandparents, siblings, children and grandchildren;
- social history, including social networks;
- history of education and achievements;
- occupational history.

It is vital, however, not to be too prescriptive and directive in obtaining such information, and steps should be taken to ask the client if there is anything they feel from their history that may have a bearing on their present experience of health and illness.

Medication

The issue of medication is of crucial importance, and a complete and comprehensive list of medication must be compiled. Information should be obtained about the use of prescribed medication and attempting to ascertain the individual's understanding and rationale for, and satisfaction with, prescribed medication. Does, for example, the client understand the effects and side-effects? Does the client know how to use their prescribed medication *smartly* if this is indicated? Such understandings are likely to be a major indicator of concordance with prescribed treatment plans. Knowledge deficits here will need to be addressed later in health-promotion strategies. In addition, the use of medical equipment such as oxygen concentrators, nebulisers and non-invasive ventilation should be noted together with the supplier.

Dissatisfaction with prescribed medication (either due to the perception of its lack of efficacy, or the client's lack of involvement in, and consent to, treatment decisions) may lead to the use of unprescribed, over-the-counter or psychoactive substances as a means to control symptoms. For example, there is evidence that some older people may use/abuse alcohol as a means of controlling pain. As such, it will be necessary to understand what steps the client has taken to self-medicate and their reasons for this.

Symptom exploration

Not every individual with a long-term disorder will require a full physical examination, particularly where there is only a single disorder and where the ability to self-care is good. However, where there are complex health and social care needs with increasing frailty and vulnerability, more comprehensive assessment will be needed. Where there are specific complaints, such as fatigue, anxiety, breathlessness and so forth, then details regarding each should be documented methodically. The mnemonic **OPQRSTU** is useful in remembering the right questions to ask as follows:

*   **O**nset – When did it start?
*   **P**rovocation/**P**alliation – What makes it worse? What relieves the symptoms?
*   **Q**uality/**Q**uantity – What is it like? How much?
*   **R**egion/**R**adiation – Where is it experienced? Does it go anywhere else?
*   **S**everity – How severe is it?
*   **T**iming – When did it start? How frequent is it? How long does it last?
*   **U**nderstanding – What do you think it means?

A risk assessment must also be undertaken in relation to what may make the condition worse; the likelihood of its occurring; the impact this may have on the individual and others; and what actions are subsequently required to reduce such impact or offset anticipated problems.

A general review of all systems from 'head to toe' is important so that the client has an opportunity to identify problems in specific areas (see Physical assessment section for systems, p. 72). It is then important to consider how reported health problems are impacting on the individual's day-to-day life, not least in being able to independently perform activities of living (see above). Each body system is reviewed systematically and questions are asked regarding current health status. Recording baseline data is particularly important when individuals are initially referred so that carers are aware of new developments. Although review of systems is often part of a planned health assessment, in many instances ongoing assessment is crucial. For example, where individuals require long-term care owing to increasing vulnerability, self-reporting of changes may not be possible and carers should be vigilant in the recognition of subtle changes from the individual's norm.

Self-assessment

Central to the subjective assessment process is the importance of the client being involved in collecting their own health-related data. Such assessments are based on what a person says about themselves and their abilities. This allows the individual to identify the issues which they see as problematic and which they are concerned about. This is the start of collaborative care and facilitates a negotiation of mutual understandings regarding the individual's needs. Of course, there will be variances in the ability and willingness to participate in this process – but self-monitoring and self-assessment is a process which should be encouraged and the client supported to collect data relating to their own health and experience of illness.

There are many techniques which could be used to facilitate self-assessment. What is crucial, however, is for the healthcare practitioner to offer a framework for such data collection which is comprehensible and not an onerous task for the person. To assist in the process there are many self-rating assessment tools which seek to capture the individual's view of a health problem, such as the Brief Pain Inventory (BPI) (Cleeland 2009) and the Medical Research Council (MRC) Breathlessness Scale (Fletcher 1960). Other methods include the keeping of a diary or journal to record not only clinical information but perhaps also thoughts, feelings and behaviours relating to their health experiences or the keeping of a chart which might include subjective experience of symptoms, for example, pain. Checklists may also be completed over the telephone where an assessor records what the service user says about their condition. This information may then be used to determine the urgency of the problem or to establish whether it can be dealt with in a different way. There are also online resources, such as the Disabled Living Foundation, which offer an online functional self-assessment for people with disabilities to give advice about equipment and services (further information is available at www.asksara.org.uk).

Functional assessments

The assessment and analysis of function provides information on a person's ability, volition and potential to live as independently as possible. Coupled with data from other assessments such as the biomedical assessment (below), the functional assessment provides an evaluation of the overall ability of the individual and identifies specific deficits which impair performance. These deficits may be of a physical nature or be aligned to cognitive or sensory impairment or related to environmental factors.

'Function' is the ability to complete the tasks which are essential to a person's well-being including personal care activities such as toileting or work-related skills such as typing. Function or occupational performance is closely influenced by the environment in which a task is performed and by the social context and other dynamics which govern all human activity: function cannot be meaningfully assessed without reference to these factors. Effective performance of a task depends on both mental and physical skills. A systematic approach to functional assessment provides a framework to identify factors which enable a person to complete a task and those which limit their ability (Law *et al.* 2005).

Assessment of function or occupational performance is a person-centred process which seeks first to establish which activities are the most important for the individual. It may also examine the person's perceptions of their performance and their insight into the problems they are experiencing. It is a dynamic process which not only identifies problems but also seeks to develop solutions to overcome those difficulties. These may include therapy or rehabilitation to improve physical ability and confidence, learning different techniques to complete the task safely, or the provision of equipment or adaptations to overcome physical barriers to independence.

Functional assessments are usually carried out by occupational therapists working in health, social services, housing or in the independent sector. However, as it provides a baseline for intervention and planning, functional assessments are also carried out by other disciplines. Physiotherapists, speech and language therapists and dieticians, for example, may also undertake assessments in their specialist areas of the assessment (such as mobility or eating). All hospital inpatients need a functional assessment prior to discharge; however, where there has been a change in physical ability a functional assessment is included as part of the discharge planning to determine what equipment and care an individual will need on their return home and to evaluate risk. An assessment of risk will consider risks to: the individual; carers; the family; and the wider community (such as the risks of driving a car after a heart attack). In addition, risk assessments should not only consider injury or damage to health but also look at factors which may impair independence, social inclusion, access to work and leisure activities, education and mental health. This process often includes a home visit by the occupational therapist.

The functional assessment of people with long-term conditions should not assume that a specific diagnosis indicates a particular disability (although of course it might) but should recognise that there may be other conditions present which also affect function. Occupational performance is also affected by features which may not be part of the initial diagnosis but are subsidiary to it. For instance, some people with long-term conditions may also be clinically depressed and this may lead to loss of confidence, low self-esteem and reduced concentration levels which may contribute to poor performance (Van Dreusen and Brunt 1997). Clear data about a person's abilities enable the therapist in partnership with the individual and their carer to plan interventions (such as rehabilitation and provision of equipment or care) which are designed to enhance performance and facilitate independence. Monitoring functional performance enables the individual and the assessor to track the progress of the condition and any changes which result from treatment and/or rehabilitation: it is perhaps the yardstick that many individuals use to assess their own health and well-being.

Elements of functional assessment may be included in the evaluation to establish eligibility for a number of benefits and resources, such as:

- equipment for personal care and assistive technology;

- wheelchair provision;
- adaptations to home;
- rehousing;
- welfare benefits such as Disabled Living Allowance, Attendance Allowance;
- travel concessions such as Disabled Parking Badge, Concessionary bus pass;
- insurance pay-outs;
- access to rehabilitation;
- social care support such as personal or residential care as identified in Community Care Assessments or discharge planning.

An initial interview will seek to identify which areas need more consideration and which do not. It is important to recognise that sometimes a person's assessment of their own abilities may not be an accurate reflection of their performance. The interview will include:

- the person's views about their own performance;
- the individual's environment;
- the needs of carers;
- past performance;
- work and leisure activities;
- informal unstructured observation of the person's abilities.

After an initial assessment where the essential or problematic tasks have been identified, the person will be asked to perform these tasks while they are observed. This may be in their own home or in an occupational therapy department in a hospital or other facility. An individual may be expected to perform better in their own home as they are familiar with the surroundings, know where things are kept and are usually more at ease within their own environment. However, in the more structured environment of an occupational therapy unit other features such as work surfaces may be at a better height and there may be more space to manoeuvre mobility equipment, enabling a person to perform better. Ultimately an individual needs to be able to do the task safely and effectively within their own environment. The therapist will not simply be watching the task but actively analysing the activity and any problems encountered. This type of assessment provides an opportunity for the therapist and individual to discuss the difficulty and solve problems together so that any solutions reached will be acceptable and therefore more likely to be sustained. Observational assessments may also include carers and may evaluate the level of a person's independence (the ability to complete tasks safely and/or unaided); any additional assistance required; any apparent risks; and the time taken to complete tasks.

The development of standardised tools for functional performance has been difficult owing to the complexity of the number of variants to be considered in each assessment and the unique nature of individuals, and the environmental and social context in which they live. However, increasingly standardised tools are being used to assess and record function. These provide a more accurate way of comparing a person's performance as the condition develops and to evaluate performance against a set of standards or norms that enables results to be quantified and measurable.

Table 5.1 Personal and Instrumental Activities of Living

Personal Activities of Living	Instrumental Activities of Living
These include:	*These include:*
• washing	• household tasks such as cleaning and laundry
• continence and use of the toilet	
• dressing	• meal preparation and clearing up
• grooming of hair and/or shaving	• shopping
• eating	• care of dependants (child, adult or pet)
• mobility and transfers from bed, chair	• communication such as use of telephone or computer
• sexual activities	
	• car-driving or use of public transport
	• money management
	• paid or voluntary work
	• leisure activities

Occupational performance is affected by a number of features which require a more in-depth assessment and so a functional assessment is often accompanied by other assessments which look at skills such as cognition and perception and at social context, and which will impact on functional performance. Activities of Living are activities which an individual has to carry out on a daily basis and which enable them to live independently. They may be classified as Personal Activities of Living (sometimes called 'basic' Activities of Living functions which are essential to well-being) and Instrumental Activities of Living (activities which are concerned with the wider community and household which may be undertaken by other people) (see Table 5.1).

However, a 'function' cannot be assessed without reference to the environment in which the task is undertaken. The layout of a room can impair or facilitate access to facilities; clutter and untidiness may be hazardous to someone with reduced mobility or confusing for someone with poor vision. Furthermore, the outdoor terrain may restrict someone's ability to walk in their garden or to reach the bus stop. All individuals are subject to the social and cultural expectations of their family and community. Most societies have clear expectations of roles based on gender, age or status and these should be taken into account when assessing function; for instance, is this a task that the person would normally undertake within their family group?

Mental health assessments

Given the psychosocial impact of long-term health problems a mental health assessment is an important part of the assessment process. In holistic health the mind, body and spirit are seen as interdependent and functioning as a whole within the environment (Jarvis 2004), and therefore a number of dimensions need to be considered. In assessing people in mental distress, the 'Five Ws' approach (What? When? Where? With? Why?) may be used (Fox and Gamble 2006). For example:

- **What?** (e.g. What do you feel are the current problems for you?)
- **When?** (e.g. When does this affect you?)
- **Where?** (e.g. In what situations?)
- **With?** (e.g. Are there people who make the problems worse? Or better?)
- **Why?** (e.g. How do you account for your current problems?)

In order to explore an issue in more detail one might use 'funnelling' questions signified by the mnemonic **FIND** (Fox and Gamble 2006):

- **F**requency (e.g. How often does this occur?)
- **I**ntensity (e.g. On a scale of 0–10 where 10 is the most you can imagine and 0 is none at all, how intense does this feel?)
- **N**umber (e.g. How many times do you experience this? Do you notice any patterns?)
- **D**uration (e.g. For how long do you experience this?)

Of course, not everyone with a long-term condition will inevitably have psychological or even psychiatric needs. However, having debilitating, chronic, painful health problems can lead to an *increased* risk of developing such problems – and this not only impacts on their overall quality of life but is likely to have a significant impact on the success of any health interventions. Furthermore, there is evidence that people with a diagnosed psychiatric problem have significantly poorer physical health than the general population. As such, there is a need to conduct a psychiatric/psychological assessment with people with long-term conditions.

Debilitating conditions with distressing symptoms and feelings of despair regarding the prognosis and/or trajectory of physical illness are often cited as a contributory factor to suicide, and it is among the older population that the highest suicide rates can be found. It is of vital importance that any client who is socially isolated; expresses feelings of hopelessness; displays symptoms of depression; has made previous suicide attempts; and has experienced recent stressors and/or bereavements (Cutcliffe and Barker 2004) is assessed for an intention and plan to commit suicide (see Chapter 15).

The various guidelines issued by the National Institute for Health and Clinical Excellence (NICE) for mental health and behavioural disorders stress the importance of a 'stepped' approach to care and treatment. The guidelines recognise, quite accurately, that most people with mental health or psychological problems are cared for in primary care. It is likely, therefore, that staff working in such settings (along with clinicians working in casualty departments or on medical or surgical admission wards) are likely to first detect symptoms of psychological, or even psychiatric, difficulties. At such times, NICE recommend that brief screening questions are used (Chapter 15) to ascertain if treatment in primary care services is warranted or if further specialist help needs to be sought. A tool which is also used widely in research and to rapidly screen for depression and anxiety in medical settings is the 'Hospital Anxiety and Depression Scale' (HADS) (Snaith 2003). The HADS Tool may be obtained from http://shop.gl-assessment.co.uk/home.php?cat=417.

We all experience symptoms of mental ill-health from time to time and not all of us will require treatment or referral to specialist services. However, help may be needed if our mental distress becomes persistent or leads to functional impairment and undermines the quality of life, or when we pose a risk to ourselves or to others. Broadly, when assessing mental ill-health the following are explored.

Affect and mood

'Affect' refers to subjective emotional experiences whereas 'mood' refers to the overall emotional state of mind of an individual. People with mood disturbances may feel anxious or sad, or experience despair, anguish and guilt (which are feelings common in depression). Alternatively, a person may feel elated, euphoric, angry or irritable (as may be the case in mania). It is possible for people to experience feelings of depression and mania alternately, such as in bipolar affective disorder (sometimes referred to as manic depression).

For some people their feelings of mental distress may be associated with persistent and disabling feelings of anxiety, worry, fear and panic. Sometimes such fear may be triggered by an environmental stimulus (such as in the case of a phobia) or may be due to internal ruminations. In extreme cases, people may experience 'derealisation' (feelings of things not being real) or 'depersonalisation' (feelings of being detached from one's own body).

Appearance and behaviour

The appearance and behaviour of a person can reveal much about the mental distress they may be experiencing but it is important not to jump to conclusions. Affective symptoms of depression are often associated with withdrawal from social situations, and such people may appear sad and downcast or be tearful. It is not uncommon for depressed people to present with a slowness of movement, known as psychomotor retardation. Alternatively, people who are elated may have an increased rate (pressure) and volume of speech, be overactive, restless or agitated, while people who are anxious may tremble or shake. Some people may also experience repetitive and ritualistic behaviours accompanied by obsessive thoughts (for example, fears of contamination leading to excessive handwashing) suggestive of an 'obsessive compulsive disorder'.

It is not uncommon for people experiencing mental distress to lack self-care or to neglect their appearance or personal hygiene (Matthews and Trenoweth 2008). This can be particularly diagnostic when someone's current behaviour is not in keeping with their usual patterns of self-care. For some people experiencing negative symptoms of schizophrenia (such as alogia (poverty of speech), apathy, lack of emotional responsiveness, social withdrawal), there may be a lack of motivation to attend to even the most basic of self-care functions and they may be extremely passive.

Cognition

Cognition refers to thinking, and there are two ways in which this is assessed. First, one is interested in the way in which someone is thinking; that is, their thinking processes. Commonly, this is referred to as the *form* of their cognition (Barker 2004). For example, a person's thought processes may be extremely fast indicated by rapidity of speech and frequent jumping between topics (flight of ideas). Alternatively, a person's thought processes may be very slow indicating impairment in the processing of information, and subsequent difficulty in decision-making and problem-solving. People who are 'thought disordered' (such as in schizophrenia) may have poor concentration and attention, and may use words that are disconnected and form sentences that make no sense to the listener, while people with dementia may be confused, have an inability to memorise recent information, and may be poorly orientated to time, person and place.

In addition, the *content* of someone's cognition (that is, what they think about) is also of interest as there may be a lack of awareness of the significance or the extent of their mental health problems. People may have 'strange' ideas that are completely impossible (delusions) or believe that public information has personal significance for them (ideas of reference). These are symptoms often associated with schizophrenia. Furthermore, some people may believe they have a superhuman ability (such as being able to control the weather) or that they are being controlled by some external force (such as the television) or have persecutory ideas (that particular people or groups of people wish to harm them, such as their neighbours).

Some people, especially those who experience depression, may harbour negative beliefs about themselves (for example, that they are worthless) or they may feel overwhelmed by their situation which may be seen as hopeless. There might be a belief that they are helpless to do anything to solve a current crisis. People may also have persistent concerns about their physical health (this is known as hypochondriasis when there is no underlying medical problem) or there may be distress and excessive concern regarding body image or physical appearance.

Perception

Hallucinations can occur in any of five senses: olfactory (smell), gustatory (taste), auditory (hearing), tactile (touch) or visual. It is important to recognise that such sensations are not beliefs or illusions but sensory perceptions which occur in the absence of corresponding external stimuli. To the person experiencing the hallucination they are perceived as real. Hallucinations are not an uncommon human experience in response to extreme or distressing circumstances. Bereaved people, for example, may report hearing the voice of, or even seeing, their loved one and visual hallucinations may occur in febrile states or during extreme fatigue. However, it becomes a mental health issue when a person regularly experiences such phenomena and when this leads to distress, increased risk or a functional impairment in the person's life. Hallucinations are one of the positive symptoms of schizophrenia and by far the most common form is auditory, such as when the person 'hears' people making derogatory comments or giving a running commentary on their actions. On occasions, the hallucinations may command the person to undertake specific actions. However, hallucinations are also not uncommon in Lewy body dementia and severe depression.

Objective assessments

'Objective' data are gathered during the assessment process by utilising various assessment skills required to perform a physical examination and also by using assessment tools to quantify data a little more effectively. By objective we do not wish to imply that such assessments always equate to a clinical truth about the individual's condition, merely that such assessments provide details of the condition which relate to a medical, psychological and functional understanding. Other than doctors and some nurses, very few carers will carry out the more complex physical examinations. Even where there is little experience in carrying out health assessments the development of observational skills during inspection can elicit a great deal of information. Indeed, observation begins during the gathering of subjective data.

How detailed physical examinations are will depend on a number of factors not least the experience of the professional carer. There are times when the focus will be on one particular area where perhaps there is only one disorder. It is impossible here to provide a detailed account of physical health assessment and only a brief overview of the key areas is possible. Where professional roles require more advanced assessment skills, the practitioner will need to reflect upon their ability, competence and confidence and seek additional resources if appropriate. The authors are mindful that there are many non-specialist carers who need to develop further their observational skills so that problems can be detected early, and the focus here will therefore be on inspection with some reference to palpation.

Physical assessments

This stage involves the use of specific clinical skills to obtain information which complements the subjective data already gathered. It begins with a general survey of the individual's state of health noting their height, weight, demeanour, facial expression and personal grooming. Specific observations such as temperature, pulse respiration, blood pressure and urinalysis should be undertaken and recorded. Additional tests such as blood tests, electrocardiogram and X-rays may also be ordered by the healthcare professional. Objective data gathering also includes a physical examination which provides a review of each system using the following assessment skills:

- **Inspection** – using our eyes to observe for possible changes;
- **Palpation** – using our hands to feel for possible changes;
- **Percussion** – using our fingers to produce a percussion note over different parts of the body which may indicate abnormalities;
- **Auscultation** – using a stethoscope to identify normal sounds and possible abnormal sounds (e.g. over the chest and abdomen).

This will also involve a more detailed review of each body system where appropriate and an assessment of symptom management, while being alert for new symptoms as a result of additional health problems. Baseline information allows future comparison and abnormalities detected during the assessment should be documented. Individual consent must always be obtained before any physical assessment which should be carried out in an area that is quiet and offers privacy. The individual should be made comfortable with any exposure kept to a minimum and explanations should be given throughout the assessment. In some instances it is appropriate to have a chaperone available and discretion should be exercised here and local policy followed. The following outlines the areas which should be reviewed.

Skin

The skin is a body system that can be directly observed and often reflects general health status. Attention should be given to the presence of any skin diseases, rashes, sores or itching and note made of any recent changes perhaps involving the hair, nails and any moles. Bruising may denote a recent injury and the location and extent of any bruising needs to be documented. There are many possible causes of bruising including side-effects of prescribed medication such as anticoagulants. Where mobility is a problem, inspection of pressure areas particularly over bony prominences is important, so that any changes indicating excessive pressure may be documented and reported. Palpation can elicit information not only about hydration status where, for example, there may be loss of skin elasticity but can also provide clues as to whether the body is too warm or too cold.

Head, eyes, ears, nose and throat (HEENT)

Although not a body system as such, it is usual to group these areas together during the initial physical assessment. When looking at the face there should be symmetry, and any abnormalities such as drooping on one side should be noted. The hair and scalp should be inspected for possible lesions and parasites. The position of the eyes and alignment is observed as well as the eyelids, sclera and conjunctiva for signs of redness, irritation and possible discharge. Both pupils should be equal in size and react to light, and muscles controlling the eyes should enable movement up, down and to the sides.

The ears should be inspected and once again any sign of irritation, inflammation and discharge documented. Hearing deficits may be initially assessed by whispering a few words behind the individual and then asking them to repeat the words, although additional tests may be carried out by more experienced professionals. The nose, including nasal mucosa, is then observed and gentle palpation over the frontal and maxillary sinuses may reveal tenderness. Inspection of the lips and oral cavity including mucosa, tongue, gums, teeth and tonsils then follows. Where individuals are not able to self-report and particularly where there are difficulties with dietary and fluid intake, inspection should be carried out regularly, as inflammation and infection can cause considerable discomfort and distress. The possibility of neck stiffness or pain should also be considered and observation made for any swollen areas.

Breasts and axillae

Breasts should be examined with the arms first relaxed and then elevated, and observation made on size, symmetry, texture and colour. Important to note is the presence of retraction, and bruising and palpation should reveal no masses or tenderness. If there is any discharge from the nipple then consistency and colour should be noted. Palpation of each axilla may reveal small, non-tender lymph nodes which are normal, but there should be no masses or enlarged, tender nodes. Whenever possible skills in breast self-examination should be taught so that any future problems can be detected early and expert opinion sought.

Respiratory

Ideally the individual should be sitting in a chair or on the side of the bed. Both the anterior and chest wall should be inspected and palpated. It is usual to stand in front of the patient initially and observe the chest movement during breathing, and movements should be equal on both sides. There should be no distress during quiet breathing at rest with the inspiratory phase slightly shorter than expiratory (1:2) with only the diaphragm being used to breathe. Respiratory rate should be approximately 12 to 20 breaths per minute at rest in an adult. Accessory muscles used, particularly those in the neck, indicate that the work of breathing is increased and may be seen in those with respiratory or cardiac problems. A bluish discolouration of the mucous membranes in the mouth and of the tongue may indicate poor oxygenation. An audible wheeze may be heard in asthma and chronic obstructive pulmonary disease. Any cough should be noted and the amount, colour and consistency of any sputum produced. Gentle palpation of the anterior and chest wall may reveal tender areas which require further investigation. Additional respiratory tests including percussion and auscultation may be carried out by experienced professionals.

Cardiovascular

Assessment of the cardiovascular system is usually detailed and involves inspection, palpation, percussion and auscultation. Observation of body build may give some indication as to risk for cardiac disease with obesity increasing risk significantly. Again, discolouration of the lips, skin, nail beds and mucous membranes of the mouth may denote poor oxygenation of the blood while pallor may suggest anaemia. Breathlessness is also a feature of some heart conditions as well as respiratory problems. In heart failure excess fluid is often retained and this may be seen around the lower legs and ankles which become swollen (oedema). As heart failure worsens and fluid retention increases, pressure in the veins increases. Evidence of this may often be seen when the individual is lying in bed at a 45-degree angle where the internal jugular vein in the neck becomes particularly prominent.

The heart rate at rest is important to note and often the apex beat is used which is usually found just under the breast on the left side (midclavicular line in the fifth intercostal space), although the position may well change where there is heart disease. One of the peripheral pulse points (e.g. the radial in the wrist) is also used to estimate the heart rate, and the volume and pattern of the beat are also important to note. Rates that are very fast or indeed very slow from what is expected for the person's age can result in problems such as confusion, faintness and loss of consciousness, needing further investigation.

Peripheral vascular

There are a number of conditions that can result in poor circulation through the peripheral blood vessels supplying the upper and lower limbs. Early signs are calf pain and cramps when walking which ease when the individual rests (intermittent claudication). Limbs should be inspected and palpated for symmetry, size, colour and warmth with major pulses palpated and compared. Inspection of each calf is particularly important where there may be tenderness, and swelling and lesions and ulcers can develop where there is a history of peripheral vascular disease.

Gastrointestinal

Individuals may present with a range of possible problems including swallowing difficulties, heartburn, nausea, vomiting, abdominal pain and changes in bowel habits. On inspection of the abdomen there may be signs of swelling and distension and note should be made of any colour changes, markings, scars, rashes or lesions. On gentle palpation of the different areas of the abdominal wall there may be tenderness elicited and increased rigidness detected. Although peristalsis can often be visible on the abdomen when viewed from the foot of the bed, normal bowel sounds can also be heard with a stethoscope placed on the abdominal wall. The silent abdomen is always a worrying sign and should be investigated. Disorders affecting the rectum and anal area can cause great discomfort and embarrassment. However, inspection may reveal skin tags, ulcers, inflammation, haemorrhoids, warts and herpes. Examination of the anus and rectum may be required and this will be carried out by an experienced health practitioner.

Genito-urinary

Individuals may present complaining of problems passing urine which may include pain, frequency, urgency, hesitancy, dribbling, incontinence and blood in the urine. Inspection may reveal changes to the external genitalia – penis, scrotum or vagina. Pubic hair has a characteristic distribution and in some individuals there may be small brown lice at the base of the hair shaft. The penis should be observed for rashes, sores or masses. The prepuce or foreskin protects the glans and, if present, should be retracted from the glans so that the area can be inspected, which again should be free of ulcers and signs of inflammation. There may be problems with a tight foreskin that makes retraction difficult if not impossible, and this may require treatment. Although a small amount of whitish material is normal under the foreskin (smegma) there should be no discharge from the urethra. During inspection of the scrotum and surrounding areas swellings and lumps may be detected as well as hernias. Whenever possible, skills in testicular self-examination should be taught so that any future problems can be detected early and expert opinion sought.

Inspection of the female external genitalia may reveal areas of irritation which may be due to the presence of lice at the base of pubic hairs. When the labia are separated it is possible to inspect the urethral and vaginal openings so that any discharge, inflammation, swelling or ulceration can be detected if present. Individuals may present with problems that require internal examination, and this will be performed by a doctor or other experienced health practitioner.

Musculoskeletal

Musculoskeletal problems resulting in stiffness and pain can occur across the life stages but become increasingly common with the passage of time. Occasionally it may be necessary to use inspection and palpation skills in this area where perhaps someone with a long-term condition complains of joint pain which is a new development or where the pain is different in character and intensity. There are of course many different joints in the body, some more stable than others, and the assessment needed will require a different approach depending on the joint involved. There should be some basic knowledge of the range of movement normally possible with individual joints so that deviation from the norm can be recognised and so that joints are not moved beyond their normal range.

Carers should be aware of what an individual is capable of doing in terms of their musculoskeletal function not least in performing various activities of living. For those individuals who are still able to mobilise, observing how they are able to stand from a sitting position can be quite useful as also can their ability to undress and dress themselves. It is useful to compare a joint on one side of the body with the same joint on the other side, observing the range of motion which is possible with each. Joints should be inspected for shape, unusual markings, bruising, redness and swelling. There may be lacerations and deformity may be obvious in affected joints. Using palpation, note should be made of any tenderness and masses present, and when attempting to move joints through a range of movement, either actively or passively, any crepitus (cracking or grating sound) and/or tenderness must be documented. Where there are problem joints with reduced movement, the associated muscle group often becomes weak and any loss of muscle strength should be noted. If these are new findings, these should be reported so that further investigation and possible treatment can be arranged.

Neurological

Neurological assessment may be required where there are problems with changes in mood, memory, swallowing, speech, smell, vision, hearing, concentration, head-aches, dizziness, fits and limb weakness or paralysis. There are many different groups of nerves including central and peripheral sensory (sensation) and motor (movement) nerves as well as cranial nerves and all can be tested during assessment. However, a detailed neurological assessment is beyond the scope of this text. Again, it is useful to think in terms of symmetry and moving from the head downward to compare each side of the face and body. Movement, strength and sensation can all be tested and the distribution of any loss can provide important clues as to which nerves are involved. Where level of consciousness is altered, the Glasgow Coma Score (GCS) (Teasdale and Jennett 1974) is universally recognised (see Table 5.2). It comprises three parameters: best eye response, best verbal response, best motor response, and is scored between 3 and 15, with 3 being the worst and 15 the best, with the total score the sum of the three parameters.

Endocrine

Endocrine glands (e.g. pituitary and thyroid) are found throughout the body and are responsible for secreting hormones, important physiological regulators which have many different functions. Sometimes these glands may become either underactive or overactive and where this is the case there may be many signs and symptoms depending on the gland involved. Weight gain or loss, fatigue, intolerance of heat or cold, nervousness and mood swings are examples of changes which can occur. Where these cannot be attributed to other disorders, tests of endocrine function may be necessary.

Table 5.2 Glasgow Coma Score

Best eye response	Best verbal response	Best motor response
4 = Spontaneous	5 = Orientated	6 = Obeys commands
3 = To verbal command	4 = Confused	5 = Localising pain
2 = To pain	3 = Inappropriate words	4 = Withdrawal from pain
1 = No eye-opening	2 = Incomprehensible sounds	3 = Flexion to pain
	1 = No verbal response	2 = Extension to pain
		1 = No motor response

Haematological (blood)

The blood can be affected by many different diseases including leukaemia, haemophilia and sickle cell disorder, and carers need to be aware if such problems have already been diagnosed. Anaemia can be a primary disorder affecting the blood alone or may be a feature of other health problems. Changes to the blood may also occur as a result of medication where, for example, anticoagulants have been prescribed. Ongoing observation is important and, where there is fatigue and breathlessness on exertion and/or excessive bruising, bleeding gums, or the passage of blood in urine or faeces, this should be reported as further investigation is required.

During the assessment of each system any abnormalities are documented carefully. These should be discussed with an experienced health professional so that there is further review and investigation.

Assessing lifestyle issues

Alcohol use

It is important to recognise the need for screening for the use and misuse of psychoactive substances in long-term conditions. However, the majority of hazardous drinkers are undiagnosed and often present with symptoms or problems that at first seem unconnected to their drinking (Trenoweth and Tobutt 2009), such as those who use alcohol as a means of pain control. The National Treatment Agency (NTA) has recently outlined an integrated model of care, involving four tiers of escalating complexity of assessment and interventions (NTA 2002, 2006). The first tier comprises assessment and interventions in non-substance misuse specific services such as primary care. Here, 'screening and referral' assessments will be undertaken acting as a possible 'gateway' to care for the person with alcohol misuse problems (DoH 2005b, 2006). Information gathered at this stage is most likely to be quite basic, comprising personal and historical data relating to the person, along with information about levels and patterns of alcohol use (Scottish Executive 2002). In support of this, the Fast Alcohol Screening Test (FAST) may be useful to structure such initial screening (Health Development Agency 2002) (see Table 5.3). FAST comprises four questions. Answers are scored from 0–4 as indicated below. Total scores range from 0–16 and a score of 3 or more indicates hazardous drinking.

If an individual's pattern of alcohol consumption is considered to be hazardous the FAST recommends a brief intervention (signified by the acronym BRIEF: see below) to offer advice, further information and to clarify the person's intentions to reduce their intake. That is, following screening the interventions may comprise (HDA 2002):

- **B**enefits: Offering information about the benefits of sensible drinking.
- **R**isk factor: Exploring the patterns of alcohol consumption as a risk factor in the individual's current situation to raise awareness of its use.
- **I**ntentions: Clarifying the client's future intentions, for example, to seek support in reducing intake.
- **E**mpathise: The practitioner should empathise and maintain a non-judgemental attitude.
- **F**eedback: Giving the client feedback on their levels of consumption.

Table 5.3 Fast Alcohol Screening Test (FAST)

1 *Men*: How often do you have *eight* or more drinks on one occasion?
   Women: How often do you have *six* or more drinks on one occasion?

   (one drink = half a pint of beer or one glass of wine or one single spirit)

0	1	2	3	4
Never	Less than monthly	Monthly	Weekly	Daily or almost daily

2 How often during the past year have you been unable to remember what happened the night before because you had been drinking?

0	1	2	3	4
Never	Less than monthly	Monthly	Weekly	Daily or almost daily

3 How often during the last year have you failed to do what was normally expected of you because of drinking?

0	1	2	3	4
Never	Less than monthly	Monthly	Weekly	Daily or almost daily

4 In the past year has a relative or friend, or a doctor or other health worker been concerned about your drinking or suggested you cut down?

0	2	4
No	Yes, on one occasion	Yes, on more than one occasion

Source: Health Development Agency (2002) Manual for the Fast Alcohol Screen Test (FAST): Fast screening for alcohol problems. London: HDA. Available from www.nice.org.uk. Reproduced with permission.

Based on the resultant discussion of this brief intervention, referral to the next tier of services may be warranted or requested by the client.

Smoking

It is important to catalogue patterns of cigarette use and to establish how many cigarettes the person smokes and under what circumstances, and what may trigger the desire for a cigarette. It is important to understand how soon after waking the person has their first cigarette as this can give an indication of the extent of physiological dependence. It is usual to calculate pack years of smoking (see Table 5.4) which is a simple way of calculating the amount a person has smoked over a period of time, where the number of cigarettes smoked per day is multiplied by the number

Table 5.4 Calculating pack years

$$\frac{\text{Number of cigarettes per day} \times \text{years smoked}}{20}$$

If the person has smoked intermittently, pack years should be calculated for each period smoked and then totalled.

20 pack years or more carries increased risk of chronic obstructive pulmonary disease (COPD).

---

of years the person has smoked. An electronic calculation tool may be found at www.smokingpackyears.com/.

In addition, for clients with long-term conditions who continue to smoke (as a preliminary for health promotion advice or smoking cessation interventions) it is important to establish their willingness, readiness and confidence in their ability to quit smoking.

Exercise and activity

An active lifestyle can be an important preventive step in the development of long-term conditions and contributes to an overall positive sense of physical and mental health. Indeed, NICE (2007) have recently recommended exercise as a preliminary treatment for depression (see Chapter 15). A general assessment of activity levels is therefore important in a comprehensive and holistic assessment. However, the assessment of exercise and activity is a complex process and caution is advised. Such assessments and advice regarding activity and exercise should only be undertaken by suitably qualified people with an understanding of long-term conditions. For example, suggested activity for one individual with a respiratory condition may not be appropriate for another who has a different respiratory problem. (More information on exercise may be found in Chapter 9.)

Weight, diet and nutrition

An assessment of nutritional intake and diet is vital in a comprehensive assessment. While an assessment of diet should be undertaken by a suitably qualified practitioner, there is much that can be done to screen for potential problems before referral to specialist dietetic services. Such assessments involve not only the quantity of food that someone is eating but also the quality. For example, someone could be taking in excess of the guideline daily amount (GDA) of 2000 calories per day for the typical woman and 2500 calories per day for the typical man, but their diet may lack sufficient nutrients and fibre. The current recommendations are that everyone should eat a variety of at least five portions of fruit and vegetables each day (DoH 2004). An assessment of how many portions of fruit and vegetables people are consuming per day (a portion is 80 grams and does not include potatoes), with basic healthy eating advice if people are not reaching the target of five a day, can be an important health promotion strategy.

Obesity and malnutrition have a significant impact on the general health of the population and the aetiology of ill-health and disease, and may complicate the trajectory and prognosis of many long-term conditions. The Body Mass Index (BMI) is a simple way of calculating a healthy weight for an individual's height. The calculation is one's height in metres squared divided by one's weight in kilograms, although there are many 'ready reckoners' available on the Internet (for example, NHS Choices:www.nhs.uk/healthprofile/Pages/BMI.aspx). If the resultant score is less than 18.5 one is underweight; between 18.5 and 25 one is of normal weight; between 25 and 30 one is overweight. Scores of 30 and over indicate obesity. However, the BMI is not suitable for older people or children. Nor is it useful for athletic people whose high muscle bulk might artificially raise their BMI score. Other assessments include a measurement of waist circumference (greater than 80 cm for women and 94 cm for men is of concern, while a measurement of more than 88 cm for women and 102 m for men represents a significantly increased health risk). Another assessment is that of the ratio of one's waist to hip (the comparison between the circumference of the narrowest and widest parts on one's abdomen respectively). If one's waist circumference exceeds one's hips then this can indicate an increased health risk. (More information on diet and nutrition may be found in Chapter 10.)

Conclusion

In this chapter we have sought to offer a systematic framework for comprehensive assessments (see Table 5.5). Comprehensive and holistic assessments are a crucial component in improving the overall quality of life of people with long-term con-

Table 5.5 A systematic framework for comprehensive assessment

Subjective information	Personal biography
	Personal and family history
	Medication
	Symptom exploration
Self-assessment	
Functional assessment	Personal activities of living
	Instrumental activities of living
Mental health assessment	Affect and mood
	Appearance and behaviour
	Cognition (form and content)
	Perception
Objective information	Skin
	Head, eyes, ears, nose and throat
	Breasts and axillae
	Respiration
	Cardiovascular
	Peripheral vascular
	Gastro-intestinal
	Genito-urinary
	Musculoskeletal
	Neurological
Lifestyle issues	Alcohol consumption
	Smoking
	Exercise and activity
	Weight, diet and nutrition

ditions. The overall aim of such assessments is to establish the type and range of support needed to maintain independent living, and to improve psychological well-being and resilience while maintaining and developing social networks and delaying deterioration in physical or mental health. Information needs to be collected systematically in order to analyse subjective and objective data. This process should be a collaborative process, involving the person, their carer and family whenever appropriate and wherever possible. Importantly, such assessments should attempt to avoid a fragmented appraisal of discrete *parts* of the individual while attempting to capture the totality of their experience.

References

Barker, P. (2004) *Assessment in Psychiatric and Mental Health Nursing* (2nd edn). Cheltenham: Nelson Thornes.

Bickley, L.S. (2007) *Bates' Guide to Physical Examination and History Taking*. London: Lippincott Williams and Wilkins.

Cleeland, C. (2009) *The Brief Pain Inventory: A User's Guide*. Online. Available at: www.mdanderson.org/pdf/bpi-userguide.pdf (accessed 1 February 2009).

Cutcliffe, J.R. and Barker, P. (2004) The Nurses' Global Assessment of Suicide Risk (NGASR): Developing a Tool for Clinical Practice. *Journal of Psychiatric and Mental Health Nursing*, 11, 393–400.

Department of Health (DoH) (2001) *National Service Framework for Older People*. Online. Available at: www.dh.gov.uk/en/Publicationsandstatistics/Publications/PublicationsPolicyAndGuidance/DH_4003066 (accessed 25 February 2009).

Department of Health (DoH) (2004) *5 A Day*. Online. Available at: www.dh.gov.uk/en/Publichealth/Healthimprovement/FiveADay/DH_4069867 (accessed 24 February 2009).

Department of Health (DoH) (2005a) *National Service Framework for Long Term Conditions*. Online. Available at: www.dh.gov.uk/en/Publicationsandstatistics/Publications/PublicationsPolicyAndGuidance/DH_4105361 (accessed 25 February 2009).

Department of Health (DoH) (2005b) *Alcohol Needs Assessment Research Project (ANARP): The 2004 National Alcohol Needs Assessment for England*. Available at: www.dh.gov.uk/en/Publicationsandstatistics/Publications/PublicationsPolicyAndGuidance/DH_4122341 (accessed 14 March 2008).

Department of Health (DoH) (2006) *Alcohol Misuse Interventions: Guidance on Developing a Local Programme of Improvement*. Available at: www.dh.gov.uk/en/Publicationsandstatistics/Publications/PublicationsPolicyAndGuidance/DH_4123297 (accessed 14 March 2008).

Fletcher, C.M. (Chairman) (1960) Standardised Questionnaire on Respiratory Symptoms: A Statement Prepared and Approved by the MRC on the Aetiology of Chronic Bronchitis (MRC Breathlessness Score). *British Medical Journal*, 2, 1665.

Fox, J. and Gamble, C. (2006) Consolidating the Assessment Process: The Semi-structured Interview. In: Gamble, C. and Brennan, G. (eds) *Working with Serious Mental Illness: A Manual for Clinical Practice*. Edinburgh: Elsevier.

Health Development Agency (HDA) (2002) *Manual for the Fast Alcohol Screen Test (FAST): Fast Screening for Alcohol Problems*. London: HDA. Available http: www.nice.org.uk (accessed 15 December 2008).

Jarvis, C. (2004) *Physical Examination and Health Assessment*. St Louis, MO: Saunders.

Launer, J. (2002) *Narrative-based Primary Care: A Practical Guide*. Abingdon: Radcliffe Medical Press.

Law, M., Baum, C. and Dunn, W. (2005) *Measuring Occupational Performance: Supporting Best Practice in Occupational Therapy*. Thorofare, NJ: Slack Incorporated.

Margereson, C. (2008) Physical Illness: Promoting Effective Coping in Clients with Co-morbidity. In: Lynch, J. and Trenoweth, S. (eds) *Contemporary Issues in Mental Health Nursing*. Chichester: John Wiley & Sons.

Matthews, J. and Trenoweth, S. (2008) Some Considerations for Mental Health Nurses Working with Patients Who Self-neglect. In: Lynch, J. and Trenoweth, S. (eds) *Contemporary Issues in Mental Health Nursing*. Chichester: John Wiley & Sons.

Miller, W. and Rollnick, S. (2002) *Motivational Interviewing: Preparing People for Change* (2nd edn). New York: The Guilford Press.

National Institute for Health and Clinical Excellence (NICE) (2007) *Depression (Amended): Management of Depression in Primary and Secondary Care*. Online. Available at: www.nice.org.uk/Guidance/CG23/NiceGuidance/pdf/English (accessed 17 January 2009).

National Treatment Agency for Substance Misuse (NTA) (2002) *Models of Care for the Treatment of Adult Drug Misusers. Part Two: Full Reference Report*. London: National Treatment Agency for Substance Misuse and the Department of Health.

National Treatment Agency for Substance Misuse (NTA) (2006) *Models of Care for Alcohol*. London: National Treatment Agency for Substance Misuse and the Department of Health.

Rollnick, S., Mason, P. and Butler, C. (1999) *Health Behaviour Change: A Guide for Practitioners*. Edinburgh: Churchill Livingstone.

Scottish Executive (2002) *Integrated Care for Drug Users: Assessments. Digest of Tools Used in the Assessment Process and Core Data Sets*. Available at: www.drugmisuse.isdscotland.org/eiu/intcare/intcare.htm (accessed 14 February 2008).

Snaith, R.P. (2003) The Hospital Anxiety And Depression Scale *Health and Quality of Life Outcomes*, 1, 29. Online. Available at: www.hqlo.com/content/1/1/29 (accessed 28 March 2009).

Teasdale, G. and Jennett, B. (1974) Assessment of Coma and Impaired Consciousness. A Practical Scale. *Lancet*, 2 (7872), 81–84.

Trenoweth, S. and Tobutt, C. (2009) Assessing Alcohol Use and Misuse in Primary Care. In: Martin, C. (ed.) *Identification and Treatment of Alcohol Dependency*. Cumbria: M&K Publishing.

Van Dreusen, J. and Brunt, D. (1997) *Assessment in Occupational Therapy and Physical Therapy*. Philadelphia, PA: W.B. Saunders.

6 Maximising symptom control

Carl Margereson, Colin Martin and Tim Duffy

Introduction

Symptom control remains a key concern for people living with long-term conditions and is a cornerstone indicator of good-quality healthcare intervention and management. However, the area is complex, multi-modal and interactional, with many factors impacting on individual experience of symptoms including the physical aspects of the pathology itself and the uniqueness of each person which will inevitably shape the experience and perceptions of symptoms. This chapter will explore the main salient dimensions influencing the experience of symptoms and identifies the elements which healthcare professionals need to be aware of in order to enhance and optimise individual mastery of health problems and reduce overall disease burden.

Significance of symptoms

Although living with a long-term condition does not necessarily mean living with ongoing symptoms, for many the experience of distressing symptoms, whether persistent or intermittent, is a reality. Our perceptions are influenced by complex physical, sociocultural and psychological factors, and the emotional experience of a symptom is considered inseparable from its physical experience and/or mechanism (Corner *et al.* 1995). For example, it is shown that peace of mind is a powerful adjuvant for relief of pain whereas fear, anger and guilt all amplify pain (Bope *et al.* 2004). Consistent with the notion that holism deals with health problems in their physical, psychological, social, cultural and existential dimensions (Gartner *et al.* 1991) it is argued that healthcare models should include spirituality. An association is also found between biopsychosocial symptoms and spiritual factors, which points to synergy between spiritual symptoms and other symptom dimensions affecting health (Katerndahl 2008).

Symptoms may be related to a diagnosed primary medical disorder and treatments can sometimes result in unpleasant side-effects, occasionally more distressing than the symptoms of the disorder itself. Being aware of possible side-effects of various treatments can contribute to early recognition and resolution of problems. In those with mental health problems antipsychotic medication can affect the gastrointestinal, hepatic, renal and circulatory systems and may result in unwanted weight gain, and there is a well-established relationship with such medication, appetite control, metabolism and weight (Vanina *et al.* 2002).

New symptoms are always a possibility and may herald the onset of additional medical problems. With polarisation of physical health and mental health, uninten-

tional bias can easily result in symptoms being missed and ongoing vigilance is important. In those with learning disabilities symptoms are often overlooked and medical
conditions untreated, and there is often a lack of uptake of generic health promotion
such as blood pressure screening (Kerr 2004). Difficulties in communication with
older adults, particularly those with cognitive impairment, often lead to an under-
treatment of symptoms such as pain, or inappropriate treatments (Amella 2003;
McMullan *et al.* 2007) and many in residential care simply cannot express their needs.

There are, of course, many symptoms associated with physical and mental health
problems. It may be extremely difficult to determine the origin of specific symptoms, and careful assessment will be necessary to differentiate between those which
are due to physical disease and those which are psychogenic. There are many cases
of individuals presenting with symptoms, where, after an exhausting period of diagnostic testing, a diagnosis cannot be made (Reid *et al.* 2001). Medically unexplained
chest pain is such an example where, even following numerous sophisticated tests a
physical defect may not be found. Yet symptoms are real to the individual, and, even
where no medical cause can be found, need to be taken seriously. No matter
whether the origin of any symptom is physical or psychogenic the resulting distress
and potential disability can be the same. Individuals who exhibit disease symptoms
or experience health-related limitations that impact on daily living have low health-
related quality-of-life scores (Giacobbi *et al.* 2008).

Physical symptoms

Three common physical symptoms which are experienced by many coping with long-
term conditions are pain, breathlessness and fatigue, either in isolation or together.
Symptom assessment and management are vital aspects of care across the entire trajectory of diagnosis, treatment, recovery and, if applicable, palliative care (Fu *et al.*
2007). Assessment of symptoms must begin by listening carefully to how symptoms are
experienced and how these are impacting on day-to-day life. Any assessment should
reflect the multidimensional nature of symptoms, and carers should also use an
appropriate tool so that baseline and outcome measures may be obtained. Despite a
great deal of evidence showing the benefit of using symptom measurement tools, in
one study a significant number of nurses had negative views about using these in practice (Young *et al.* 2006). With symptoms being very subjective, such attitudes can result
in failure to recognise symptom severity and under-treatment. A systematic approach
should be adopted and appropriate assessment frameworks may be found in Chapter
5. A variety of assessment tools are available and, where there is a single symptom, the
selection and use of an appropriate tool is relatively straightforward. Many people,
however, may experience multiple symptoms resulting in a great deal of distress. What
should not be ignored is the impact of symptoms on activities of living and any resulting disability needs to be assessed. Table 6.1 outlines examples of various assessment
scales that are available for measuring symptoms.

Chronic pain

Pain is probably the most common reason why people seek medical advice (Turk
1994) and chronic pain affects about 20 per cent to 30 per cent of the adult population in Western countries (Verhaak *et al.* 1998). Pain results in unpleasant physical,

Table 6.1 Examples of assessment tools

Assessment tool	Type of scale	Source
New York Heart Association (NYHA) functional classification scale	Classification of disability in heart failure	Criteria Committee of the New York Heart Association Inc (1979)
Medical Research Council (MRC) breathlessness scale	Grades degree of breathlessness (1–5) related to activities in chronic respiratory disease	Fletcher (1960)
Visual analogue scale (VAS) for breathlessness (can be used for pain also)	100-mm horizontal line with verbal anchors – 'no pain/breathlessness' and 'as bad as can be'. Vertical VAS available also	Gift (1989)
Abbey pain scale	Used in end-stage dementia. A one-minute numerical indicator	Abbey *et al.* (2004)
Brief pain inventory	0–10 numeric rating scales across various dimensions measuring severity and functional impact	Cleeland (2009)
Fatigue symptom inventory	14-item measure of severity, frequency, variation and perceived interference with quality of life	Hann *et al.* (1998)
Fatigue assessment scale	10 items: 5 assessing physical fatigue 5 assessing mental fatigue	Michielson *et al.* (2003)

sensory and emotional experiences, and although it is often the result of tissue damage this may not always be the case. It can be defined as acute or chronic where acute pain is of recent onset and limited duration, and chronic pain lasts for long periods (usually at least six months) often beyond the time of any tissue injury. Chronic pain can be malignant or non-malignant in origin and can also appear in the absence of identifiable pathology (Ross and Hahn 2008). There has been a rapid growth of research in the association between psychiatric morbidity and long-term medical illnesses, and depression has been particularly linked to pain (Carrol *et al.* 2004; Jackson 2004; Blay *et al.* 2007).

Pain receptors (nociceptors) are distributed throughout the body and, once activated by events such as trauma or inflammation, result in pain impulses being transmitted along sensory nerves into the spinal cord and brain. This results in nocioceptive pain arising from skin, muscles, joints, arteries and internal organs (McCance and Huether 2006), and is often sharp and intense. For example, where joints are inflamed as in arthritic conditions, pain receptors can be activated by prostaglandin, a chemical released by inflammatory cells. Once pain impulses have been generated, transmission can be increased by many different neurotransmitters released along the sensory nerves.

Chronic pain (neuropathic) is not initiated by nociceptor stimulation but from damage and dysfunction of the peripheral nerves and the dorsal horn of grey matter in the spinal cord. This often results in excessive pain impulse activity in the spinal cord where only minimal stimuli (e.g. gentle touch) can trigger excruciating pain which can be very difficult to eradicate. Such pain is often described as burning, tingling or 'electric shock-like' and is unrelieved by traditional pain medications (McCaffrey *et al.* 2003). Table 6.2 lists some causes of neuropathic pain.

Both nociceptive and neuropathic pain can of course occur together. Following spinal cord injury and stroke, for example, neuropathic pain can be experienced as a result of spinal cord damage, but there can be additional musculoskeletal problems resulting in nociceptive pain (Goldstein 2000; Ehde *et al.* 2003). The transmission of pain impulses through the spinal cord is complex and a 'gating mechanism' has been described where various factors can open the 'gate', thus increasing impulse transmission and pain. Similarly there are factors that can close the 'gate' resulting in less pain (Melzack and Wall 1965). Improved knowledge of pain physiology has led to multi-modal models of pain relief recognising that different sites need to be targeted including pain receptor sites, the spinal cord and the brain where pain impulses are processed. Anti-inflammatory agents, for example, act at receptor sites whereby opiates such as morphine have a more central effect in the spinal cord and brain.

As well as pain sensory impulses being transmitted through the spinal cord, there are also different sensory nerves transmitting touch and pressure impulses. When both types of sensory nerve are being stimulated, touch/pressure impulses are transmitted through the spinal cord in preference to the pain impulses. That is, the 'gate' in the spinal cord is closed to pain impulses, and techniques such as therapeutic massage have been found to have this effect (Ganong 1999).

The brain and spinal cord can also release 'morphine-like' molecules (e.g. endorphins) which can bind to receptors and close the 'gate' to pain impulses. Conversely, stress and anxiety can cause the release of neurotransmitters (e.g. Substance P), which can increase pain impulse transmission. This illustrates the complexity of the 'mind–body' connection and Western health professionals, in an attempt to become more effective in managing chronic pain, are looking to complementary approaches (Pike 2008). More information on complementary and alternative therapies may be found in Chapter 11.

Table 6.2 Causes of neuropathic pain

Diabetic neuropathy
Following amputation (phantom limb pain)
Drug induced (e.g. chemotherapy)
Following shingles (post-herpetic neuralgia)
Trigeminal neuralgia
Alcoholism
Post surgery (e.g. chest surgery)
Spinal cord injury
Multiple sclerosis
Tumours
HIV infection

Assessment of pain

If management is to be effective, comprehensive holistic assessment is important and chronic pain needs to be assessed regularly and systematically. With acute pain there are often signs that pain is being experienced including pallor, sweating, restlessness, increased heart rate and obvious signs of distress. However, with chronic pain these signs may be absent and it should not be assumed that the individual is pain-free. This is where simple pain assessment tools can be used and individuals are asked to simply score their pain where '0' is no pain and '10' is the very worse pain possible. Used in isolation these simple scales may be inadequate as level of disability is not taken into account. The Brief Pain Inventory (Cleeland 2009) uses a numerical scale across a number of dimensions including impact on activities (see Box 6.1). Care needs to be taken where there is cognitive impairment, and the Abbey Pain Scale was developed to measure pain as accurately as possible in dementia so that individuals are neither over-treated nor under-treated (Abbey *et al.* 2004).

Drug therapy for chronic pain

Traditional pain killers can be useful for chronic pain and include paracetamol, non-steroidal anti-inflammatory drugs (NSAID) as well as codeine and morphine. In 1968 the World Health Organisation (WHO) published a stepped approach to pain relief in cancer called the WHO analgesic ladder which guides pain management in many different conditions. *Step 1* where pain is mild may involve taking a simple non-opioid pain killer (paracetamol, aspirin, diclofenac or ibuprofen). Where pain is moderate *Step 2* requires prescription of an opioid analgesic combination, usually codeine with either paracetamol or aspirin. In *Step 3* where pain is reported as severe (rated '7' to '10' on a '0' to '10' scale) the doctor may prescribe a much more powerful pain killer such as morphine (an opioid). There are additional drugs which, when prescribed for other conditions, have also been found to have pain-relieving qualities. At any of the three steps these so-called adjuvant therapies may be prescribed and include anti-depressant and anticonvulsant drugs.

Adjuvant agents can take several weeks to achieve optimum pain control and encouragement is needed to facilitate concordance. Side-effects can be troublesome and can also lead to non-concordance. The indigestion and potential risk of gastric ulceration and bleeding associated with NSAIDs can be reduced by taking these drugs with meals. Opioids can result in constipation, nausea, vomiting, sedation and possible confusion, although as tolerance builds up over a few days these side-effects often disappear. Constipation, however, is common and although stool softeners are often required, maintaining adequate hydration is important. Where prescribed pain killers do not result in good pain control then referral to the doctor for review is necessary so that alternative or additional drugs may be considered. Additional physical therapies may also be required including physiotherapy, acupuncture, nerve blocks and Transcutaneous Electrical Nerve Stimulation (TENS).

The control of neuropathic pain is often challenging with drug therapy alone often inadequate. Although therapeutic approaches have resulted in significant

Box 6.1 Brief pain inventory

1 Throughout our lives, most of us have had pain from time to time (such as minor headaches, sprains and toothaches). Have you had pain other than these everyday kinds of pain today?

Yes/No

2 On the diagram, shade in the areas where you feel pain. Put an X on the area that hurts the most.

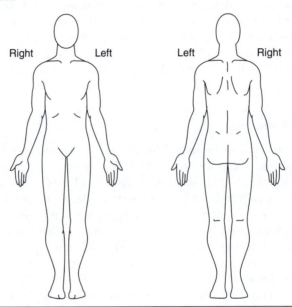

Right   Left   Left   Right

3 Please rate your pain by circling the one number that best describes your pain at its **worst** in the past 24 hours.

0   1   2   3   4   5   6   7   8   9   10
No pain   Pain as bad as
                                                                  you can imagine

4 Please rate your pain by circling the one number that best describes your pain at its **least** in the past 24 hours.

0   1   2   3   4   5   6   7   8   9   10
No pain   Pain as bad as
                                                                  you can imagine

5 Please rate your pain by circling the one number that best describes your pain on the **average**.

0   1   2   3   4   5   6   7   8   9   10
No pain   Pain as bad as
                                                                  you can imagine

6 Please rate your pain by circling the one number that tells how much pain you have **right now**.

| 0 | 1 | 2 | 3 | 4 | 5 | 6 | 7 | 8 | 9 | 10 |

No pain   Pain as bad as
                                                                                 you can imagine

---

7 What treatments or medications are you receiving for your pain?

---

8 In the past 24 hours, how much **relief** have pain treatments or medications provided? Please circle the one percentage that most shows how much.

| 0% | 1% | 2% | 3% | 4% | 5% | 6% | 7% | 8% | 9% | 10% |

No relief   Complete relief

---

9 Circle the one number that describes how, during the past 24 hours, **pain has interfered** with your:

a. General activity

| 0 | 1 | 2 | 3 | 4 | 5 | 6 | 7 | 8 | 9 | 10 |

Does not   Completely
interfere   interferes

b. Mood

| 0 | 1 | 2 | 3 | 4 | 5 | 6 | 7 | 8 | 9 | 10 |

Does not   Completely
interfere   interferes

c. Walking ability

| 0 | 1 | 2 | 3 | 4 | 5 | 6 | 7 | 8 | 9 | 10 |

Does not   Completely
interfere   interferes

d. Normal work (includes both work outside the home and housework)

| 0 | 1 | 2 | 3 | 4 | 5 | 6 | 7 | 8 | 9 | 10 |

Does not   Completely
interfere   interferes

e. Relations with other people

| 0 | 1 | 2 | 3 | 4 | 5 | 6 | 7 | 8 | 9 | 10 |

Does not   Completely
interfere   interferes

f. Sleep

| 0 | 1 | 2 | 3 | 4 | 5 | 6 | 7 | 8 | 9 | 10 |

Does not   Completely
interfere   interferes

g. Enjoyment of life

| 0 | 1 | 2 | 3 | 4 | 5 | 6 | 7 | 8 | 9 | 10 |

Does not   Completely
interfere   interferes

Note
Used with permission. Source: Dr. Charles Cleeland, Anderson Cancer Center, Pain Research Group, 1100 Holcombe, Houston, TX 77030.

improvements, the most potent drugs only reduce pain by 30 to 40 per cent in fewer than 50 per cent of patients (Turk 2002). Pain impulses which terminate in the brain are interpreted by different areas, based not only on the stimulus itself but on psychological and sociocultural factors which influence the perception and expression of pain. Perception of pain may therefore be modified not only by drugs affecting higher centres in the brain but by the use of various psychological techniques. Psychological treatments in pain management have included hypnosis, relaxation training, operant behavioural, cognitive behavioural approaches, psychopharmacological treatment, and multidisciplinary pain management programs (Tunks *et al.* 2008). In a study of 171 people with chronic pain, both pain-related and psychosocial variables contributed to quality of life of sufferers (Lee *et al.* 2008), and while medication and other physical modalities were important, understanding of the client's perception of how pain affected daily functioning was equally important. For instance, if someone is experiencing challenges in basic self-care skills, referral to an occupational therapist may reduce levels of disability and distress as well as increasing perceived control.

Breathlessness

Normally, breathing is something we do not have to think about as it is an automatic activity that takes place without any conscious effort. In many disorders, however, the awareness of increasing difficulty with each breath can be frightening and result in significant distress. Breathlessness may be defined as a subjective experience consisting of qualitatively distinct sensations varying in intensity (American Thoracic Society 1999) and which may not correlate with physical symptoms or biochemical parameters (Williams 2006), so that minor physiological impairment can sometimes result in intense breathlessness and distress.

The physiological mechanisms of breathlessness are complex and not understood fully, but receptors in blood vessels, brain, airways, lung and chest wall are all involved (Beach and Schwartzstein 2006; Spector *et al.* 2007). In respiratory disorders, awareness of respiratory effort is more often than not increased because the airways are narrower than usual (e.g. in asthma or chronic bronchitis), or the lungs are stiffer and more difficult to expand (e.g. in pneumonia, rib fractures and fibrotic lung disorders). Both narrowed airways and stiff lungs may be the cause in some disorders but in either case the work of breathing is increased, and greater pressure and effort must be generated to ensure that air enters and leaves the lungs. This increased work of breathing is evident through the distress exhibited and the additional muscles employed to breathe. In severe breathlessness, additional muscle use can lead to a tenfold increase in calories, and poor diet will further compromise respiratory status and result in fatigue and lack of energy.

As with many other symptoms breathlessness needs to be thought of as a multidimensional phenomenon with physiological, psychological, social and environmental factors all contributing. For many there may be a known cause, and two-thirds of cases are due to either a respiratory or cardiac problem (Gillespie and Staats 1994) but other causes may include anaemia, neuromuscular problems, hyperventilation syndrome (associated often with anxiety) as well as end-stage disease. This chapter assumes that breathlessness is an accompanying symptom of an already diagnosed disorder resulting in ongoing health problems.

Assessment of breathlessness

Assessment data regarding breathlessness should be obtained and recorded, and compared with usual respiratory status. It is important to establish what is 'normal' and therefore acceptable for each individual, and this can only be done if there are documented baseline data. How comprehensive the respiratory assessment is will depend on the care setting and experience of individual care providers. As with pain, the use of an assessment tool can help to measure how breathlessness is impacting on daily activities and allows useful comparison when evaluating care. Individual expression of breathlessness severity is difficult and there may be an inability to describe the sensation. Unlike pain, where many different descriptive terms can be used, the language of breathlessness is poorly developed and there may be cultural differences influencing individual narrative and experience (Schwartzstein 1998; Fraser *et al.* 2006). There are many different breathlessness scales available and selection will depend on context and purpose. The Medical Research Council (MRC) Breathlessness Scale (Fletcher 1960) (Table 6.3) is often used with respiratory conditions such as chronic obstructive pulmonary disease (COPD) and helps to determine impact on exercise tolerance.

Assessment should include observations of respiratory rate and depth, and while respiratory rate is often increased to compensate for a decrease in depth, this utilises a great deal of energy which can easily lead to fatigue and exhaustion. Although breathing is usually diaphragmatic only, where there is increasing breathlessness additional muscle contraction is necessary with even more energy expenditure. The degree of distress associated with breathing should also be noted together with the position adopted to breathe, which is often sitting up and leaning forward. Inability to complete a sentence in one breath also denotes severe breathlessness. During such times effective oxygenation may be compromised and blue discoloration of the skin (e.g. fingers and ear lobes) and mucous membranes inside the mouth (called cyanosis) is a worrying trend which should be reported if this is a new development. Additional elements of respiratory assessment may be reviewed in Chapters 5 and 18.

Management of breathlessness

How breathlessness is managed will depend on the pathophysiological mechanisms responsible as well as the stage of the illness. Where breathlessness is caused by a respiratory disease, time should be taken in ensuring that all prescribed medication

Table 6.3 Medical Research Council (MRC) breathlessness scale

Degree of breathlessness related to activities

1 = Not troubled by breathlessness except on strenuous exercise
2 = Short of breath when hurrying or walking up a slight hill
3 = Walks slower than contemporaries on level ground because of breathlessness, or has to stop for breath when walking at own pace
4 = Stops for breath after walking about 100 metres or after a few minutes on level ground
5 = Too breathless to leave the house or breathless when dressing or undressing

Source: Fletcher CM (Chairman) (1960). Reproduced with permission.

and treatments are administered effectively and the effects monitored carefully. Relief of breathlessness and individual comfort should focus on the mechanisms contributing to this symptom and on pharmacological and non-pharmacological measures (Williams 2006). Holistic care must involve collaboration with other professionals with experience in palliative care settings supporting this (Syrett and Taylor 2003). Where the desired outcomes are not achieved and disability marked with or without confusion, referral to the doctor or specialist team is important so that the treatment plan may be reviewed and modified if necessary. Admission to hospital or an intermediate care facility may be indicated.

Positioning can affect breathing and, when sitting and leaning forward, there is often less diaphragmatic pressure and better chest expansion with reduced breathlessness. Breathing exercises involving controlled breathing and chest expansion can result in a number of beneficial physiological changes which can reduce the work of breathing. Initially it may be appropriate for a physiotherapist to be involved but carers should be able to reinforce and encourage ongoing practice of taught breathing techniques. A physiotherapist will also be able to work with individuals in performing exercises, initially low intensity, which will improve muscle strength and reduce breathlessness which in turn will improve performance of activities in living (Jantarakupt and Porock 2005). Close collaboration with both physiotherapists and occupational therapists can result in improved exercise tolerance and self-care ability.

Calm surroundings and care minimise panic and anxiety and are important when caring for someone who is breathless. Panic is easily communicated and this can result in loss of confidence in carers and cause even greater distress. A well-ventilated area is crucial, restrictive clothing should be loosened, and positioning near an open window if possible can offer great relief. Similarly the use of a fan or facial cooling can be very soothing by reducing the intensity of breathlessness (Schwartzstein *et al.* 1987; Thompson 2001).

Oxygen therapy

Some people with breathing difficulties may require long-term oxygen therapy (LTOT) and standards are available to guide assessment and prescription (British Thoracic Society (BTS) Working Group on Home Oxygen Services 2006). Assessment by a respiratory specialist is usual although general practitioners often prescribe oxygen for palliative care. Long-term oxygen used continuously is usually for chronic respiratory failure where there is difficulty in maintaining arterial oxygen pressures (hypoxaemia) resulting in low oxygen levels in tissues (hypoxia). However, administering oxygen therapy where there is no hypoxaemia is considered an expensive placebo and other non-pharmacological interventions should be used first (Booth *et al.* 2004). Sometimes oxygen may only be necessary during exercise and small portable devices are available which can enable individuals to leave home for longer periods. Similarly, there may be benefit from short bursts of oxygen for around ten to 20 minutes to relieve breathlessness. This method is only prescribed where there is documented improvement in breathlessness and/or exercise tolerance, and guidance should be sought from a specialist health professional.

Inhalers

Handheld inhalers are commonly used to deliver drugs into the lungs in a number of respiratory diseases particularly in asthma and chronic obstructive pulmonary disease. Bronchodilators are taken by many with respiratory problems and these are best administered using a handheld inhaler. Users should be able to demonstrate satisfactory technique, and ability to use a particular device should be regularly assessed by a competent healthcare professional (NICE 2004). Where technique is faulty perhaps due to poor coordination, treatment may be suboptimal with poor symptom control and use of a volume spacer can aid drug delivery. Often it is simply a case of choosing the right device, and a practice nurse or respiratory nurse specialist will be able to offer advice.

Where there is distressing and perhaps disabling breathlessness despite maximal therapy using inhalers, or where the individuals are too ill or incapable of using an inhaler, a nebuliser may be prescribed (Muers 1997) generating a fine mist from a liquid drug which can then be inhaled through a mask. Drugs which are commonly nebulised are bronchodilators to dilate the airways (e.g. salbutamol and ipratropium bromide). In palliative care settings where breathlessness is a distressing symptom, morphine may be prescribed and occasionally administered through a nebuliser although this remains controversial. Nebulisers may also be used to help clear secretions where there is difficulty removing these from the airways.

Recent research has shown that in acute asthma and exacerbations of COPD, in order to avoid nebulisation, high-dose bronchodilators can be delivered equally efficiently by giving multiple 'puffs' from a pressurised metered dose inhaler through a large volume spacer (Dewar *et al.* 1999; Brocklebank *et al.* 2001). This should be demonstrated in the promotion of self-management so that individuals and carers are confident is doing this when necessary. Devices can be a prime source of infection and there should be a spare mask or cannulae so that these can be washed. Volume spacers should be washed and rinsed well and left to dry, which reduces static. Similarly, masks and jet nebulisers should be washed in soapy water, rinsed and dried carefully with disposable units changed every three months if used regularly (Booker 2007).

Fatigue

Tiredness and fatigue are common in people living with long-term health problems (Small and Lamb 1999); yet perhaps of all symptoms they are more likely to be overlooked or even dismissed by healthcare workers (Trendall 2000). Lack of motivation and low energy are features of many chronic physical disorders as well as psychiatric problems such as depression, and can impact significantly on disability level and quality of life with feelings of helplessness, loss of control and frustration (Droegemueller *et al.* 2008).

Fatigue has been defined as a subjective feeling of tiredness, weakness or lack of energy, and although there are qualitative differences between fatigue in those with cancer and health controls, it is thought that such differences are only an expression of the overwhelming intensity of cancer-related fatigue (Radbruch *et al.* 2008). In one study of people with cancer, fatigue was ranked higher over nausea, depression and pain in terms of affecting everyday life the most (Curt *et al.* 2000). Most of us feel fatigued at some point in our lives but it is estimated that 20 per cent of the population experience troublesome fatigue, with women experiencing fatigue more than men (Sharpe and Wilks 2002). Yet, although fatigue may be due primarily to a physical health problem, there are many factors that can contribute to prolonged tiredness and lack of energy. Complaints of fatigue or decreased ability to undertake usual activities may be signs of anaemia, thyroid problems, depression or neurological and cardiac problems (Amella 2006). In a number of chronic progressive diseases there are molecules produced by the body called cytokines which can result in loss of appetite, muscle wasting, sleepiness, fever and aching joints (Dantzer and Kelley 2007). The root cause of fatigue may be unknown, but individual habits and routines as well as environmental factors can contribute significantly.

Assessment of fatigue

Assessment of fatigue is an important first step in identifying a possible cause, with consideration given to the social, emotional and spiritual realms of the person's life, as well as physical symptoms, so that advice can be offered to assist self-care (Kralik *et al.* 2005). Listening carefully to individual experiences with fatigue will lead to a better understanding of the factors that can contribute to successful self-regulation and better fatigue management strategies (Droegemueller *et al.* 2008).

Psychosocial issues

Biomedical aspects of care are of course important and prescribed treatments including medication need to be delivered timely and effectively so that any pathophysiological causes of symptoms are addressed and good control achieved. It should not be assumed, however, that symptoms are only driven by the disease process. Many additional factors will influence symptom presentation and health outcome. We live in a culture where physical symptoms are often seen as more legitimate than emotional difficulties and many people tend to tell stories of their distress in terms of somatic rather than mental manifestations (Launer 2002). The stories that individuals bring to health encounters with professionals are often not well formed and clearly articulated, and Launer suggests that initial narratives are often hesitant, disjointed, fragmented, complicated or full of elements that puzzle, and that new narratives must provide a better kind of explanation and coherence for what is happening.

Anxiety and emotional distress is common in a significant number with ongoing health problems. The illness trajectory will sometimes involve periods of crisis precipitated perhaps by negative life events resulting in personal loss and distress. Indeed, distress may be so profound that individuals experience mental or physical pain on a scale associated with personal suffering. Attempts have been made to explore the construct of suffering which is considered to be multidimensional and strongly linked with physical symptoms. In a study of 381 patients with advanced cancer where suffering was experienced, this was not only as a result of psychological distress but of existential concerns and social–relational worries (Wilson *et al.* 2007). In a recent audit of NHS Direct, data were collected on individuals in Hampshire and the Isle of Wight who had contacted the service the preceding year before suicide (Bessant *et al.* 2008). Out of 278 suicides in the area 30 people had contacted NHS Direct: 17 (57 per cent) of these had reported physical problems and nine (30 per cent) had reported mental health problems. The reporting of physical symptoms was an unexpected finding and illustrates how emotional suffering with suicidal intention can often be masked by somatic presentation such as physical pain.

Differentiating between physical and mental symptoms is not always easy, and there may be complex personal histories further influenced by co-morbidity and gender. More than half of women with severe mental illness report a history of childhood sexual abuse where the rate of depression is doubled. These women are twice as likely to have gynaecological problems and seek care in primary care settings for insomnia, gastrointestinal problems, chronic pain and multiple problems (Vandiver 2007). This is particularly the case for women with mental illness who are in relationships that are abusive and exploitative, and Vandiver suggests that these women often find it difficult to participate and engage in healthcare. Neither is it easy for some women with mental illness to recognise or describe physical symptoms, and psychosis may contribute to this difficulty as well as to communication problems with healthcare providers.

Individual illness representations and personal meanings attributed to symptoms need careful exploration. Where a symptom is perceived to be important and a source of potential threat, the symptom is attended to (attentional bias) and cognitive–emotional processes activated, thereby influencing behaviours and judgements (Beck and Clark 1997; Snider *et al.* 2000). In chronic pain, for example, attentional bias can promote anxiety and avoidant behaviours, increasing pain still further. Emotional distress with negative emotions including sad mood can also increase attentional bias towards symptoms (Poon and Knight 2009). There may be enhanced attentional bias to symptoms in some older people where cognitions attribute physical symptoms to old age (Leventhal and Crouch 1997), and increased symptom focus may be due to belief patterns based on stereotyping where poorer health is automatically linked to old age. Conversely, potentially serious and life-threatening symptoms may not be taken seriously and where these are ignored can have serious consequences. Ongoing education is important so that individuals can be involved in self-monitoring of symptoms and are able to recognise significant change and take appropriate action.

Mental health problems and recovery

From a medical perspective, the control of mental illness may be seen as being focused on the abatement of psychiatric symptoms (Cohen 2005) and as such one may be perceived as being mentally ill, and in need of psychiatric care, until pronounced 'cured' (Corrigan and Phelan 2004). For people with a diagnosed mental health problem there can be no doubt that psychiatric symptoms can be a major source of mental distress, undermining their quality of life and subjective well-being. Chapter 15, for example, describes some of the ways in which medication can assist the person with symptoms of moderate to severe depression. However, in modern mental healthcare it is more common to focus on an individual's recovery in a holistic sense rather than an explicit focus on controlling psychiatric symptoms (Corrigan and Phelan 2004).

For the National Institute of Mental Health for England (NIMHE 2005) recovery is a process of returning to an optimum state of wellness and the achievement of a quality of life which is personally acceptable to the individual. Such non-medical perceptions of recovery are subjective and the identification of 'end goals' that individuals wish to strive for and the meaning they attach to their experiences, along with their hopes, aspirations and fears is important (Rethink 2005; Matthews and Trenoweth 2008). Recovery in this sense 'is not about regaining a problem-free life – whose life is? It is about living life more resourcefully, living a satisfying and contributing life, in spite of limitations caused by a continuing vulnerability to disabling distress' (Watkins 2001, 45). This implies that a more expansive vista is needed for assessing the sources of distress in people's lives than the purely biomedical, important though this may be. It also implies that the response of the professional helper to such distress requires emphasis to be placed on the psychological, social, emotional, physical and existential dimensions of self. As such, recovery is supported when

> Hope is encouraged, enhanced and/or maintained; Life roles with respect to work and meaningful activities are defined; Spirituality is considered; Culture is understood; Educational needs as well as those of families/significant others are identified; Socialisation needs are identified; [and when people] are supported to achieve their goals.
>
> (NIMHE 2005, 4)

In this sense, helping people to regain some control over their lives in the face of mental distress can be as important in the recovery process as medical interventions (Coodin-Schiff 2004; Matthews and Trenoweth 2008).

To enable recovery, emphasis is placed on supporting a person to move on, in a climate of optimism, acceptance, hope and positive determination by all those involved in the process (Kelly and Gamble 2005). Furthermore, people who engage with support mechanisms around them often have a greater chance of improving their quality of life, and seem to be less limited by their health problems (Cunningham *et al.* 2005). This can reveal significant improvements in an individual's subjective well-being and quality of life (Ochocka *et al.* 2005) while assisting in the achievement of personal goals despite experiencing 'psychiatric symptoms'.

Facilitating effective symptom management

Medical treatment, while important, is only part of the overall management of ongoing symptoms. Indeed, there may be limited benefit from orthodox medical approaches, and individuals desperate for relief from distressing symptoms may consider less traditional therapies. While some complementary approaches may offer benefit (see Chapter 11) there are many therapies where evidence is weak. For some long-term conditions there are well-organised services focusing on disease management using programmes involving multidisciplinary teams, regular monitoring and patient education, and underpinned by National Service Frameworks (Pascoe *et al.* 2004). These principles, however, need to be applied across all groups with long-term conditions, particularly those vulnerable groups where poor uptake of healthcare services is well documented. For example, individuals with learning disabilities can benefit from health promotion opportunities to reduce the incidence and severity of secondary conditions that further limit their participation in society (Ravesloot *et al.* 2007).

Promotion of health and general well-being should be an important objective for those with long-term conditions. Studies show how rehabilitation programmes can improve quality of life by addressing non-medical problems including exercise reconditioning, relative social isolation, altered mood states, muscle wasting and weight loss (Stephenson and McHugh 2004). Benefits have been demonstrated in a number of groups including those with cardiac problems, pulmonary problems, neurological problems and musculoskeletal problems. Organised rehabilitation programmes in terms of availability can be a little patchy but there are elements of rehabilitation which may be incorporated into the individual's daily routine whatever the care setting, which can have a significant impact on performance and quality of life.

Physical activity

Rehabilitation includes not only symptom management but should incorporate a range of health promotion activities and there is greater success when psychoeducational strategies are employed. A number of areas should be considered including regular exercise within the limits of the individual's functional abilities, dietary aspects, and the promotion of adequate sleep. Many symptoms, particularly pain, breathlessness and fatigue, can result in inactivity and deconditioning where the longer the inactivity persists the more tired the individual feels, reducing further the capacity for physical exercise (Casaburi 2006). Nutritional deficits can also contribute to symptom experience and appropriate changes to diet and eating habits may result in significant benefits. It may be necessary to seek advice from a dietician where ongoing fatigue and weight loss are problematic (further information on nutrition may be found in Chapter 10).

There are a number of studies which support the idea that being physically active can offer major health benefits including reduced physical disability and promotion of psychological well-being (Berger 2004; Smith *et al.* 2007) as well as being a buffer against age-related cognitive decline in older people (Weuve *et al.* 2004). Nor is it only objective measures of physical fitness or function that are of importance, but also more subjective measures including self-reports of pain, self-efficacy, and satisfaction with physical function (Biddle and Ekkekakis 2005). This is particularly relevant in long-term conditions where even very low levels of activity may result in improved self-report measures. Activity needs to be enjoyable, and it is important that exercise history is taken into account and activity is selected which is appropriate for any pre-existing medical condition or physical limitation (Pearce 2008).

Self-management

The principles of self-management may also be incorporated into practice and the five core skills which need to be developed if confidence is to be increased include:

- problem-solving;
- decision-making;
- resource utilisation;
- developing effective partnerships with healthcare providers;
- taking action.

These core skills are elaborated on in the Expert Patients Programme (EPP) (DoH 2001) which is explored in other chapters of this book. Symptom management is a key component of any EPP. Collaborative relationships with healthcare providers are important and are effective when individuals with long-term conditions and care providers have shared goals, a sustained working relationship, mutual understanding of roles and responsibilities and the requisite skills for carrying out these roles (Von Korff *et al.* 1997).

Pacing activities to conserve energy

Yet despite the importance of collaborative goal-setting and follow-up support activities for people with long-term conditions these are conducted significantly less often than other actions (Glasgow *et al.* 2005). Each day may offer new challenges for individuals with ongoing symptoms and care providers must work collaboratively in identifying appropriate coping strategies. Pacing of activities where there are physical symptoms such as pain, breathlessness and/or fatigue is one such strategy, and time is needed to explore factors that precipitate symptoms. This is where the use of a diary can be helpful and a log may be kept of when symptoms are most troublesome during a 24-hour period, together with the specific activities or other factors (antecedents) resulting in symptoms. In cancer where fatigue can be particularly intense, recommendations have included diary-keeping on daily activities and counselling for energy conservation principles, so that individuals learn to do the most important things when their energy levels are highest (Portenoy and Itri 1999; Radbruch *et al.* 2008).

For many people symptoms fluctuate throughout a 24-hour cycle and there may be times of the day when symptoms are particularly severe. It may be necessary to rethink and plan daily routines differently so that self-care activities are not executed during vulnerable periods. This can be quite hard where, for example, personal hygiene activities have always been completed in the morning. Yet clustering of self-care activities in the morning can result in severe exhaustion and worsening of other symptoms for many people, and minor adjustments to daily routines can result in significant benefits. It is unlikely that any single care provider will possess the requisite expertise to care for all individuals with disability, as the range of conditions is considerable (Lawthers *et al.* 2003). However, care providers must be knowledgeable about how and where to access professional expertise across medical, nursing, social and vocational services.

Conclusion

Symptom control is a vital area of concern for individuals with long-term conditions and healthcare professionals responsible for care planning and interventions. There is little doubt that improvement in symptom control and the development of individual mastery in this area can promote both self-efficacy and affect outcome in a number of areas. Quality of life is becoming an increasingly important domain in the evaluation of healthcare experience across the long-term condition trajectory. Awareness of the constellation of factors that impact on symptom control is essential in devising the most effective strategies to reduce unpleasant and distressing symptom intrusion and enhance quality of life.

References

Abbey, J., Piller, N., De Bellis, A. *et al.* (2004) The Abbey Pain Scale: A 1-minute Numerical Indicator for People with End-stage Dementia. *International Journal of Palliative Nursing*, 10, 6–13.

Amella, E. (2003) Geriatrics and Palliative Care. Collaboration for Quality of Life until Death. *Journal of Hospice and Palliative Nursing*, 5(1), 40–48.

Amella, E.J.A. (2006) Presentation of Illness in Older Adults: If You Think You Know What You're Looking For, Think Again. *AORN Journal*, 83, 372–389.

American Thoracic Society (1999) Dyspnea: Mechanisms, Assessment and Management: A Consensus Statement. *American Journal of Respiratory and Critical Care Medicine*, 159, 321–340.

Beach, D. and Schwartzstein, R.M. (2006) The Genesis of Breathlessness – What Do We Understand? In: Booth, S. and Dudgeon, D. (eds) *Dyspnoea in Advanced Disease: A Guide to Clinical Management* (pp. 1–18). Oxford: Oxford University Press.

Beck, A.T. and Clark, D.A. (1997) An Information Processing Model of Anxiety: Automatic and Strategic Processes. *Behaviour Research and Therapy*, 35, 49–58.

Berger, B.G. (2004) Subjective Well Being in Obese Individuals: The Multiple Roles of Exercise. *Quest*, 56, 50–76.

Bessant, M., King, E.A. and Peveler, R. (2008) Characteristics of Suicides in Recent Contact with NHS Direct. *Psychiatric Bulletin*, 32, 92–95.

Biddle, S.J.H. and Ekkekakis, P. (2005) Physically Active Lifestyles and Well-being. In: Huppert, F.A., Baylis, N. and Keverne, B. (eds) *The Science of Well-being* (pp. 141–168). Oxford: Oxford University Press.

Blay, S.L., Andreoli, S.B., Dewey, M.E. *et al.* (2007) Co-occurrence of Chronic Physical Pain and Psychiatric Morbidity in a Community Sample of Older People. *International Journal of Geriatric Psychiatry*, 22, 902–908.

Booker, R. (2007) Correct Use of Nebulisers. *Nursing Standard*, 22, 39–41.

Booth, S., Wade, R. and Johnson, M. (2004) The Use of Oxygen in the Palliation of Breathlessness. A Report of the Expert Working Group of the Scientific Committee of the Association of Palliative Medicine. *Respiratory Medicine*, 98, 66–77.

Bope, E.T., Douglass, A.B. and Gibovsky, A. (2004) Pain Management by the Family Physician: The Family Practice Pain Education Project. *Journal of the American Board of Family Medicine*, 17, S1–12.

British Thoracic Society (BTS) Working Group on Home Oxygen Services (2006) *Clinical Component for the Home Oxygen Service in England and Wales.* London: British Thoracic Society.

Brocklebank, D., Ram, F., Wright, J. *et al.* (2001) Comparison of the Effectiveness of Inhaler Devices in Asthma and Chronic Obstructive Airways Disease: A Systematic Review of the Literature. *Health Technology Assessment*, 5, 1–149.

Carrol, L.J., Cassidy, J.D. and Cote, P. (2004) Depression as a Risk Factor for Onset of an Episode of Troublesome Neck and Low Back Pain. *Pain*, 107, 134–139.

Casaburi, R. (2006) Impacting Patient-centred Outcomes in COPD: Deconditioning. *European Respiratory Review*, 15, 42–46.

Cleeland, C. (2009) *The Brief Pain Inventory: A User's Guide.* Online. Available at: www.mdanderson.org/pdf/bpi-userguide.pdf (accessed 1 February 2009).

Cohen, O. (2005) How Do We Recover? An Analysis of Psychiatric Survivor Oral Histories. *Journal of Humanistic Psychology*, 45, 333–354.

Coodin-Schiff, A. (2004) Recovery and Mental Illness: Analysis and Personal Reflections. *Psychiatric Rehabilitation Journal*, 27, 212–218.

Corner, J., Plant, H. and Warner, L. (1995) Developing a Nursing Approach to Managing Dyspnoea in Lung Cancer. *International Journal of Palliative Nursing*, 1, 5–11.

Corrigan, P.W. and Phelan, S.M. (2004) Social Support and Recovery in People with Serious Mental Illnesses. *Community Mental Health Journal*, 40, 513–523.

Criteria Committee of the New York Heart Association Inc. (1979) *Nomenclature and Criterion for the Diagnosis of the Heart and Great Vessels* (8th edn). Boston: Little, Brown & Co.

Cunningham, K., Wolbert, R., Graziano, A. and Slocum, J. (2005) Acceptance and Change: The Dialectic of Recovery. *Psychiatric Rehabilitation Journal*, 29, 146–148.

Curt, G.A., Breitbart, W. and Cella, D. (2000) Impact of Cancer Related Fatigue on the Lives of Patients: New Findings from the Fatigue Coalition. *The Oncologist*, 5, 353–360.

Dantzer, R. and Kelley, K.W. (2007) Twenty Years of Research on Cytokine Induced Sickness Behaviour. *Brain Behavior Immunology*, 21, 153–160.

Department of Health (DoH) (2001) *The Expert Patient. A New Approach to Chronic Disease Management for the 21st Century*. London: The Stationery Office.

Dewar, A.L., Stewart, A., Cogswell, J.J. *et al.* (1999) A Randomised Controlled Trial to Assess the Relative Benefits of Large Volume Spacers and Nebulisers to Treat Acute Asthma in Hospital. *Archives of Disease in Childhood*, 80, 421–423.

Droegemueller, C.J.M., Brauer, D.J.P. and Van Buskirk, D.J.M. (2008) Temperament and Fatigue Management in Persons With Chronic Rheumatic Disease. *Clinical Nurse Specialist*, 22, 19–27.

Ehde, D.M., Jensen, M.P. and Engel, J.M. (2003) Chronic Pain Secondary to Disability: A Review. *The Clinical Journal of Pain*, 19, 3–17.

Fletcher, C.M. (Chairman) (1960) Standardised Questionnaire on Respiratory Symptoms: A Statement Prepared and Approved by the MRC Committee on the Aetiology of Chronic Bronchitis (MRC Breathlessness Score). *British Medical Journal*, 2, 1665.

Fraser, D.D., Kee, C.C. and Minick, P. (2006) Living with Chronic Obstructive Pulmonary Disease: Insiders' Perspectives. *Journal of Advanced Nursing*, 55, 550–558.

Fu, M.R., McDaniel, R.W. and Rhodes, V.A. (2007) Measuring Symptom Occurrence and Symptom Distress: Development of the Symptom Experience Index. *Journal of Advanced Nursing*, 59, 623–634.

Ganong, W.F. (1999) *Review of Medical Physiology*. New York: McGraw-Hill.

Gartner, J., Allen, G.D. and Larson, D.B. (1991) Religious Commitment and Mental Health – a Review of the Empirical Literature. *Journal of Psychology Theology*, 19(1), 6–25.

Giacobbi, J., Stancil, M., Hardin, B. *et al.* (2008) Physical Activity and Quality of Life Experienced by Highly Active Individuals with Physical Disabilities. *Adapted Physical Activity Quarterly*, 25, 189–207.

Gift, A.G. (1989) Validation of a Vertical Visual Analogue Scale as a Measure of Clinical Dyspnoea. *Rehabilitation Nursing*, 14(6), 323–325.

Gillespie, D. and Staats, B.A. (1994) Unexplained Dyspnea. *Mayo Clinical Proceedings*, 69, 657–663.

Glasgow, R.E., Wagner, E., Schaefer, J. *et al.* (2005) Development and Validation of the Patient Assessment of Chronic Illness Care (PACIC). *Medical Care*, 43, 436–444.

Goldstein, B. (2000) Musculoskeletal Conditions after Spinal Cord Injury. *Physical Medicine and Rehabilitation of Clinics of North America*, 11, 91–108.

Hann, D.M., Jacobsen, P.B., Azzarello, L.M. *et al.* (1998) Measurement of Fatigue in Cancer Patients: Development and Validation of the Fatigue Symptom Inventory. *Quality of Life Research*, 7, 301–310.

Jackson, J.L. (2004) Somatic and Vegetative Symptoms in Depression. *Depression Mind Body*, 1, 42–49.

Jantarakupt, P. and Porock, D. (2005) Dyspnea Management in Lung Cancer: Applying the Evidence from Chronic Obstructive Pulmonary Disease. *Oncology Nursing Forum*, 32, 785–797.

Katerndahl, D.A. (2008) Impact of Spiritual Symptoms and their Interactions on Healthy Services and Life Satisfaction. *Annals of Family Medicine*, 6(5), 412–442.

Kelly, M. and Gamble, C. (2005) Exploring the Concept of Recovery in Schizophrenia. *Journal of Psychiatric and Mental Health Nursing*, 12, 245–251.

Kerr, M. (2004) Improving the General Health of People with Learning Disabilities. *Advances in Psychiatric Treatment*, 10, 200–206.

Kralik, D.P., Telford, K.B., Price, K.P.R. *et al.* (2005) Women's Experiences of Fatigue in Chronic Illness. *Journal of Advanced Nursing*, 52, 372–380.

Launer, J. (2002) *Narrative-based Primary Care. A Practical Guide.* Oxford: Radcliffe Medical Press.

Lawthers, A.G., Pransky, G.S., Peterson, L.E. *et al.* (2003) Rethinking Quality in the Context of Persons with Disability. *International Journal for Quality in Health Care*, 15, 287–299.

Lee, G.K., Chronister, J. and Bishop, M. (2008) The Effects of Psychosocial Factors on Quality of Life Among Individuals with Chronic Pain. *Rehabilitation Counseling Bulletin*, 51, 177–189.

Leventhal, E.A. and Crouch, M. (1997) Are there Differences in Perception of Illness Across the Lifespan? In: Petrie, K.J. and Weinman, J.A. (eds) *Perceptions of Health and Illness* (pp. 76–77). Amsterdam: Harwood Academic Press.

Matthews, J. and Trenoweth, S. (2008) Some Considerations for Mental Health Nurses Working with Patients Who Self-neglect. In: Lynch, J. and Trenoweth, S. (eds) *Contemporary Issues in Mental Health Nursing* (pp. 239–252). Chichester: John Wiley & Sons.

McCaffrey, R., Frock, T.L. and Garguilo, H. (2003) Understanding Chronic Pain and the Mind–Body Connection. *Holistic Nursing Practice*, 17, 281–287.

McCance, K.L. and Huether, S.E. (2006) *Pathophysiology. The Biologic Basis for Disease in Adults and Children* (5th edn). St Louis, MI: Elsevier Mosby.

McMullan, D., White, C. and Jackson, N. (2007) Psychiatric Issues in Palliative Medicine. *Medicine*, 36(2), 88–90.

Medical Research Council Working Party (MRC) (1981) Long Term Domiciliary Oxygen Therapy in Chronic Hypoxic Cor Pulmonale Complicating Chronic Bronchitis and Emphysema. *Lancet*, I, 681–686.

Melzack, R. and Wall, P.D. (1965) Pain Mechanism: A New Theory. *Science*, 150, 971–979.

Michielsen, H.J., DeVries, J. and VanHeck, G.L. (2003) Psychometric Qualities of a Brief Self Rated Fatigue Measure: The Fatigue Assessment Scale. *Journal of Psychosomatic Research*, 54, 345–353.

Muers, M.F. (1997) Overview of Nebuliser Treatment. *Thorax*, 52, S25–S30.

National Institute for Clinical Excellence (NICE) (2004) Chronic Obstructive Pulmonary Disease: National Clinical Guideline for the Management of Chronic Obstructive Pulmonary Disease in Primary and Secondary Care. *Thorax* (supple. 1), 1–232.

National Institute for Mental Health in England (NIMHE) (2005) *NIMHE Guiding Statement on Recovery.* Online. Available at: www.psychminded.co.uk/news/news2005/feb05/nimherecovstatement.pdf (accessed 4 April 2009).

Nocturnal Oxygen Therapy Trial Group (1980) Continuous or Nocturnal Oxygen Therapy in Hypoxic Chronic Obstructive Pulmonary Disease: A Clinical Trial. *Annals of International Medicine*, 93, 391–398.

Ochocka, J., Nelson, G. and Janzen, R. (2005) Moving Forward: Negotiating Self and External Circumstances in Recovery. *Psychiatric Rehabilitation Journal*, 28, 315–322.

Pascoe, S.W., Neal, R.D., Allgar, V.L. *et al.* (2004) Psychosocial Care for Cancer Patients in Primary Care? Recognition of Opportunities for Cancer Care. *Family Practice*, 21, 437–442.

Pearce, P.Z. (2008) Exercise is Medicine. *Current Sports Medicine Reports*, 7, 171–175.

Pike, A.J. (2008) Body-mindfulness in Physiotherapy for the Management of Long-term Chronic Pain. *Physical Therapy Reviews*, 13, 45–56.

Poon, C.Y.M. and Knight, B.G. (2009) Influence of Sad Mood and Old Age Schema on Older Adults' Attention to Physical Symptoms. *The Journals of Gerontology Series B: Psychological Sciences and Social Sciences*, 64B, 41–44.

Portenoy, R.K. and Itri, L.M. (1999) Cancer-related Fatigue: Guidelines for Evaluation and Management. *Oncologist*, 4, 1–10.

Radbruch, L., Strasser, F., Elsner, F. *et al.* (2008) Fatigue in Palliative Care Patients – An EAPC Approach. *Palliative Medicine*, 22, 13–32.

Ravesloot, C.H., Seekins, T., Cahill, T. *et al.* (2007) Health Promotion for People with Disabilities: Development and Evaluation of the Living Well with a Disability Program. *Health Education Research*, 22, 522–531.

Regnard, C., Matthews, D. and Gibson, L. (2003) Difficulties in Identifying Distress and its Causes in People with Severe Communication Problems. *International Journal of Palliative Nursing*, 9(3), 173–176.

Reid, S., Wessely, S., Crayford, T. *et al.* (2001) Medically Unexplained Symptoms in Frequent Attenders of Secondary Health Care: Retrospective Cohort Study. *British Medical Journal*, 322, 767.

Rethink (2005) *A Report On The Work Of The Recovery Learning Sites And Other Recovery-orientated Activities And Its Incorporation Into The Rethink Plan 2004–08*. Online. Available at: www.rethink.org/living_with_mental_illness/recovery_and_self_management/recovery/index.html (accessed 4 April 2009).

Ross, E.L. and Hahn, K. (2008) Kadian (Morphine Sulfate Extended-release) Capsules for Treatment of Chronic, Moderate-to-severe, Nonmalignant Pain. *International Journal of Clinical Practice*, 62, 471–479.

Schwartzstein, R.M. (1998) The Language of Dyspnea. In Mahler, D.A. (ed.) *Dyspnea* (pp. 35–62). New York: Marcel Dekker.

Schwartzstein, R.M., Lahive, K., Pope, A. *et al.* (1987) Cold Facial Stimulation Reduces Breathlessness Induced in Normal Subjects. *American Review of Respiratory Disease*, 136, 58–61.

Sharpe, M. and Wilks, D. (2002) ABC of Psychological Medicine: Fatigue. *British Medical Journal*, 325, 480–483.

Shee, C.D. and Green, M. (2003) Non-invasive Ventilation and Palliation: Experience in a District General Hospital and a Review. *Palliative Medicine*, 17, 21–26.

Small, S. and Lamb, M. (1999) Fatigue in Chronic Illness: The Experience of Individuals with Chronic Obstructive Pulmonary Disease and with Asthma. *Journal of Advanced Nursing*, 30, 469–478.

Smith, P.J., Blumenthal, J.A., Babyak, M.A. *et al.* (2007) Effects of Exercise and Weight Loss on Depressive Symptoms among Men and Women with Hypertension. *Journal of Psychosomatic Research*, 63, 463–469.

Snider, B.S., Asmundson, G.J.G. and Weiss, K.C. (2000) Automatic and Strategic Processing of Threat Cues in Patients with Chronic Pain: A Modified-stroop Evaluation. *Clinical Journal of Pain*, 16, 144–154.

Spector, N., Connolly, M.A. and Carlson, K.K. (2007) Dyspnea: Applying Research to Bedside Practice. *AACN Advanced Critical Care*, 18(1), 45–60.

Stephenson, D. and McHugh, A. (2004) The Non-pharmacological Nursing Management of Dyspnoea in End-stage Respiratory Disease and Palliative Care Populations. *Collegian*, 11, 37–41.

Syrett, E. and Taylor, J. (2003) Non-pharmacological Management of Breathlessness: A Collaborative Nurse-physiotherapist Approach. *International Journal of Palliative Nursing*, 9, 150–156.

Thompson, C.L. (2001) Dyspnea with and without Fan Blowing on Face of Hospitalised Adults. *Critical Care Medicine*, 29 (suppl), A148.

Trendall, J. (2000) Concept Analysis: Chronic Fatigue. *Journal of Advanced Nursing*, 32, 1126–1131.

Tunks, E.R., Crook, J. and Weir, R. (2008) Epidemiology of Chronic Pain with Psychological Co-Morbidity: Prevalence, Risk, Course, and Prognosis. *Canadian Journal of Psychiatry*, 53, 224–234.

Turk, D. (1994) Perspectives on Chronic Pain: The Role of Psychological Factors. *Current Directions in Psychological Science*, 3, 45–48.

Turk, D.C. (2002) Clinical Effectiveness and Cost-effectiveness of Treatments for Patients with Chronic Pain. *Clinical Journal of Pain*, 18, 355–365.

Vandiver, V. (2007) Health Promotion as Brief Treatment: Strategies for Women with Co-morbid Health and Mental Health Conditions. *Brief Treatment and Crisis Intervention*, 7, 161–175.

Vanina, Y., Podolskaya, A., Sedky, K. *et al.* (2002) Body Weight Changes Associated with Psychopharmacology. *Psychiatric Services*, 53(7), 842–847.

Verhaak, P.F., Kerssens, J.J., Dekker, J. *et al.* (1998) Prevalence of Chronic Benign Pain Disorder Among Adults: A Review of the Literature. *Pain*, 17, 231–239.

Von Korff, M., Gruman, J., Schaefer, J. *et al.* (1997) Collaborative Management of Chronic Illness. *Annals of Internal Medicine*, 127(12), 1097–1102.

Watkins, P. (2001) *Mental Health Nursing: The Art of Compassionate Care*. Edinburgh: Butterworth Heinemann.

Weuve, J., Kang, J., Manson, J. *et al.* (2004) Physical Activity Including Walking and Cognitive Function in Older Women. *JAMA*, 292, 1454–1461.

Williams, C.M. (2006) Dyspnea. *Cancer Journal*, 12, 365–373.

Wilson, K.G., Chochinov, H.M., McPherson, C.J. *et al.* (2007) Suffering with Advanced Cancer. *Journal of Clinical Oncology*, 25, 1691–1697.

Woodrow, P. (2007) Caring for Patients Receiving Oxygen Therapy. *Nursing Older People*, 19, 31–36.

Young, J.L., Horton, F.M. and Davidhizar, R. (2006) Nursing Attitudes and Beliefs in Pain Assessment and Management. *Journal of Advanced Nursing*, 53, 412–421.

7 Facilitating, supporting and maintaining recovery

Tim Duffy, Colin Martin and Tim Anstiss

Introduction

The concept of recovery in long-term conditions is both paradoxical and contested; paradoxical in that long-term conditions are those from which people are not expected to recover. Yet there are plenty of ways in which people with long-term conditions can and do recover. People can recover from exacerbations and complications of the condition; from the psychological impact of the diagnosis; from associated mental health problems such as depression or anxiety; from associated physical health problems such as overweight and obesity; and from chronic pain syndrome. Lifestyle changes can reverse some of the pathological changes in coronary heart disease (CHD), and exercise programmes can stop people experiencing angina – even if the underlying disease remains untouched. People with long-term conditions can recover their sense of meaning, purpose and self-worth when these are affected by their condition. And finally, of course, some people can and do recover from the condition itself.

The concept of recovery is also contested in that within mental health discourse the concept of recovery has multiple meanings – being a journey people experience, a process, a movement, an approach, a philosophy, a set of values and a paradigm (Turner 2002). In a recent review of the British literature Bonney and Stickley (2008) identified six main, somewhat interweaving themes to do with recovery and mental health: identity; the service provision agenda; the social domain; power and control; hope and optimism; and risk and responsibility. A range of recovery models are in existence (May *et al.* 1999; Heather 2002; NICE 2002; Repper and Perkins 2003; Fisher 2005) and many organisations are implementing a recovery approach. In mental healthcare, a key policy document has been the National Institute for Mental Health in England (NIMHE) (2005) *NIMHE Guiding Statement on Recovery* which seeks to place emphasis on recovery being related to the person achieving a life of optimum personal value rather than a focus on the reduction of medical symptoms of mental distress (see Chapter 15). For an excellent discussion of how the recovery approach can and should be used to inform policy and service redesign, see *A New Vision for Mental Health* (Future Vision Coalition 2008).

Earlier chapters have identified the range and extent of long-term conditions. Consideration has been given to assessing people with such conditions and assisting them with appropriate symptom control. In this chapter the focus will be on ways in which holistic care can be structured and enhanced by using specific therapeutic approaches. Specifically, this chapter will provide an overview of some key psychological and therapeutic strategies. The main focus will be on brief interventions, motivational interviewing, problem-solving, cognitive behavioural therapy and applied positive psychology.

Psychosocial interventions and recovery

In recent years, there has been a developing awareness of the effectiveness of non-pharmacological psychosocial interventions for people experiencing difficulty with alcohol and drug, mental health and many other behavioural problems. A growing body of research evidence supports the application of psychosocial interventions across a wide range of long-term conditions; for example, Peyrot and Rubin note the benefits of these interventions for people with diabetes including acceptance of, and adherence to, treatment regimens as well as dealing more effectively with diabetes-related stress and depression (Peyrot and Rubin 2007). Further, interventions seen to be effective in one area are being shown to be helpful in other settings and contexts. Motivational interviewing, which originated in the context of assisting people with alcohol problems, is now used to help clients deal with diabetes, fibromyalgia, cardiovascular disease, in addition to assisting people with a range of mental health difficulties (Miller and Rollnick 2002). Similarly, problem-solving techniques and cognitive behavioural therapies have been adopted for use across a range of clinical areas. In many instances these psychosocial interventions are delivered alongside and in harmony with already planned medical interventions, possibly enhancing their effectiveness by increasing client exposure to the effective ingredients.

The therapeutic relationship

Within each psychosocial intervention the client–therapist relationship is important. Zetzel (1956) considered a conscious, collaborative, rational agreement between therapist and client as required to help bring about a successful treatment outcome (Zetzel 1956). Rogers (1959) famously considered and evaluated key counsellor skills for facilitating natural changes and identified the importance of accurate empathy, non-possessive warmth and genuineness (Rogers 1959). The client's perception of the therapeutic relationship is also a strong indicator of treatment success (Connors *et al.* 1997). Miller and Rollnick (2002) note that the characteristics of the counsellor may be associated with successful treatment outcomes and may account for up to 7 per cent of the outcome variance (Project MATCH Research Group 1998). The relationship between therapist and client can be enhanced by therapists' expression of warmth, friendliness, openness, good eye contact, expression of empathy and facial expressions (see Chapter 8).

In addition to therapists' attributes, Horvath *et al.* (1993) identify three further aspects which can impact on the effectiveness of a therapeutic relationship. These include the clients' view of how relevant the intervention is to them and how effective it is likely to be, and second, the clients' agreement with the counsellor as what seems to be reasonable and relevant healthcare outcomes both in the short and long term. Finally, Horvath *et al.* note the importance of the development of a personal bond between clients and therapists with the latter presenting as caring, sensitive and willing to help (Horvath *et al.* 1993).

Brief interventions

The provision of psychosocial interventions to clients with long-term conditions does not have to be a time-consuming activity although it commonly requires specialist training to be skilfully delivered. Many counsellors and therapists believe the service they deliver helps bring about change in clients' health-related behaviour, with their knowledge, skills and personality helping people to change. However, people often change without any professional help or outside intervention whatsoever. For this reason, Miller and Rollnick (2002, 4) suggest that 'Treatment can be thought of as facilitating what is a natural process of change.'

A wide range of studies from different countries have shown the effectiveness of brief interventions on behaviour change – so-called because these interventions are often short in duration focusing on specific problems including health behaviour change. Bien *et al.* (1993) summarised the key elements of brief interventions using the acronym FRAMES as follows:

- **FEEDBACK** on assessment results;
- **RESPONSIBILITY** – changing is up to the client;
- **ADVICE** to reduce or stop problematic behaviour;
- **MENU** of options in the process of change;
- **EMPATHY** features in most descriptions in some form, although some appear confrontational;
- **SELF-EFFICACY** is promoted to reduce feelings of helplessness and increase empowerment to undertake change.

Duffy (1994) has suggested that brief or minimal interventions can take the form of a single interview, a series of interviews, or the provision of a self-help manual with little or even no personal contact, and states that 'Minimal interventions, assuming they are well planned and executed, can have quite an impact, often as significant as that offered by more extensive intervention' (Duffy 1994, 4) (for example, see Chapter 5 for the Fast Alcohol Screening Test (FAST) (Health Development Agency (HDA) 2002). Within the context of caring for people with long-term conditions within busy surgeries, hospitals and specialist units, the use of effective, brief interventions has a significant time-saving advantage. As Miller and Rollnick remark, 'The fascinating point is that so much change occurs after so little counselling' (Miller and Rollnick 2002, 5).

Stages of change

Prochaska and Di Clemente (1982) considered how people change their behaviour, either with or without assistance from a therapist or counsellor. Initially their model consisted of five stages: contemplation, determination, action, maintenance and relapse. Later developments identify six stages with the sixth being a pre-contemplation stage (see Figure 7.1). In this model, there is the recognition that people may go around the cycle from pre-contemplation to relapse perhaps several times before successfully changing their behaviour. Individuals may stay in each stage for differing amounts of time. Individuals are likely to be assisted to change by differing external forces, depending on the particular stage of change.

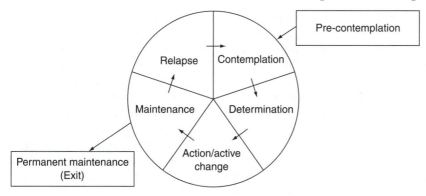

Figure 7.1 The stages of change (source: Prochaska and Di Clemente (1982)).

For example, someone at the pre-contemplation stage may benefit from a conversation that raises their awareness of the risks associated with not changing their behaviour, and the benefits of changing. That is, therapeutic work at this stage often involves discussing and highlighting the need for change. For example, someone recently diagnosed with diabetes may need support to raise awareness regarding changes they may need to make to their lifestyle behaviours (particularly if they smoke, drink alcohol excessively or have a diet high in sugar and fat) and how specific treatment regimes will help to keep them healthy. This can be assisted by providing accurate information on their diagnosis and treatment, and a subsequent discussion where any subsequent uncertainties can be clarified and the person's concerns aired. In having this discussion with someone who started the conversation in pre-contemplation (not thinking about change), the counsellor has moved them into the contemplation stage – in that they may now be thinking about (contemplating) whether or not to change. Rushing in and providing a person with assistance in developing a plan to change may have little impact at this level of readiness, as the person has not yet decided to change – and indeed may not even perceive the existence of a problem, let alone the need to change it.

When a person is in the contemplation stage they are ambivalent about the need to either change their lifestyle, follow a recommended treatment regime or both. Ambivalence is natural and common, and is simply feeling two ways about something, being unsure as to whether to change or stay the same. The person may be weighing up the need for change with the desire to remain as they are. Helping the patient explore and resolve this ambivalence in a non-judgemental way is the very heart of motivational interviewing, and a range of strategies are available to help with this exploration of ambivalence – including exploring the good things and less good things about changing, and exploring two possible futures (one with change and one without). Merely providing the client with information about diabetes at this stage is likely to be insufficient, and telling the client what to change and how to change may trigger resistance. The client may already have enough information to indicate they have a problem, but may not necessarily have considered sufficiently why there is a need for change. At this stage the client may benefit from talking about the difficulties they may experience if they do not change, and the benefits likely to flow from changing aspects of lifestyle and treatment. The role of the therapist may be to tip the balance so that the client recognises the need to change and argues in favour of change.

A client at the determination stage of the model has decided to change but may lack the confidence or skills to carry out the change and to stay changed. At this stage the therapist may focus on increasing self-confidence and self-efficacy in behaviour change. Clients in the action stage may benefit from skills training to help them carry out changes they have decided to make – for instance, taking more exercise, eating more healthily, better at managing stress, coping with urges to smoke and so forth. Providing someone at this stage only with information about their diagnosis would be considered inefficient and possibly counterproductive, since the stage matched approach suggests that what may be required is assistance in carrying out a planned lifestyle change. Of course many people with long-term conditions just need help deciding what to do. Once they have decided, no further help may be necessary – apart, perhaps, from a mutually agreed review.

This model of behaviour change suggests that providing the same therapeutic assistance to all people is not appropriate – that specific types of intervention and help should be provided to people at different stages of change, or levels of readiness. This is, in part, what individually tailoring the care plan is all about. The approach requires some skill, however. Some people may stay in the same stage of change for some time, and this may be easily identifiable – others may progress from one stage to another quite rapidly, sometimes within a single session. Identifying the clients' readiness to change is therefore crucial as it helps guide the therapist response and focus. Two aspects of client speech greatly assist the counsellor in this task: resistance and change talk (Rollnick *et al.* 2008). Table 7.1, adapted from Miller and Rollnick (1991), summarises the external motivational tasks most suitable at each stage of change.

Table 7.1 The stages of change and motivational tasks

Stage of change	Motivational task
Pre-contemplation	The therapist should aim to increase the clients' view of problems they are currently experiencing and the risks of maintaining the status quo
Contemplation	The therapist should aim to elicit from the clients reasons to change and difficulties anticipated if no change is made. A further aim is to strengthen self-efficacy for change
Determination	The therapist should aim to assist clients in determining the best course of action to take in seeking change
Action	The therapist should aim to assist clients to take steps towards change
Maintenance	The therapist should aim to assist clients to identify and implement strategies to prevent relapse, or breakdown of change process
Relapse/breakdown of change process	The therapist should assist clients to renew their commitment to change

Motivational interviewing

Motivational interviewing (MI) has increased in popularity since the 1980s and is now used by therapists in a wide range of clinical and non-clinical settings. In 2002, Miller and Rollnick stated that 'Motivational interviewing is a client-centred, directive method for enhancing intrinsic motivation to change by exploring and resolving ambivalence' (Miller and Rollnick 2002, 25). More recently they have defined motivational interviewing as 'a person-centred method of guiding to elicit and strengthen personal motivation for change' (Miller and Rollnick 2009, 25). The approach is supported by a growing research base and over 100 controlled trials (see e.g. Burke *et al.* 2002; Heather 2005; Rubak *et al.* 2005) and has been recognised by many as improving the quality of the client–therapist relationship. It is now widely used to assist clients with health promotion activity, dietary change (Vanwormer and Boucher 2004) and weight loss (Carels *et al.* 2007), physical activity promotion (Bennett *et al.* 2007), medication adherence (Cooperman *et al.* 2007), diabetes (Channon *et al.* 2007), mental health (Arkowitz *et al.* 2008), chronic pain (Rau *et al.* 2008) and stroke rehabilitation (Watkins *et al.* 2007), among others.

While this approach shares many characteristics with humanistic approaches including the emphasis on non-judgemental listening and the development of accurate empathy, Miller and Rollnick note that the approach is more focused (on behaviour change issues) and goal directed (towards the exploration and resolution of ambivalence) than non-directive counselling. The focus is on helping people to explore and resolve their ambivalence about change as being undecided may be the main barrier to change for most people (Miller and Rollnick 1991).

The spirit of MI has been described as collaborative, autonomy-supporting and evocative. Clinicians aim to work alongside and in harmony with the patient, rather than arguing with them due to a mismatch of agendas and needs. Clinicians remember that the patient is the active decision-maker (autonomy), and seek to 'evoke' both concerns and solutions from the patient rather than telling the patient what they should be concerned about, why they should be concerned, and what they should do about it. How well a clinician manifests this spirit seems to predict both increased client responsiveness and treatment outcome (Moyers and Martin 2006; Gaume *et al.* 2008).

Helping people explore and resolve their ambivalence about changing is best done in a detached manner where the therapist has 'no clear attachment to or recommendation for one resolution more than another' (Miller and Rollnick 2002, 91). This is not to be confused with detachment from the experience and feelings of the client. This approach is sometimes called the 'equipoise', where the therapist is indifferent to the direction of the outcome of the intervention.

MI practitioners use a range of tools, strategies and exercises to manifest the spirit of the approach, deploy the principles and ultimately help their patients explore and resolve their ambivalence about behaviour change – including: setting the scene; agreeing on the agenda; exploring a typical day; assessing importance and confidence; exploring two possible futures; looking back and looking forwards; exploring options; agreeing goals and agreeing to a plan. For more information about how to use these approaches in clinical practice, see Rollnick *et al.* (2008). Furthermore, MI practitioners pay particular attention to two key aspects of client speech: 'change talk' and 'resistance'. Change talk comprises client speech indicating desire, ability, reasons, need or commitment to change (Amrhein *et al.* 2003) and may be predictive of future behaviour change (Gollwitzer 1999). Resistance – a state of oppositional, angry, irritable or suspicious patient behaviour – bodes poorly for treatment effectiveness (Beutler *et al.* 2002) and so MI practitioners use a range of strategies to avoid triggering resistance in the first place and to 'roll' with resistance as and when it is observed (Moyers and Rollnick 2002). Paying attention and appropriately responding to what the client says may help determine client outcome, and motivational interviewing may significantly increase change talk and reduce resistance relative to other approaches (Miller *et al.* 1993).

Finally, MI practitioners use their 'OARS' to help bring about health behaviour change – four key communication skills identified as critically important (Miller and Rollnick 2002):

1   Using of **O**pen-ended questions such as 'Why might this be a good time for you to change?' or 'What would be the main benefits for you if you did decide to become more active?' Such open questions are more likely to get the client talking, and reduce the chance of falling into the 'yes, but...' trap (where the patient finds ways to ignore or dismiss suggestions from the clinician).
2   Making episodic, accurate and honest **A**ffirmations of the client's strengths and abilities, to help build client confidence and commitment to change. For example, 'It's really good that you have managed to talk about these issues, despite all the stress you are under right now.'
3   **R**eflective listening in which the clinician really listens to what the client is saying, and communicates this by reflecting back part of what the client has said in a way which encourages them to continue speaking while feeling understood.
4   Using **S**ummaries which allow the listener to demonstrate his or her interest in an individual's story and their understanding of what has been said. Summaries are very helpful in communicating accurate empathy and building rapport, and can help bring key issues to the foreground before possibly moving the focus of the discussion.

Training the workforce in motivational interviewing is likely to deliver significant improvements in the effectiveness and efficiency of care delivered to people with long-term conditions. A recent article (Anstiss 2009) outlines several ways in which MI can help healthcare systems become more integrated and deliver improved personalisation, care and outcomes for people with long-term conditions, including:

• Helping leaders, service managers and clinicians deliver core elements of the Chronic Illness Care Model.
• Helping contribute to the task of building more integrated teams working within a shared approach.
• Helping clinicians integrate evidence-based medicine with patient-centred care and shared decision-making.
• Helping integrate physical and mental healthcare.
• Helping clinicians integrate treatment with prevention.
• Helping integrate substance abuse detection and treatment into primary care settings.
• Helping integrate treatment approaches with wellness and well-being approaches.
• Helping integrate clinician care with self-care.

Problem-solving technique

It is unusual for motivational interviewing to be conducted in its purest form. Frequently Adaptations of Motivational Interviewing (AMIs) are made available with other counselling approaches or techniques. Problem-solving techniques, while often used as a stand-alone intervention, are also often used as an adjunct to motivational interviewing. This combination may also be defined as an adaptation of motivational interviewing (Miller and Rollnick 2002).

There are many different approaches to problem-solving. Some have developed in the areas of management and business, others in the area of counselling people with personal or family difficulties. Most people can learn the skills and processes involved in the problem-solving techniques outlined in this chapter (Whetten and Cameron 2002). However, there is some evidence that individuals who are severely cognitively impaired may have difficulty with this approach and as such it should be used with caution with this client group (Sanchez-Craig and Walker 1982).

It is also believed that many people already know how to use problem-solving techniques but do not always apply their knowledge and skills when facing difficult situations. Whetten and Cameron (2002, 166) note that sometimes people have 'developed certain conceptual blocks in their problem solving activities of which they are not even aware. These blocks inhibit them from solving certain problems effectively.'

According to Adair (1997), problem-solving is based on three premises:

1   All problems have a solution (though the solution is not always immediately visible).
2   Most problems have more than one solution, some acceptable, some not. It is useful therefore to generate a wide range of alternative solutions, some of which are likely to be acceptable and possibly also desirable. This principle is supported by March (1999).
3   Analytical problem-solving techniques are transferable across a range of aspects of our lives. When people develop problem-solving techniques they will be able to apply these successfully to control most areas of their lives including work, personal and family life (Adair 1997).

Some versions of problem-solving techniques have a four-stage process (Whetten and Cameron 2002) while others advocate six key areas (Adair 1997). The Adair version is used more widely in the counselling of people attempting to make changes in their personal lives. The six stages identified by Adair (1997) are:

1   Orientate yourself. Before starting, try to stand back and be objective.
2   Clearly define the problem accurately and unambiguously.
3   Brainstorm for solutions. 'Much research on problem solving supports the prescription that the quality of solutions can be significantly enhanced by considering multiple alternatives' (Whetten and Cameron 2002, 162). A minimum of ten possible options should therefore be identified.
4   Decide on the best option(s). Bearing in mind the problem identified, delete poor options and identify preferred options.
5   Set realistic achievable goals. To increase the chances of success, goals should

be clear, specific relevant, realistic, achievable, measurable and feasible within an agreed timeframe (Velleman 1991).

6   Review if it works. Assuming that realistic goals are set within agreed timeframes, it is imperative that they are reviewed as they progress. If the goals have not been achieved, reflect on why they have not been achieved and perhaps revise them accordingly.

Cognitive behavioural therapy

Cognitive behavioural therapy (CBT) has its origins in cognitive and behavioural therapy and builds on the strengths of both. CBT is an overarching term for a wide range of empirically supported approaches sharing a common focus on helping people set goals for themselves as well as changing aspects of their thinking, feeling and behaving. Similar to the other psychosocial interventions outlined in this chapter, CBT involves close collaboration between the client and the therapist with the emphasis on the client owning and experimenting with changes in aspects of their lifestyle and mental life.

The approach has proved helpful in a wide range of long-term conditions such as cancer, heart disease, obesity, diabetes, dermatology, chronic pain and the treatment and management of mental health conditions including depression and schizophrenia (White 2001; Turkington *et al.* 2003; Whitfield and Williams 2003). In addition to directly treating some conditions, CBT is effective at helping people cope with, adapt to and maintain a good quality of life while living with a long-term condition, not least by helping them change the way they think about and interpret their symptoms including pain. In the case of the latter symptom, Novy (2004) states that CBT 'focuses on providing clients with techniques to gain a sense of control over the effects of pain on daily living as well as modifying the affective, behavioural, cognitive and sensory-physical dimensions of the experience' (Novy 2004, 284).

While there is considerable variation of different types of CBT, key elements of the approach include the following:

• Education about the rationale for CBT, including helping the client see how the environment, thinking, feeling and behaving are interrelated, and how making changes to one aspect can bring about helpful changes in another. During this educational process clients (and sometimes their partners) are encouraged to become active collaborators in the process.
• Skill acquisition and development, including in-session and between session practice and rehearsal. For instance, in recognising and changing unhelpful thinking patterns, disputing unhelpful beliefs (Padesky and Greenberger 1995), managing and reducing anxiety, or practising acceptance and mindfulness approaches to reduce the amount of distress associated with certain thoughts and symptoms (Hayes *et al.* 1999; Teasdale *et al.* 2000).
• Generalisation and maintenance processes to help prevent or reduce the risk of a relapse – including problem-solving techniques to deal with difficulties in carrying out agreed tasks and high-risk situations where clients may have difficulty coping. Where a lapse or relapse occurs, clients are encouraged to review progress made in a positive manner and to set revised goals and strategies for the future.

CBT is a very flexible approach to helping people. It can be conducted by clinicians with individuals, couples or groups, or used by individuals on themselves using self-help books or the Internet.

Applied positive psychology

Positive psychology is the scientific study of positive emotional states, character strengths, lives that go well, optimum human development and the institutions which foster and enable the same. A wide range of 'positive psychology interventions' exist which seem to improve health, well-being, happiness and even clinical outcomes in a range of settings (Seligman *et al.* 2005; Snyder 2005; Lyubomirsky 2007).

Applied positive psychology can help people with long-term conditions identify their strengths, reconnect with their values and experience positive emotions on their journey towards improved physical and psychological health. The ability of positive psychology interventions to increase the frequency, intensity and duration of positive emotional states may be one of the mechanisms which explains their effectiveness in bringing about physical healing, psychological health and human flourishing (Lyubomirsky 2007). This may be especially true in the case of the positive emotion of hope, known to be of critical importance in the process of recovery in long-term mental health conditions (Kylmä *et al.* 2006; Koehn and Cutcliffe 2007). Applying the insights and exercises from the emerging field of positive psychology in routine front-line practice promises to deliver improved outcomes for people with long-term conditions, and should be in the therapeutic and wellness toolkit of the holistic practitioner.

Conclusion

Motivational interviewing, cognitive behavioural therapy, problem-solving and applied positive psychology techniques are brief, effective interventions which may be applied in a range of clinical and non-clinical settings across a range of health-related difficulties including long-term conditions such as stroke, mental health problems and diabetes. A strong focus of each of these psychosocial interventions is to put the client central as the decision-maker in the therapeutic process. Each intervention supports the client in identifying what they see as their main concern, the opportunities and what they plan to do to help themselves in partnership with the clinician or therapist. The therapist adopts a guiding, not a telling style, helping the client define and make sense of their problem, explore options and ways forward, and take practical steps on the road to recovery, improved health, improved well-being and improved quality of life. These approaches may be used to complement and increase the effectiveness of other approaches (e.g. exercise, dietary change, medication taking), can be conducted within a relatively short space of time, and can be supported by self-help booklets and web-based exercises.

References

Adair, J. (1997) *Decision Making and Problem Solving, Training Extras*. Institute of Personnel and Development.

Amrhein, P.C., Miller, W.R., Yahne, C.E. *et al.* (2003) Client Commitment Language During Motivational Interviewing Predicts Drug Use Outcomes. *Journal of Consulting and Clinical Psychology*, 71, 862–878.

Anstiss, T. (2009) Motivational Interviewing in Primary Care. *Journal of Clinical Psychology in Medical Settings*, 16(1), 87–93.

Arkowitz, H., Westra, H.A., Miller, W.R. and Rollnick, S. (eds) (2008) *Motivational Interviewing in the Treatment of Psychological Problems*. New York: Guilford Press.

Bennett, J.A., Lyons, K.S., Winters-Stone, K. *et al.* (2007) Motivational Interviewing to Increase Physical Activity in Long-term Cancer Survivors: A Randomized Controlled Trial. *Nursing Research*, 56, 18–27. doi:10.1097/00006199–200701000–00003.

Beutler, L.E., Moleiro, C. and Talebi, H. (2002) Resistance in Psychotherapy: What Conclusions are Supported by Research? *Journal of Clinical Psychology*, 58, 207–217.

Bien, T.H., Miller, W.R. and Tonigan, J.S. (1993) Brief Interventions for Alcohol Problems: A Review. *Addiction*, 88(3), 315–335.

Bonney, S. and Stickley, T. (2008) Recovery and Mental Health: A Review of the Literature. *Journal of Psychiatric and Mental Health Nursing*, 15, 140–153.

Burke, B.L., Arkowitz, H. and Dunn, C. (2002) The Efficacy of Motivational Interviewing and its Adaptations. What we Know So Far. In: Miller, W.R. and Rollnick, S. *Motivational Interviewing. Preparing People for Change*. New York: Guilford Press.

Carels, R.A., Darby, L., Cacciapaglia, H.M. *et al.* (2007) Using Motivational Interviewing as a Supplement to Obesity Treatment: A Stepped-care Approach. *Health Psychology*, 26, 369–374. doi:10.1037/0278–6133. 26.3.369.

Channon, S.J., Huws-Thomas, M.V., Rollnick, S. *et al.* (2007) A Multicenter Randomized Controlled Trial of Motivational Interviewing in Teenagers with Diabetes. *Diabetes Care*, 30, 1390–1395. doi:10.2337/dc06–2260.

Connors, G.J., Carroll, K.M., Diclemente, C.C. *et al.* (1997) The Therapeutic Alliance and its Relationship to Alcoholism Treatment Participation and Outcome. *Journal of Consulting and Clinical Psychology*, 65(4), 588–598.

Cooperman, N.A., Parsons, J.T., Chabon, B. *et al.* (2007) The Development and Feasibility of an Intervention to Improve HAART Adherence Among HIV-positive Patients Receiving Primary Care in Methadone Clinics. *Journal of HIV/AIDS and Social Services*, 6, 101–120. doi:10.1300/J187v06n01_07.

Cuijpers, P., van Straten, A. and Andersson, G. (2008) Internet-administered Cognitive Behavior Therapy for Health Problems: A Systematic Review. *Journal of Behavioral Medicine*, 31:169–177 DOI 10.1007/s10865–007–9144–1.

Duffy, T. (1994) Brief Interventions and Their Role in Relation to More Intensive Treatment of Alcohol Problems. *Addictions Update*. Health Promotion Department, Greater Glasgow Health Board, Scotland.

Fisher, D. (2005) *The Empowerment Model of Recovery: Finding Our Voice and Having a Say*. National Empowerment Centre, Lawrence, MA. Online. Available at: www.power2u.org/articles/recovery/new_vision.html (accessed 15 April 2009).

Future Vision Coalition (2008) *A New Vision for Mental Health: Discussion Paper*. Online. Available at: www.newvisionformentalhealth.org.uk/ (accessed 15 December 2008).

Gaume, J., Gmel, G. and Daeppen, J.B. (2008) Brief Alcohol Interventions: Do Counsellors' and Patients' Communication Characteristics Predict Change? *Alcohol and Alcoholism*, 43, 62–69.

Gollwitzer, P.M. (1999) Implementation Intentions: Simple Effects of Simple Plans. *American Psychologist*, 54, 493–503.

Hayes, S., Strosahl, K. and Wilson, K. (1999) *Acceptance and Commitment Therapy: An Experiential Approach to Behavior Change*. New York: Guilford Press.

Health Development Agency (2002) *Manual for the Fast Alcohol Screen Test (FAST): Fast Screening for Alcohol Problems*. London: HDA. Available at: www.nice.org.uk (accessed 31 March 2009).

Heather, F. (2002) Promotion: A Positive Way Forward for Clients with Severe and Enduring Mental Health Problems Living in the Community, Part 1. *British Journal of Occupational Therapy*, 65, 551–558.

Heather, N. (2005) Motivational Interviewing: Is It All Our Clients Need? *Addiction Research and Theory*, 13(1), 1–18.

Horvath, A.O., Gaston, L. and Luborsky, L. (1993) The Therapeutic Alliance and its Measures. In: Miller, L., Luborsky, L., Barber, J. *et al.* (eds) *Psychodynamic Treatment and Research* (pp. 247–273). New York: Basic Books.

Jensen, M.P., Turner, J.A. and Romano, J.M. (1994) Correlates of improvement in multidisciplinary treatment of chronic pain. *Journal of Consulting and Clinical Psychology*, 62, 172–179.

Keefe, F.J., Caldwell, D.S., Williams, D.A. *et al.* (1990a) Pain Coping Skills Training in the Management of Osteoarthritic Knee Pain: A Comparative Study. *Behavior Therapy*, 21, 49–62.

Koehn, C. and Cutcliffe, J. (2007) Hope and Interpersonal Psychiatric/Mental Health Nursing: A Systematic Review of the Literature – Part One. *Journal of Psychiatric and Mental Health Nursing*, 14, 134–140.

Kylmä, J., Juvakka, T., Nikkonen, M. *et al.* (2006) Hope and Schizophrenia: An Integrative Review. *Journal of Psychiatric and Mental Health Nursing*, 13, 651–664.

Lyubomirsky, S. (2007) *The How of Happiness. A Scientific Approach to Getting the Life You Want.* New York: Penguin.

May, R., Risman, J., Kidder, K. *et al.* (1999) *Recovery Advisory Group Recovery Model. A Work in Process. Recovery Advisory Group.* Online. Available at: www.mhsip.org/recovery/ (accessed 15 April 2009).

Miller, W.R. and Rollnick, S. (1991) *Motivational Interviewing, Preparing People to Change Addictive Behaviour.* New York: Guilford Press.

Miller, W.R. and Rollnick, S. (2002) *Motivational Interviewing. Preparing People for Change.* New York: Guilford Press.

Miller, W.R. and Rollnick, S. (2009) Ten Things that Motivational Interviewing is not. *Behavioural and Cognitive Psychotherapy*, 37, 129–140.

Miller, W.R., Benefield, R.G. and Tonigan, J.S. (1993) Enhancing Motivation for Change in Problem Drinking: A Controlled Comparison of Two Therapist Styles. *Journal of Consulting and Clinical Psychology*, 61, 455–461.

Moyers, T. and Martin, T. (2006) Therapist Influence on Client Language During Motivational Interviewing Sessions: Support for a Potential Causal Mechanism. *Journal of Substance Abuse Treatment*, 30, 245–251.

Moyers, T. and Rollnick, S. (2002) A Motivational Interviewing Perspective on Resistance in Psychotherapy. *Journal of Clinical Psychology*, 58, 185–193.

National Institute for Clinical Excellence (NICE) (2002) *Core Interventions in the Treatment and Management of Schizophrenia in Primary and Secondary Care. Clinical Practice Algorithms and Pathways to Care.* London: NICE.

National Institute for Mental Health in England (NIMHE) (2005) *NIMHE Guiding Statement on Recovery.* Online. Available at: www.psychminded.co.uk/news/news2005/feb05/nimherecovstatement.pdf (accessed 9 January 2009).

Newton, C.R. and Barbaree, H.E. (1987) Cognitive Changes Accompanying Headache Treatment: The Use of a Thought-sampling Procedure. *Cognitive Therapy and Research*, 11, 635–652.

Novy, D.M. (2004) Psychological Approaches for Managing Pain. *Journal of Psychopathology and Behavioural Assessment*, 26(4), 279–288.

Padesky, C. and Greenberger, D. (1995) *Mind over Mood: Change How You Feel By Changing the Way You Think.* New York: Guilford Press.

Peyrot, M. and Rubin, R.R. (2007) Behavioral and Psychosocial Interventions in Diabetes. A Conceptual Review. *Diabetes Care*, 30(10), 2443–2440.

Prochaska, J.O. and Di Clemente, C.C. (1982) Transtheoretical Theory: Towards a More Integrated Model of Change. *Psychotherapy: Theory, Research and Practice*, 19, 276–288.

Project MATCH Research Group (1998) Therapist Effects in Three Treatments for Alcohol Problems. *Psychotherapy Research*, 8, 455–474.

Rau, J., Ehlebracht-Konig, I. and Peterman, F. (2008) Impact of a Motivational Intervention on Coping with Chronic Pain: Results of a Controlled Efficacy Study. *Schmerz*, 22, 575–578, 580–585 (in German).

Repper, J. and Perkins, R. (2003) *Social Inclusion and Recovery: A Model for Mental Health Practice.* London: Baillière Tindall.

Rogers, C.R. (1959) A Theory of Therapy, Personality and Interpersonal Relationships as Developed in the Client-centred Framework. In: Keoch, S. (ed.) *Psychology, The Study of a Science. Formulations of the Person and the Social Context*, 3 (pp. 184–256). New York: McGraw-Hill.

Rollnick, S. and Miller, W.R. (1995) What is MI? *Behavioural and Cognitive Psychotherapy*, 23, 325–334.

Rollnick, S., Miller, W. and Butler, C. (2008) *Motivational Interviewing in Health Care. Helping Patients Change Behaviour.* New York: Guilford Press.

Rubak, S., Sandbæk, A., Lauritzen, T. *et al.* (2005) Motivational Interviewing. A Systematic Review and Meta-analysis. *British Journal of General Practice*, 55, 305–312.

Sanchez-Craig, M. and Walker, K. (1982) Teaching Coping Skills to Chronic Alcoholics in a Coeducational Halfway House: I. Assessment of Program Effects. *British Journal of Addiction*, 77, 35–50.

Seligman, M., Steen, T. and Peterson, C. (2005) Positive Psychology Progress: Empirical Validation of Interventions. *American Psychologist*, 60, 410–421.

Snyder, C. and Lopez, S. (2005) *Handbook of Positive Psychology.* Oxford: Oxford University Press.

Teasdale, J.D., Segal, Z.V., Williams, J.M.G. *et al.* (2000) Prevention of Relapse/Recurrence in Major Depression by Mindfulness-based Cognitive Therapy. *Journal of Consulting and Clinical Psychology*, 68(4), 615–623.

Turkington, D., Kingdon, D. and Chadwick, P. (2003) Cognitive-behavioural Therapy for Schizophrenia: Filling the Therapeutic Vacuum. *British Journal of Psychiatry*, 183, 98–99.

Turner, D. (2002) Mapping the Routes to Recovery. *Mental Health Today*, July, 29–30.

Vanwormer, J. and Boucher, J.L. (2004) Motivational Interviewing and Diet Modification: A Review of the Evidence. *Diabetes Educator*, 30, 404–419.

Velleman, R. (1991) Alcohol and Drug Problems. In: Dryden, W. and Rentoul, R. (eds) *Clinical Problems: A Cognitive-behavioural Approach.* London: Routledge.

Watkins, C.L., Auton, M.F., Deans, C.F. *et al.* (2007) Motivational Interviewing Early after Acute Stroke: A Randomized, Controlled Trial. *Stroke*, 38, 1004–1009.

Whetten, D. and Cameron, K. (2002) *Developing Management Skills.* Upper Saddle River: Prentice Hall.

White, A. (2001) *Cognitive Behaviour Therapy for Chronic Medical Problems.* Chichester: John Wiley & Sons.

Whitfield, G. and Williams, C. (2003) The Evidence Base for Cognitive-behavioural Therapy in Depression: Delivery in Busy Clinical Settings. *Advances in Psychiatric Treatment*, 9(1), 21–30.

Zetzel, E. (1956) Current Concept of Transference. *International Journal of Psychoanalysis*, 37, 365–375.

Part III

Caring for the mind, body and spirit

Introduction

Part III explores the multifaceted nature of holistic care. While evidence-based and effective medical care is of course crucial in responding to the needs of those with long-term conditions, holistically we are also interested in caring for the person's mind, body and spirit.

A holistic approach to long-term conditions requires professional helpers to be focused on the skills of engagement, and of developing the quality and depth of their clinical relationships with clients. In Chapter 8, Jacqueline Sin and Steve Trenoweth consider how one might psychologically care for individuals who experience mental distress regardless of clinical context. As such, this chapter outlines how interpersonal and counselling skills and psychosocial approaches can create a therapeutic and positive psychological climate to emotionally support those with long-term conditions. Attention is paid to essential counselling skills to assist in relating to, and understanding, the person in need, recognising that the development of a therapeutic alliance has been found consistently to be associated with positive clinical outcomes across many conditions.

There is good psychological and biochemical evidence for the positive role of exercise as both stand-alone and adjunctive therapy in a variety of mental and physical health conditions. Chapter 9 looks, in a practical and evidence-based way, at how and why physical activity can promote not only physical health and improve mental well-being but can in a broad sense lead to positive clinical outcomes in a variety of long-term conditions. Similarly, good nutrition is an important component of both subjective and objective perceptions of health and overall physical and psychological well-being. Taking an integrative and evidence-based approach, Chapter 10 considers this issue and how practitioners may develop their knowledge and skills in assisting clients to meet their essential nutritional requirements. The chapter identifies the principles of nutritional medicine and naturopathic practice as a biological process, and of using nutritional measures to promote health and build resistance to disease.

The increased use of complementary medicine by the general public and the rapid growth in its provision can and will have a dramatic effect on healthcare. The lack of awareness of complementary medicine in the education of doctors and nurses was highlighted in the House of Lords' Select Committee Report on Complementary and Alternative Medicine (CAM) in November 2000. This has had a huge impact on education and research. The report has facilitated the movement of training and education in complementary medicine into a university framework and, with it, independent accreditation and self-regulation, and has led to an increased awareness of the value of such approaches. Chapter 11 illustrates how CAM can form an important and valuable adjunct to 'traditional' medicine.

The topic of spirituality is not only something which is of interest to ministers of religion. Spirituality, in the sense of personal meanings we attach to our lives and life experiences, is central to holistic care. Assessments of spirituality require an understanding of more than one's religious views, important though these may be. It also requires an understanding regarding the meanings that an individual attaches to their personal experiences and an appreciation of the individual's internal frame of reference. The importance of affirming the worth of the individual and finding ways in which life can be lived to the full, celebrating the past, the present and what is to come, cannot be underestimated. Confirmation of who we are through the expression of a personal narrative which is clearly listened to and valued is vital in holistic care. Chapter 12 gives an overview of the dimensions of spirituality as they relate to both the individual with a long-term condition and those who are undertaking their care, and provides a rationale which enables the person to celebrate their life.

8 Caring for the mind

Jacqueline Sin and Steve Trenoweth

Introduction

When we become unwell with a long-term health problem, it is not just our physical body that suffers. All aspects of our world are potentially affected – our mood, social circumstances, relationships, finances, work performance, confidence and so forth may well be impacted upon. A diagnosis of a long-term condition can leave the individual struggling to make sense of the world. It can be a time of much stress and uncertainty as the individual considers what the future may hold for them and speculates about the course the illness may take. This is very much a personal experience, as people inevitably have different tolerances for, and perceptions of, similar symptoms and subsequently individualised ways of interpreting and coping with the symptoms. A steep learning curve is often called for as the individual is presented with a new lexicon of diagnoses, medical symptoms, services, treatments and interventions while trying to make sense of the advice given by the respective healthcare practitioners. All this can understandably have a major impact on our psychological health and well-being.

In this chapter, we consider the psychological and emotional impact of long-term conditions and the subsequent need for caring for the mind. By this we do not wish to restrict ourselves necessarily to the care and treatment of people with diagnosed mental health problems, important though this is, but more broadly to consider our psychological and emotional worlds and the implications this might have for the trajectory of health and illness.

Coping

As we have seen from earlier chapters, our ability to cope with life events varies as a function of many factors. Resources, such as our personal values, beliefs and thinking patterns (including our ability to solve problems); our previous experiences; our immediate circumstances (such as financial security) and extensive social support networks (including supportive employers) can act to scaffold our appraisal of life events and our ability to cope with adverse circumstances (Holahan *et al.* 1996; Mueser *et al.* 1998; Mortensen *et al.* 1999).

When faced with stressful situations, there seems to be a number of coping strategies we may adopt (Zeidner and Elder 1996). We may temporarily disengage from the problem in an attempt to manage a stressful situation: this may be helpful if in the short term but can be unhelpful if one avoids such problems in the long term.

For example, studies have found that for some people distraction can be helpful as a short-term coping strategy, especially when facing painful medical interventions (Carr 2004). Alternatively, we may be focused on attempting to solve problems associated with our long-term condition. For example, we may take control and assume responsibility for our ill-health and develop realistic plans to improve the situation based on relevant health information. We may seek out advice and support to help us enact such strategies. That is, we may become 'problem-focused' in response to our healthcare needs, and this approach appears to contribute positively to our overall physical health, ability to cope with stress and psychological adjustment to illness (Heppner and Petersen 1982; Carr 2004).

Positive coping strategies often involve seeking and maintaining social support and confiding personal relationships. In caring for the mind, we aim to understand someone's reaction to, and coping with, long-term illness and to offer emotional support and assistance when a person's coping style has become dysfunctional or unhelpful. 'Emotion-focused' coping involves using such support in a positive way to allow the person to express the intense emotional impact that their health status may have upon them. For some people such strategies might lead to a positive and cathartic release of pent-up emotions. For others, professional support may be required to assist the person to *reframe* their thinking which may have been locked in a negative or destructive downward spiral, or to develop techniques for managing stress (Carr 2004). At such time, caring for the mind may involve offering hope and support to the person in their attempts to adjust, respond to and make sense of their world.

Hope and recovery

Hope is seen as an essential ingredient in recovery from long-term and chronic illness and thus the ability to inspire hope is paramount in healthcare activities (Cutcliffe and Koehn 2007; Koehn and Cutcliffe 2007). Hope is also important in mitigating stigmatisation and social exclusion. To support emotion-focused coping, a hopeful, recovery-focused style is needed along with enthusiasm and skills to generate encouragement and optimism, and practitioners and carers can inspire hope by promoting interpersonal connectedness, the feeling of being cared for and respected (Cutcliffe and Grant 2001).

Much has been written about recovery which has gained momentum over the past decade and is an important part of contemporary mental healthcare, both in policy terms and clinical practice (Repper and Perkins 2003; Kelly and Gamble 2005) (see Chapter 15). A holistic approach to recovery sees beyond the presentation of medical symptoms recognising psychological, social, emotional, spiritual as well as biological factors in the aetiology, trajectory, treatment, care and even prognosis of health problems. Caring for the mind requires practitioners to focus not just on the immediate physical suffering from medical symptoms, but on the difficulties people may encounter in the adjustment process along the road of recovery.

Psychosocial interventions

Psychosocial interventions (PSI) is an umbrella term used to describe a broad range of therapeutic activities based on psychological and social principles, carried out in collaboration with clients and their families and others important in their social network (Sin and Scully 2008). PSI is often used for people with severe and enduring mental ill-health, but may facilitate coping and support recovery from long-term conditions across physical and mental health settings. The key characteristics of the PSI approach include:

- systematic assessments conducted collaboratively with patients (and carers) to explore both needs and strengths;
- psychoeducation (that is, a process of educating individuals so as to improve their understanding and knowledge of health problems and mental health issues (Cordwell and Bradley 2008) – such as the links between mood and the experience of pain (Gureje 2007), symptoms of mental distress, the links between thoughts, emotions and behaviours, treatment options and the implications that such problems may have on an individual's life, such as in their interpersonal functioning);
- cognitive therapy to facilitate personal adjustment and processing unresolved emotions (for example, restructuring of distorted, unhelpful or dysfunctional thinking so as to view a situation differently particularly where the person feels helpless in the face of their symptoms);
- psychological management of symptoms, especially those resistant and/or unresponsive to medication treatment (for example, management of stress, such as relaxation techniques, mindfulness and meditation);
- working with the families and carers in order to enhance their understanding and coping (such interventions may range from psychoeducation to family therapy);
- medication management to optimise the medication regimen and promote concordance to therapy (such as ensuring informed consent, identifying and exploring negative attitudes towards treatment regimens).

All these interventions have an ultimate aim to optimise self-management through increased knowledge of the illness and increased sense of empowerment (Repper and Perkins 2003).

Developing therapeutic alliances

The term 'therapeutic alliance' denotes a partnership between the healthcare practitioner and the client which is healing, beneficial, remedial and salutary in nature (Repper and Perkins 2003). The therapeutic alliance has proved to be an established predictor of psychotherapy outcome, including general quality of life, symptomatology, attitudes towards medication concordance and satisfaction with mental health treatment (Marland and Cash 2005; Nolan and Badger 2005). A therapeutic alliance is also predictive of the positive clinical outcomes in a wide range of interventions and conditions across a variety of clinical settings, for example, for treatment of people with schizophrenia (Solomon *et al.* 1995); in case management of people with learning disability (Frank and Gunderson 1990); in treating depression in primary care (Nolan and Badger 2005; Zuroff and Blatt 2006) as well as interventions for people who overuse alcohol and illicit substances (Ilgen *et al.* 2006). In particular, Zuroff and Blatt's study (2006), using data from the National Institute of

Mental Health Treatment for Depression Collaborative Research Program, examined the impact on treatment outcome of the patient's perception of the quality of the therapeutic relationship and contribution to the therapeutic alliance. Independent of the type of treatment and early clinical improvement, the therapeutic relationship contributes directly to positive therapeutic outcome. This was also confirmed by Cloitre *et al.* (2004) in their study of the treatment of childhood abuse related to post-traumatic stress disorder.

A crucial aspect of developing such alliances is the creation of a safe, trusting therapeutic climate within which people feel safe to voice their concerns. Such engagement forms the prerequisite for any effective psychosocial interventions. The traditional therapeutic triad described by Rogers (1951) in his seminal work on humanistic psychotherapeutic approaches, *Client-centred therapy*, contributes to the development of a therapeutic alliance (Repper 2000) (see Gamble (2006) or Perkins and Repper (1996) for a recent account). These three essential qualities are:

1   Empathy – understanding the client from his or her own shoes in a sensitive and accepting manner.
2   Non-judgemental warmth or unconditional positive regard – accepting and valuing the client as a human being who is entitled to respect and dignity.
3   Genuineness – is reflected in being open and having an honest and hopeful approach, with the practitioner having the therapeutic optimism in the client's abilities and potential (Rogers 1951, 1957, 1983).

In a survey of 500 people with mental health problems, Rogers and Pilgrim (1994) identified empathy, tolerance, caring and personal respect as being qualities perceived as being particularly helpful. In the most recent review of mental health nursing led by the Chief Nursing Officer of England (DoH 2006), building and maintaining positive interpersonal relationships with patients and carers is, once again, identified as the cornerstone for successful mental health practice. Similar accounts are often written by users of mental health services such as is illustrated below:

> In my own history of mental health service use, the nurses who have been most help to me have been those who have had the ability to respond both humanely and professionally to my distress ... the importance of relationship between nurses and service users bodes well for quality user-centred care.
> (Excerpt by Ian Light, service user and lecturer, DoH 2006.10)

In another study of people seeking help in primary care for depression by Nolan and Badger (2005), similar qualities and behaviours are identified by the patients as helpful. These include:

*   being listened to and understood;
*   optimistic attitude from healthcare workers with reference to treatment options; honesty from practitioners in relation to prognosis and outlook;
*   practitioners being supportive, nurturing and understanding;
*   continuity of care;

- knowledge of the specialty of care in relation to providing information and offering treatment;
- genuine interests and efforts to monitor the progress.

These behaviours and qualities identified from recent studies on patients receiving specialised mental health services and more general healthcare services in primary care settings restate the core elements outlined by Rogers (1951) and set the context for developing therapeutic alliances.

However, while such qualities are important there is also a need to utilise knowledge and skills to release and optimise these human qualities through their communications and interventions (Rogers 1974). Modern healthcare service also demands that care is cost-effective, efficient as well as patient-focused (DoH 2004a, 2004b, 2006). That is, such humanistic qualities are not sufficient in themselves to assist in caring for the mind and a combination of a therapeutic alliance *and* evidence-based technical therapeutic skills (for example, cognitive behavioural techniques) is often required to effectively support coping and adjustment (Hewitt and Coffey 2005).

Interpersonal and counselling skills to enhance clinical encounters

While, as Langer (1999) argues, there are naturally occurring therapeutic alliances between practitioners and patients, interpersonal skills need to be developed in order to enhance and promote such clinical encounters. That is, there is much that can be done to build a trusting therapeutic alliance rather than leaving it to chance. The essential human qualities described previously are, of course, the foundation upon which any therapeutic encounter is built and, as mentioned above, those who seek to offer psychological support and help will still need to develop technical interpersonal and counselling skills and knowledge in order to assist the person to address and resolve troubling issues that they may be facing.

The terms 'interpersonal' and 'counselling skills' are often used to denote those communication skills and techniques which enable practitioners to effectively talk to clients in order to gather information, problem-solve and, at times, give information and advice. Counselling may be viewed as an intensive and personal process with a key aim of promoting personal development or growth (Ivey 1994). Development and growth in this sense denotes an enhanced understanding of oneself – one's ill-health, one's strengths, one's adjustment and adaptation – in the context of recovery from long-term illness. It is understandable that some people find talking about coping with, and adjusting to, their long-term illness difficult, and some people may not realise or acknowledge the difficulties they are facing. Interpersonal and counselling skills, built on qualities of being genuine, warm, non-judgemental and empathetic, along with a structured framework which is used to guide therapeutic talk and expression, can assist in identifying and developing strategies to resolve such problems.

There are many theories and approaches which inform the counselling discipline (Ivey 1994; Nelson-Jones 2002) but the focus here is on those common interpersonal communication and counselling skills drawn upon universally agreed approaches. A structured interview is commonly defined as having five stages:

1 Establishing rapport

Rapport is an essential part of the counselling process and for Rollnick, Mason and Butler (1999, 57), 'If you have a good rapport with someone, you can talk about any subject.' For Nelson-Jones (2002, 2009) the initial stage of helping involves relating to others. Indeed, establishing a rapport is a process which facilitates disclosure, demonstrated by, for example, showing attention and interest in the person. Effective communication skills (both verbal and non-verbal) are required. Throughout the counselling or interviewing sessions, attending behaviour (for example, using a firm and confident voice in which words are articulated at a rate that can be easily understood, body language which emphasises interpersonal warmness, such as eye contact with appropriate smiling and gestures) should be actively used by those seeking to help. Of course, such a psychological climate is undermined by an inappropriate physical space within which the talk takes place. Of importance here also is the creation of a quiet, private and relaxing environment.

2 Information gathering

For Nelson-Jones (2009), information gathering is an essential component of understanding the person's frame of reference and the helping process. Understanding the person is facilitated by encouraging talk through using verbal and non-verbal prompts. Using open and closed questions but doing so sparingly is important in information gathering and here it is vital that the person is 'allowed' to do most of the talking; and active listening, summarising and reflection of feelings. As such, the role of the helper is to provide a structure to the talk, encouraging the person to share their experiences, thoughts and feelings.

In cognitive behavioural therapy (CBT), the information-gathering process is often highly structured in order to assist the therapist to have a clearer understanding of the nature of the person's problem (see Chapter 7). Here, issues are assessed which relate to the person's past history, precipitants of and triggers to psychological distress; factors which help the person to cope; the nature, degree and extent of psychological symptoms the person is experiencing – physical, thoughts, feelings and behaviour; and what may perpetuate the problems the person is experiencing (Simmons and Griffiths 2009).

3 Defining outcomes/goals

At this stage, it is important that a negotiated and joint understanding of the person's problems is reached. With counselling in general, partnership working and collaboration with the client in identifying and addressing problems is paramount (Watkins 2001; Barker 2004). In CBT, for example, therapists will routinely discuss with the client their 'formulation' of the client's problem so as to arrive at a shared understanding of what the problem may be so as to develop a treatment or action plan (Simmons and Griffiths 2009). This is also crucial in clarifying goals and defining outcomes – if a client does not agree with such formulations they are unlikely to be willing to work towards addressing such problems, and are even less likely to agree that such problems have improved. We are, after all, more likely to be motivated by our own goals rather than those which have been imposed upon us.

Similarly, unrealistic goals regarding recovery from ill-health, care and treatment can have a negative impact on the client's perception of, and satisfaction with, health services. Defining outcomes and goals can also be useful in clarifying such expectations.

4 Generating alternatives and potential solutions/actions

There are many possible options and potential solutions to psychological problems. This process involves actively encouraging the client to identify and choose a possible solution to their problems which seems most appropriate to them (Rollnick *et al.* 1999; Miller and Rollnick 2002). The therapist can, of course, make constructive suggestions that would help improve the situation based on their knowledge and experience but the client is in a better position often to judge which option is best for them. Indeed, this is very much in keeping with the spirit of the *Expert Patient* programme (DoH 2001) where people are facilitated to develop knowledge, confidence and self-efficacy to manage their condition better and be more in control of their lives.

5 Implementation of actions in daily life

The implementation stage is focused on assisting the client to achieve specific goals and on offering support during the change process (such as meeting regularly to review progress and offer encouragement) (Nelson-Jones 2009). In CBT, this may involve assisting the client to develop adaptive behavioural responses to situations or cognitive strategies to change maladaptive thinking processes (Simmons and Griffiths 2009). The helper or therapist may also set some tasks (or homework) in support of their goals which are subsequently reviewed in future therapy sessions.

The five-stage interviewing cycle and interpersonal communications skills stated here are commonly used in a variety of circumstances. In the context of offering support to people with long-term conditions, the process and techniques need to be amalgamated with the therapeutic values and philosophy of recovery to deliver the psychosocial interventions (outlined earlier), and will need to be modified by the helper to address the specific needs and presentation of individuals. For instance, in the information-gathering stage, the helper should make explicit efforts to guide the client in appraising their own strengths, pre-existing coping mechanisms, support systems, in addition to symptoms and illness impediment, in order to support and encourage hope. The same considerations should be put into generating alternatives and exploring choices in the implementation stages to ensure that the patient is placed in the centre of the plan. These structured processes and skills should not be prescriptive, but assist in providing a systematic and goal-directed framework within which therapeutic talk may occur.

Collaboration and partnership

Studies have consistently identified a positive correlation between the extent to which people feel able to discuss concerns and treatment options with helpers and to subsequent concordance with treatment regimens across a wide variety of long-term health conditions (Attree 2001; Randall *et al.* 2002; Broody 2003). Hence, collaboration is more than 'mere' good practice; it may also have an impact on promoting the involvement of individuals in their own care and adherence to suggested treatment interventions (NICE 2009). Furthermore, a collaborative therapeutic alliance appears to improve satisfaction with overall care, as clients consistently state that they wish to feel informed, supported and encouraged to participate and collaborate in their care (Geddes *et al.* 2003; Marland and Cash 2005). Indeed, it is important to note that many clinical issues raised by clients relate to their psychosocial needs, and these appear over and above the original health concerns that brought them in touch with the health services from the outset. As such, satisfaction with health services does not rely purely on the quality of medical treatment important though this is, but also on care processes and communication with healthcare professionals.

However, in a recent survey undertaken with just over a quarter of a million of patients using the NHS in England, across a variety of clinical settings in mental health services, local primary care services, outpatient departments and emergency departments, the Healthcare Commission (2006) identified three main issues from the patients' experiences. A total of 282,631 patients using 535 NHS organisations and services in the survey (Healthcare Commission 2006) overwhelmingly gave a negative response regarding their involvement and collaboration in decisions about their own care and recovery. Many patients cited the experiences of medical staff and clinical practitioners talking in front of them as if they were not there. Another area in need of improvement as identified by patients in the survey is the development of cultural competence and sensitivities which should be taken into account when caring for patients.

Clinical supervision and reflection

Establishing and sustaining a therapeutic relationship with an individual with a long-term condition requiring psychological care is a combined form of art and science, requiring the use of oneself and one's personal qualities and skills, along with the process of implementing evidence-based psychological interventions. It can be a demanding and draining experience. Clinical supervision provides practitioners with space for personal and professional development, seeking support and observing boundaries and standards in both personal and professional fronts (Kirby and Cross 2002; Repper and Perkins 2003; Townend 2005).

Clinical supervision is 'a process that enables increased knowledge, increased skills, appropriate attitude and values to maintain clinical and professional competence' (Townend 2005, 586), and thus ultimately aims to enhance and protect the welfare of patients. It is not surprising to note that clinical supervision works best when there is a trusting and durable relationship between the supervisor and the supervisee (Loxley 1997). An effective clinical supervision session has three aims to address, through which the practitioners can honestly and openly reflect on their practice and experiences, in order to:

- identify lessons learned;
- develop the skills and knowledge as indicative;
- seek support to alleviate the stress and emotions.

However, clinical supervision, like counselling styles and techniques, needs to be flexible and integrative in addressing the clinical circumstances.

In addition to the one-to-one support between supervisor and supervisee (which is by far the commonest and most effective supervision framework (Townend 2008)), peer group supervision attended by a group of practitioners having a similar level of expertise and a common focus or set of issues is also a frequently used forum of supervision. If a structured and focused approach is used, helpers can find peer group supervision as useful as one-to-one and may even enhance formative development by learning through one another's practice experiences and shared reflection.

Ultimately, helpers themselves need to feel supported to offer psychological care and treatment for their clients. If recovery and hope are the ultimate goals that helpers need to aspire to when caring for people with long-term illness, they themselves need to be hopeful and positive to inspire hope and recovery in those with whom they are working collaboratively.

Summary and conclusion

When faced with a long-term condition, all aspects of our world are potentially affected – our mood, social circumstances, relationships, finances, work performance, confidence and so forth may well be impacted upon. A diagnosis of a long-term condition can leave the individual struggling to make sense of the world. In caring for the mind, we aim to understand someone's reaction to, and coping with, long-term illness and to offer emotional support and assistance when a person's coping style has become dysfunctional or unhelpful. A crucial aspect of developing such alliances is the creation of a safe, trusting, therapeutic climate within which people feel safe to voice their concerns. Such humanistic qualities are not sufficient in themselves to assist in caring for the mind and a combination of a therapeutic alliance *and* evidence-based technical therapeutic skills is often required to effectively support coping and adjustment. That is, interpersonal and counselling skills, built on qualities of being genuine, warm, non-judgemental and empathetic, along with a structured framework which is used to guide therapeutic talk and expression, can assist in identifying and developing strategies to assist in caring for the mind.

References

Attree, M. (2001) Patients' and Relatives' Experiences and Perspectives of 'Good' and 'Not So Good' Quality Care. *Journal of Advanced Nursing*, 33(4), 456–466.

Barker, P. (2004) *Assessment in Psychiatric and Mental Health Nursing* (2nd edn). Cheltenham: Nelson Thornes.

Broody, H. (2003) *Stories of Sickness*. Oxford: Oxford University Press.

Carr, A. (2004) *Positive Psychology*. Hove: Routledge.

Cloitre, M., Chase Stovall-McClough, K., Miranda, R. and Chemtob, C.M. (2004) Therapeutic Alliance, Negative Mood Regulation, and Treatment Outcome in Child Abuse-related Post-traumatic Stress Disorder. *Journal of Consulting and Clinical Psychology*, 72(3), 411–416.

Cordwell, J. and Bradley, L. (2008) Enhancing Effective Multi-disciplinary Team-working: A Psycho-educational Approach. In: Lynch, J. and Trenoweth, S. (eds) *Contemporary Issues in Mental Health Nursing*. Chichester: John Wiley & Sons.

Cutcliffe, J.R. and Grant, G. (2001) What Are the Principles and Processes of Inspiring Hope in Cognitively Impaired Older Adults Within a Continuing Care Environment? *Journal of Psychiatric and Mental Health Nursing*, 8, 427–436.

Cutcliffe, J.R. and Koehn, C.V. (2007) Hope and Interpersonal Psychiatric/Mental Health Nursing: A Systematic Review of the Literature – Part II. *Journal of Psychiatric and Mental Health Nursing*, 14, 141–147.

Deegan, P. (1989) A Letter to my Friend who is Giving Up. In: *Proceedings of the Connecticut Conference on Supported Employment, Connecticut Association of Rehabilitation Facilities, Cromwell, CT, USA.* Burlington, VT: Centre for Community Change Through Housing and Support, Trinity College.

Department of Health (DoH) (2001) *The Expert Patient: A New Approach To Chronic Disease Management For The 21st Century.* Online. Available at: www.dh.gov.uk/en/Publication sandstatistics/Publications/PublicationsPolicyAndGuidance/DH_4006801 (accessed 12 October 2008).

Department of Health (DoH) (2004a) *The 10 Essential Shared Capabilities – A Framework For The Whole Of The Mental Health Workforce.* London: Department of Health.

Department of Health (DoH) (2004b) *Organising And Delivering Psychological Therapies.* London: Department of Health.

Department of Health (DoH) (2006) *From Values to Action: The Chief Nursing Officer's Review of Mental Health Nursing.* London: HMSO.

Frank, A.F. and Gunderson, J.G. (1990) The Role of the Therapeutic Alliance in the Treatment of Schizophrenia. Relationship to Course and Outcome. *Archives of General Psychiatry*, 47(3), 228–236.

Gamble, C. (2006) Building Relationships: Lessons To Be Learnt. In: Gamble, C. and Brennan, G. (eds) *Working with Serious Mental Illness – A Manual for Clinical Practice* (2nd edn). Edinburgh: Elsevier.

Geddes, J.R., Freemantle, N., Mason, J. *et al.* (2003) *SSRIs Versus Other Antidepressants for Depressive Disorder.* The Cochrane Library, 2. Update Software.

Gureje, O. (2007) Psychiatric Aspects of Pain. *Current Opinion in Psychiatry*, 20, 42–46.

Healthcare Commission (2006) *Variations in the Experiences of Patients Using the NHS Services in England.* London: Commission for Healthcare, Audit and Inspection.

Heppner, P.P. and Petersen, C.H. (1982) The Development and Implications of a Personal Problem-solving Inventory. *Journal of Counselling Psychology*, 29(1), 66–75.

Hewitt, J. and Coffey, M. (2005) Therapeutic Working Relationships with People With Schizophrenia: Literature Review. *Journal of Advanced Nursing*, 52(5), 561–570.

Holahan, C.J., Moos, R.H. and Schaefer, J. (1996) Coping, Resilience, and Growth: Conceptualizing Adaptive Functions. In: Zeidner, M. and Endler, N. (eds) *Handbook of Coping: Research, Theory, and Application* (pp. 24–43). New York: John Wiley & Sons.

Ilgen, M., Tiet, Q., Finney, J. *et al.* (2006) Self-efficacy, Therapeutic Alliance, and Alcohol-use Disorder Treatment Outcomes. *Journal of Studies on Alcohol*, 67(3), 465–472.

Ivey, A.E. (1994) *Intentional Interviewing and Counselling – Facilitating Client Development in a Multicultural Society* (3rd edn). California: Brooks/Cole.

Kelly, M. and Gamble, C. (2005) Exploring the Concept of Recovery in Schizophrenia. *Journal of Psychiatric and Mental Health Nursing*, 12, 245–251.

Kirby, S.D. and Cross, D. (2002) Socially Constructed Narrative Interventions: A Foundation for Therapeutic Alliances. In: Kettles, A.M., Woods, P. and Collins, M. (eds) *Therapeutic Interventions for Forensic Mental Health.* London: Jessica Kingsley.

Koehn, C.V. and Cutcliffe, J.R. (2007) Hope and Interpersonal Psychiatric/Mental Health Nursing: A Systematic Review of the Literature – Part I. *Journal of Psychiatric and Mental Health Nursing*, 14, 134–140.

Langer, N. (1999) Culturally Competent Professionally Therapeutic Alliances Enhance Patient Compliance. *Journal of Healthcare for the Poor and Underserved*, 10(1), 19–26.

Loxley, A. (1997) *Collaboration in Health and Welfare*. London: Jessica Kingsley.

Marland, G.R. and Cash, K. (2005) Medicine Taking Decisions: Schizophrenia in Comparison to Asthma and Epilepsy. *Journal of Psychiatric and Mental Health Nursing*, 12, 163–172.

McQueen, A. (2000) Nurse–Patient Relationships and Partnership in Hospital Care. *Journal of Clinical Nursing*, 9, 723–731.

Miller, W.R. and Rollnick, S. (2002) *Motivational Interviewing: Preparing People for Change* (2nd edn). New York: Guilford Press.

Mortensen, P.B., Pedersen, C.B., Westergaard, T. *et al.* (1999) Effects of Family History and Places and Season of Birth on the Risk of Schizophrenia. *New England Journal of Medicine*, 25, 645–647.

Mueser, K.T., Goodman, L.B., Trumbetta, S.L. *et al.* (1998) Trauma and Post-traumatic Stress Disorder in Psychosis. *Journal of Consulting and Clinical Psychology*, 66, 493–499.

National Institute for Health and Clinical Excellence (NICE) (2009) *Medicines Adherence*. Online. Available at: www.nice.org.uk/guidance/index.jsp?action=download&o=43042 (accessed 1 March 2009).

National Institute for Mental Health in England (NIMHE) (2005) *NIMHE Guiding Statement on Recovery*. Online. Available at: www.psychminded.co.uk/news/news2005/feb05/nimherecovstatement.pdf (accessed 12 October 2008).

Nelson-Jones, R. (2002) *Essential Counselling and Therapy Skills: The Skilled Client Model*. London: Sage.

Nelson-Jones, R. (2009) *Introduction to Counselling Skills: Text and Activities* (3rd edn). London: Sage.

Nolan, P. and Badger, F. (2005) Aspects of the Relationship Between Doctors and Depressed Patients that Enhanced Satisfaction with Primary Care. *Journal of Psychiatric and Mental Health Nursing*, 12, 146–153.

Perkins, R. and Repper, J.M. (1996) *Working Alongside People with Long Term Mental Health Problems*. Cheltenham: Stanley Thornes.

Procter, B. (1987) A Co-operative Exercise in Accountability. In: Marken, M. and Payne, M. (eds) *Enabling and Ensuring – Supervision in Practice*. Leicester: National Youth Bureau Council for Education and Training in Youth and Community Work.

Randall, F., Wood, P., Day, J. *et al.* (2002) Enhancing Appropriate Adherence with Neuroleptic Medication: Two Contrasting Approaches. In Morrison, A.P. (ed.) *A Casebook of Cognitive Therapy for Psychosis*. New York: Brunner-Routledge.

Repper, J. (2000) Adjusting the Focus of Mental Health Nursing: Incorporating Service Users' Experiences of Recovery. *Journal of Mental Health*, 9, 575–587.

Repper, J. and Perkins, R. (2003) *Social Inclusion and Recovery – A Model for Mental Health Practice*. Edinburgh: Baillière Tindall.

Rogers, A. and Pilgrim, D. (1994) Service Users' Views of Psychiatric Nurses. *British Journal of Nursing*, 3, 16–18.

Rogers, C. (1951) *Client-Centred Therapy: Its Current Practice, Implications and Theory*. Boston, MA: Houghton Mifflin.

Rogers, C. (1957) The Necessary and Sufficient Conditions of Therapeutic Personality Change. *Journal of Counselling Psychology*, 21(2), 95–103.

Rogers, C. (1974) In Retrospect: Forty-six Years (Editorial). *American Psychologist*, 29(2), 115–123.

Rogers, C. (1983) *Freedom to Learn for the 80s*. Columbus, OH: Merrill.

Rollnick, S., Mason, P. and Butler, C. (1999) *Health Behaviour Change; A Guide for Practitioners*. Edinburgh: Churchill Livingstone.

Simmons, J. and Griffiths, R. (2009) *CBT For Beginners*. London: Sage.

Sin, J. and Scully, E. (2008) An Evaluation of Education and Implementation of Psychosocial Interventions Within one UK Mental Healthcare Trust. *Journal of Psychiatric and Mental Health Nursing*, 15, 161–169.

Sloan, G., White, C. and Coit, F. (2000) Cognitive Therapy Supervision as a Framework for Clinical Supervision in Nursing: Using Structure to Guide Discovery. *Journal of Advanced Nursing*, 32(3), 515–524.

Solomon, P., Draine, J. and Delaney, M.A. (1995) The Working Alliance and Consumer Case Management. *Journal of Mental Health Administration*, 22(2), 126–134.

Townend, M. (2005) Interprofessional Supervision from the Perspectives of both Mental Health Nurses and other Professionals in the Field of Cognitive Behavioural Psychotherapy. *Journal of Psychiatric and Mental Health Nursing*, 12, 582–588.

Townend, M. (2008) Clinical Supervision in Cognitive Behavioural Psychotherapy: Development of a Model for Mental Health Nursing Through Grounded Theory. *Journal of Psychiatric and Mental Health Nursing*, 15, 328–339.

Watkins, P. (2001) *Mental Health Nursing: The Art of Compassionate Care.* Edinburgh: Butterworth-Heinemann.

Zeidner, M. and Endler, N. (1996) *Handbook of Coping: Theory, Research and Applications.* New York: John Wiley & Sons.

Zuroff, D.C. and Blatt, S.J. (2006) The Therapeutic Relationship in the Brief Treatment of Depression: Contribution to Clinical Improvement and Enhanced Adaptive Capacities. *Journal of Consulting and Clinical Psychology*, 74(1), 130–140.

9 Exercise

Tim Anstiss and Paul Bromley

> All parts of the body which have a function if used in moderation and exercised in labors in which each is accustomed, become thereby healthy, well developed and age more slowly, but if unused they become liable to disease, defective in growth and age quickly.
>
> Hippocrates

> Lack of activity destroys the good condition of every human being, while movement and methodical physical exercise save it and preserve it.
>
> Plato

> A bear, however hard he tries, grows tubby without exercise.
>
> A.A. Milne

Exercise as medicine

Exercise is effective medicine. If it were a drug it would be the most powerful poly-pill in the world, with a unique and unusually extensive beneficial side-effect profile. In an excellent review and recommendation Haskel *et al.* (2007) list how regular physical activity reduces the risk of cardiovascular disease, thromboembolic stroke, hypertension, type 2 diabetes mellitus, osteoporosis, obesity, colon cancer, breast cancer, anxiety and depression while reducing the risk of falls and injuries from falls (American Geriatric Society (AGS) 2001), preventing or mitigating functional limitations (Keysor 2003 Nelson *et al.* 2004; LIFE Study Investigators 2006), possibly preventing or delaying cognitive impairment (Tseng *et al.* 1995; Larson *et al.* 2006) and disability (Penninx *et al.* 2001) and improving sleep (King *et al.* 1997).

Exercise is effective therapy for many chronic diseases and clinical practice guidelines identify substantial therapeutic roles for physical activity in coronary heart disease (Fletcher *et al.* 2001; Pollock *et al.* 2000), hypertension (Chobanian *et al.* 2003; Thompson 2003; American College of Sports Medicine (ACSM) 2004), peripheral vascular disease (Stewart *et al.* 2002; McDermott 2006), type 2 diabetes (Sigal *et al.* 2004), obesity (US Preventive Services Task Force 2003), elevated cholesterol (Thompson *et al.* 2003), osteoporosis (Going *et al.* 2003), osteoarthritis (American College of Rheumatology 2000), claudication (Stewart *et al.* 2002), chronic obstructive pulmonary disease (Pauwells *et al.* 2001), the management of depression and anxiety disorders (Brosse *et al.* 2002), dementia (Doody *et al.* 2001), pain (AGS Panel 2002), congestive heart failure (Remme and Swedberg 2001), syncope (Brignole *et al.* 2001), stroke (Gordon *et al.* 2004), prophylaxis of venous thromboembolism (SIGN 2002), back pain (Hagen *et al.* 2002), and constipation (Pemberton and Phillips 2001). For another excellent review of the health effects of exercise, see the UK Chief Medical Officer's Report *At Least Five a Week: Evidence on the Impact of Physical Activity and its Relationship to Health* (DoH 2004).

Exercise not only delivers benefits to people of all ages, with and without disease, but also delivers benefits at multiple levels: social health and well-being; psychological health and well-being; system health (e.g. cardiovascular system, musculoskeletal system); organ health (e.g. heart, intestine); tissue health (e.g. muscle, bone); cellular health (e.g. muscle cells (myocytes)); and molecular health (e.g. protein synthesis and anti-oxidants).

Few individuals with long-term conditions will not derive some (probably considerable), benefit from increasing their level of exercise or physical activity.

Principals of exercise prescription and programming

The knowledge base around how much and what type of exercise is likely to deliver what type of benefit in which individuals over which timeframe (and with what risk, and how to reduce this risk) is extensive, growing and accessible. We do not necessarily need more knowledge about the health benefits of exercise to deliver large volumes of individual and population health gain. Big improvements in the health and well-being of people with long-term conditions are much more likely to follow from health and social care professionals (and others) using what we already know to help people with long-term conditions become more active. Individually tailoring a physical activity/exercise programme to the needs, wishes and interests of the patient, while simultaneously increasing their readiness to become more active and their confidence about being able to maintain a physically active lifestyle, is a skill set which could and should be in the toolkit of most health and social care professionals.

Three basic principles of exercise programming with which health and social care professionals should be familiar are progressive overload, specificity and individual tailoring.

Progressive overload

This is the gradual increase of the stress placed upon the body during exercise training. Progressive overload stimulates ongoing beneficial physiological adaptation in people with and without disease. Once the body has adapted to a particular exercise programme, more stress is required to induce further beneficial adaptations, and this increased stress may be achieved by changing either the intensity, duration, frequency, speed, recovery, total volume or type of exercise undertaken.

Specificity

The physiological adaptations from exercise are specific to the training stimulus provided. The most effective and motivating programmes are designed to reliably achieve specific functional goals determined by the individual. For instance, if a person wants to be able to bathe independently for as many years as possible, a resistance training programme targeting the shoulders (especially anterior deltoid), chest, triceps, thighs, buttocks and abdominal musculature would be helpful, combined with a flexibility programme to maintain or increase the range of motion around the shoulder joint.

Individual tailoring

It doesn't matter how 'good' an exercise programme is if the person will not follow it. Exercise programmes need to be designed to be effective and efficient at helping people reach their health, well-being and quality-of-life goals, but they also need to be engaging for the individual and tailored to their resources, experience, desires and preferences. (For more information about how to tailor health behaviour change interventions to the needs of the individual while increasing the chance that they will be followed see Rollnick *et al.* 2008.)

The key variables to be taken into consideration when crafting an individually tailored exercise programme can be remembered by the acronym FITT: Frequency, Intensity, Type and Time.

- **Frequency:** How often the person should exercise. Daily? Three to four times per week? Two sessions of resistance training (with at least 24 hours' rest between sessions) plus three cardiovascular sessions and two flexibility sessions per week?
- **Intensity:** How hard the person should exercise during the session. Below the threshold at which speech becomes uncomfortable for aerobic fitness sessions, or such that ten to 15 repetitions can be completed in good form for resistance training?
- **Type:** The types or forms of exercise that the person should engage in. Walking? Aerobic exercise in a gym environment? Resistance training? Balance training? Flexibility exercises? A combination of the above?
- **Time:** How long the person should exercise for. So that a session in a facility lasts less than an hour to maximise adherence? A 30-minute walk? A 15-minute stretching session?

So, generally speaking, how much and what type of exercise should people with long-term conditions do? The ACSM and American Heart Association (AHA) (Nelson *et al.* 2007) recommendations for adults over 65 years of age and adults aged 50 to 64 with chronic conditions is that they should:

- undertake moderately intense aerobic exercise 30 minutes a day, five days a week, or vigorously intense aerobic exercise 20 minutes a day, three days a week;
- perform eight to ten strength-training exercises, ten to 15 repetitions of each exercise twice to three times per week;
- perform balance exercises if the person is at risk of falling;
- have a physical activity plan.

Strength development

Strength, the ability to exert force, is a key determinant of quality of life in people with long-term conditions. Maintaining and developing strength is vital. Loss of strength will partly determine when a person can no longer shop for themselves, bathe themselves, get up from a chair or walk safely from one place to another. Strength also contributes to a person's level of endurance, allowing them to continue with key tasks for longer as the relative effort required is reduced. The good news is that strength can be increased safely and reliably in most individuals regardless of age or starting condition.

For resistance training for optimal strength in older adults, the American College of Sports Medicine (ACSM 2004) recommends performing at least one set of ten to 15 repetitions of eight to ten different exercises that train the major muscle groups, and recommends that this be done two to three days each week with at least 24 hours between sessions. Once the person can perform one to two repetitions above this number, the resistance should be increased by 2 to 10 per cent to ensure continued healthy adaptation and strength development.

Risk and safety considerations

The main risk associated with exercise is not doing enough of it. Insufficient physical activity is a major cause of several long-term conditions, and contributes to the rate at which people with long-term conditions lose health, functional capacity and quality of life. That being said, transient rises in risk occur when people with long-term conditions start an exercise programme. These risks are relatively well understood and can be managed in a number of ways, including:

- avoiding prescribing vigorous intensity exercise;
- patient education;
- risk stratification and further testing;
- patient monitoring;
- facility and programme readiness.

A key way to reduce the risk of an untoward event is to keep intensity low at the start of the programme. The main risk of triggering acute myocardial infarction during exercise is associated with vigorous exertion (six METS or metabolic equivalents in adults with a capacity of eight to ten METS) in individuals with pre-existing heart disease (Mittleman *et al.* 1993; Willich *et al.* 1993; Albert *et al.* 2000). The energy used during an activity is measured in units called METS and these are multiples of an individual's basal metabolic rate.

Foster *et al.* (2008) argue that the low rates of complications in patients with known cardiac disease in cardiac rehabilitation programmes may be the result of careful use of intensity, and that the low risk of exercise in healthy individuals may be contributed to by the tendency to walk rather than run at the beginning of a programme. Keeping exercise intensity low at the start of the programme may also be associated with improved compliance, as the intensity of exercise is the variable most strongly associated with its discomfort.

Two well-validated subjective methods help clinicians guide patients towards exercising at a safe intensity – RPE or ratings of perceived exertion scales (Borg 1998) and the talk test (Goode *et al.* 1998). The highest intensity at which speech is still 'comfortable' is close to the ventilator threshold in both the healthy and patients with cardiovascular disease (Dehart-Beverley *et al.* 2000) and below the intensity at which patients with exertional ischaemia develop symptoms (Cannon *et al.* 2004).

Summary

Helping someone living with a long-term condition to become more active is one of the most beneficial things a health and social care professional can do to improve the person's physical and mental health, well-being, risk profile for complications, rate of deterioration, functional capacity and quality of life. Tailoring the programme to the person's health status, goals, needs, resources and preferences is key to success. An abundance of guidelines and high-quality resources exist to help health and social care professionals with this task, including the American College of Sports Medicine (2003) and Jonas and Phillips (2009). The following ACSM website is also useful: www.exerciseismedicine.org/. Being insufficiently active is a much greater risk to a person's health than the transient and manageable risk associated with becoming more active.

References

Abbott, R., White, L., Ross, G. *et al.* (2004) Walking and Dementia in Physically Capable Elderly Men. *JAMA*, 292(12), 1447–1453.

Albert, C., Mittleman, M., Chae, C. *et al.* (2000) Triggering of Sudden Death from Cardiac Causes by Vigorous Exertion. *New England Journal of Medicine*, 343, 1355–1361.

American College of Rheumatology (2000) Recommendations for the Medical Management of Osteoarthritis of the Hip and Knee: 2000 Update. *Arthritis and Rheumatism*, 43, 1905–1915.

American College of Sports Medicine (ACSM) (2003) *Exercise Management for Persons with Chronic Diseases and Disabilities* (2nd edn). Champaign, IL: Human Kinetics.

American College of Sports Medicine (2004) Position Stand. Exercise and Hypertension. *Medical Science Sports Exercises*, 36, 533–553.

American Geriatric Society (AGS) (2001) Exercise Prescription for Older Adults with Osteoarthritis Pain: Consensus Practice Recommendations. Supplement to the AGS Clinical Practice Guidelines on the Management of Chronic Pain in Adults. *Journal of the American Geriatric Society*, 9(6), 808–823.

AGS Panel on Persistent Pain in Older Persons (2002) The Management of Persistent Pain in Older Persons. American Geriatric Society. *Journal of the American Geriatric Society*, 50(6), 1–20.

American Geriatric Society, British Geriatric Society and American Academy of Orthopaedic Surgeons Panel on Falls Prevention (2001) Guideline for the Prevention of Falls in Older Persons. *Journal of the American Geriatric Society*, 49, 664–672.

Borg, G. (1998) *Borg's Perceived Exertion and Pain Scales*. Champaign, IL: Human Kinetics.

Brignole, M., Alboni, P., Benditt, D. *et al.* (2001) Guidelines on Management Diagnosis and Treatment of Syncope. *European Heart Journal*, 22, 1256–1306.

Brosse, A., Sheets, E., Lett, H. *et al.* (2002) Exercise and the Treatment of Clinical Depression in Adults: Recent Findings and Future Directions. *Sports Medicine*, 32, 741–760.

Cannon, C., Foster, C., Porcari, J. *et al.* (2004) The Talk Test as a Measure of Exertional Ischaemia. *American Journal of Medical Sports*, 6, 52–56.

Chobanian, A., Bakris, G., Black, H. *et al.* (2003) The Seventh Report of the Joint National Committee on Prevention, Detection, Evaluation, and Treatment of High Blood Pressure: The JNC 7 Report. *JAMA*, 289, 2560–2572.

Dehart-Beverley, M., Foster, C., Porcari, J. *et al.* (2000) Relationship Between the Talk Test and the Ventilatory Threshold. *Clinical Exercise Physiology*, 2, 34–38.

Department of Health (DoH) (2004) *At Least Five a Week: Evidence on the Impact of Physical Activity and its Relationship to Health.* A Report from the Chief Medical Officer. London: Department of Health.

Doody, R., Stevens, J., Beck, C. *et al.* (2001) Practice Parameter: Management of Dementia (An Evidence-Based Review). Report of the Quality Standards Subcommittee of the American Academy of Neurology. *Neurology*, 56, 1154–1166.

Fletcher, G., Balady, G., Amsterdam, E. *et al.* (2001) Exercise Standards for Testing and Training: A Statement for Healthcare Professionals from the American Heart Association. *Circulation*, 104, 1694–1740.

Foster, C., Porcari, J., Battista, R. *et al.* (2008) The Risk in Exercise Training. *American Journal of Lifestyle Medicine*, 2, 279–284.

Franklin, B., Whaley, M. and Howley, E. (2000) *ACSM's Guidelines for Exercise Testing and Prescription* (6th edn). London: Lippincott Williams & Wilkins.

Geliebter, A., Maher, M., Gerace, L. *et al.* (1997) Effects of Strength or Aerobic Training on Body Composition, Resting Metabolic Rate, and Peak Oxygen Consumption in Obese Dieting Subjects. *American Journal of Clinical Nutrition*, 66, 557–563.

Going, S., Lohman, T., Hooutkooper, L. *et al.* (2003) Effects of Exercise on Bone Mineral Density in Calcium-replete Postmenopausal Women with and without Hormone Replacement Therapy. *Osteoporosis International*, 14(8), 637–643.

Goode, R., Mertens, R., Shaiman, S. *et al.* (1998) Breathing and the Control of Exercise Intensity. *Advances in Experimental Medicine and Biology*, 450, 223–229.

Gordon, N., Gulanick, M., Costa, F. *et al.* (2004) Physical Activity and Exercise Recommendations for Stroke Survivors: An American Heart Association Scientific Statement from the Council on Clinical Cardiology, Subcommittee on Exercise, Cardiac Rehabilitation, and Prevention; the Council on Cardiovascular Nursing; the Council on Nutrition, Physical Activity, and Metabolism; and the Stroke Council. *Circulation*, 109, 2031–2041.

Hagen, K., Hilde, G., Jamtvest, G. *et al.* (2002) The Cochrane Review of Advice to Stay Active as a Single Treatment for Low Back Pain and Sciatica. *Spine*, 27, 1736–1741.

Haskell, W., Lee, I., Pate, R. *et al.* (2007) Physical Activity and Public Health. Updated Recommendation for Adults From the American College of Sports Medicine and the American Heart Association. *Circulation*, 116, 1081–1093.

Jonas, S. and Phillips, E. (2009) *ACSM's Exercise is Medicine™ A Clinician's Guide to Exercise Prescription.* London: Lippincott Williams & Wilkins.

Keysor, J. (2003) Does Late-life Physical Activity or Exercise Prevent or Minimize Disablement? A Critical Review of the Scientific Evidence. *American Journal of Preventive Medicine*, 25(3 Suppl 2), 129–136.

King, A., Oman, R., Brassington, G. *et al.* (1997) Moderate-intensity Exercise and Self-rated Quality of Sleep in Older Adults. A Randomized Controlled Trial. *JAMA*, 277, 32–37.

Larson, E., Wang, L., Bowen, J. *et al.* (2006) Exercise is Associated with Reduced Risk for Incident Dementia Among Persons 65 years of Age and Older. *Annals of Internal Medicine*, 144, 73–81.

LIFE Study Investigators (2006) Effects of a Physical Activity Intervention on Measures of Physical Performance: Results of the Lifestyle Interventions and Independence for Elders Pilot (LIFE-P) Study. *Journal of Gerontology Series A – Biological Sciences and Medical Sciences*, 61A(11), 1157–1165.

Mcdermott, M., Liu, K., Ferrucci, L. *et al.* (2006) Physical Performance in Peripheral Arterial Disease: A Slower Rate of Decline in Patients who Walk More. *Annals of Internal Medicine*, 144, 10–20.

Mittleman, M., Maclure, M., Tofler, G. *et al.* (1993) Triggering of Acute Myocardial Infarction by Heavy Physical Exertion: Protection Against Triggering by Regular Exertion: Determinants of Myocardial Infarction Onset Study Investigators. *New England Journal of Medicine,* 329, 1677–1683.

Nelson, M., Layne, J., Bernstein, M. *et al.* (2004) The Effects of Multidimensional Home-based Exercise on Functional Performance in Elderly People. *Journal of Gerontology Series A – Biological Sciences and Medical Sciences,* 59A(2), 154–160.

Nelson, M., Rejeski, J., Blair, S. *et al.* (2007) Physical Activity and Public Health in Older Adults. Recommendation From the American College of Sports Medicine and the American Heart Association. *Circulation,* 116, 1094–1105.

Pauwells, R., Buist, A., Calverley, M. *et al.* (2001) GOLD Scientific Committee. Global Strategy for the Diagnosis, Management, and Prevention of Chronic Obstructive Pulmonary Disease. NHLBI/WHO Global Initiative for Chronic Obstructive Lung Disease (GOLD) Workshop Summary. *American Journal of Respiratory and Critical Care Medicine,* 163, 1256–1276.

Pemberton, J. and Phillips, S. (2001) American Gastroenterological Association Medical Position Statement: Guidelines on Constipation. *Gastroenterology,* 119, 1761–1766.

Penninx, B., Messier, S., Rejeski, W. *et al.* (2001) Physical Exercise and the Prevention of Disability in Activities of Daily Living in Older Persons with Osteoarthritis. *Archives of Internal Medicine,* 161, 2309–2316.

Pollock, M., Franklin, B., Balady, G. *et al.* (2002) AHA Science Advisory. Resistance Exercise in Individuals with and without Cardiovascular Disease: Benefits, Rationale, Safety, and Prescription: An Advisory from the Committee on Exercise, Rehabilitation, and Prevention, Council on Clinical Cardiology, American Heart Association; Position Paper Endorsed by the American College of Sports Medicine. *Circulation,* 101, 828–833.

Remme, W. and Swedberg, K. (2001) Guidelines for the Diagnosis and Treatment of Chronic Heart Failure. *European Heart Journal,* 22, 1527–1560.

Rollnick, S., Miller, W. and Butler, C. (2008) *Motivational Interviewing in Health Care. Helping Patients Change Behaviour.* New York: Guilford Press.

Scottish Intercollegiate Guidelines Network (SIGN) (2002) *Prophylaxis of Venous Thromboembolism. A National Clinical Guideline.* Edinburgh: SIGN Publication No. 62.

Sigal, R., Kenny, G., Wasserman, D. *et al.* (2004) Physical Activity/Exercise and Type 2 Diabetes. *Diabetes Care,* 27, 25, 18–2539.

Stewart, K., Hiatt, W., Regensteiner, J. *et al.* (2002) Exercise Training for Claudication. *New England Journal of Medicine,* 347, 1941–1951.

Thompson, P., Buchner, D., Pin, I. *et al.* (2003) Exercise and Physical Activity in the Prevention and Treatment of Atherosclerotic Cardiovascular Disease: A Statement from the Council on Clinical Cardiology (Subcommittee on Exercise, Rehabilitation, and Prevention) and the Council on Nutrition, Physical Activity, and Metabolism (Subcommittee on Physical Activity). *Circulation,* 107, 3109–3116.

Tseng, B., Marsh, D., Hamilton, M. *et al.* (1995) Strength and Aerobic Training Attenuate Muscle Wasting and Improve Resistance to the Development of Disability with Aging. *Journal of Gerontology Series A – Biological Sciences and Medical Sciences,* 50 (Spec. No), 113–119.

U.S. Preventive Services Task Force (2003) Screening for Obesity in Adults: Recommendations and Rationale. *Annals of Internal Medicine,* 139, 930–932.

Weuve, J., Kang, J., Manson, M. *et al.* (2004) Physical Activity, Including Walking, and Cognitive Function in Older Women. *JAMA,* 292, 1454–1461.

Willich, S., Lewis, H., Lowel, H. *et al.* (1993) Physical Exertion as a Trigger of Acute Myocardial Infarction: Triggers and Mechanisms of Myocardial Infarction Study Group. *New England Journal of Medicine,* 329, 1677–1683.

10 Nutrition

Michele Wood, Smita Hanciles and Shoela Detsios

Introduction

Nutrition is a powerful tool for rectifying imbalance within the body, and by correcting nutritional deficiency or excess, significant intervention can be made into disease and healing processes. This chapter will outline the key food groups and discuss creating a balanced diet, show how cooking and processing methods can influence nutrient status, and will consider the emotional factors affecting food choices and the motivation to eat.

It is well recognised that inadequate nutrition can play a part in the disease process, while optimal nutrition promotes health and healing. Some strategies have been widely recommended for decades, such as reducing salt to lower blood pressure. Other nutritional benefits, like the use of Omega 3 fatty acids to improve brain function, have been publicised more recently. The specific nutritional needs of each patient will differ depending on the exact condition, and the purpose of this chapter is to provide general nutritional advice rather than to suggest treatment strategies for particular diseases. Where specific conditions are mentioned they are examples for illustrative purposes only, and thus should not be taken to be a recommendation for any patient with that condition.

The holistic approach

One of the key principles of holistic healthcare is that the body is inherently self-healing. This means that by correcting nutrient deficiencies or excesses, biochemical imbalance may be corrected, homeostasis is restored, cellular function becomes more effective, and healing can occur. Promoting optimal nutritional status allows the body to restore balance by giving the best possible conditions to encourage healing, rather than targeting treatment towards the management of existing symptoms.

Many non-dietary factors may influence a person's nutritional status, and should be considered in order to treat a patient holistically. For example, exposure to foreign substances, chemicals and pollutants from the atmosphere increases the requirement for antioxidants – since antioxidant nutrients are required to render these foreign substances harmless. Emotional state may affect the digestive function, and digestive disorders such as irritable bowel syndrome (IBS) are noted by some to be aggravated by stress. The efficiency by which a patient is able to absorb nutrients from food is also relevant, since if absorption is poor even a good diet will not give maximum benefit.

Essential nutrition

Nutrition and chronic illness

People with long-term conditions usually have altered metabolism which can affect the nutritional requirements for protein, carbohydrate, fat, vitamins and minerals (Schattner and Shike 2006). For example, cancer treatment can cause symptoms such as anorexia, early satiety, changes in taste and smell, and disturbances of the gastrointestinal tract, and lead to inadequate nutrient intake and subsequent malnutrition (Nitenberg and Raynard 2000; Doyle *et al.* 2006).

Depending on the condition and treatments undergone, priorities may be either to prevent or achieve weight loss, as well as optimise nutritional status to assist the body to reverse the disease process or delay further progression. Surgery and chemotherapy can alter eating habits and affect digestion and absorption of nutrients, possibly necessitating a change in normal eating patterns which in itself can prove stressful. Dietary counselling and individualised nutritional support can result in improved appetite and better dietary intake (Rock 2005; Schattner and Shike 2006).

Energy intake and body weight

The energy (calorie) contributors to the diet are carbohydrate, fat and protein which are all present in a wide variety of foods. Smaller, more frequent meals without liquids may help to increase food intake and some may need to use meal supplements to increase energy and nutrient intake. Others may need to reduce weight, since evidence indicates that being overweight can reduce immunity and the likelihood of survival in many cancers (Chandra 1997; Calle *et al.* 2003). Abdominal obesity, particularly in women defined by a large waist circumference (≥ 76.2 cm) or high waist to hip ratio (≥ 0.76), is a stronger risk factor for heart disease, stroke and type 2 diabetes (Clifton *et al.* 2004).

Safe weight loss should be achieved through a well-balanced diet and increased physical activity at an appropriate level for the specific individual. Reducing the energy density of the diet by increasing the proportion of low-energy density foods (e.g. cooked wholegrains, soups, vegetables, fruits, water) and limiting the intake of fat and sugars helps promote healthy weight control (Rolls *et al.* 2005). This approach avoids hunger and a feeling of deprivation since volume of food is not reduced. Limiting portion sizes of energy-dense foods can accompany this strategy for greater effect (Rolls *et al.* 2002; Nielson and Popkin 2003).

Carbohydrates

Carbohydrates provide the greatest proportion of the daily energy requirement. The recommended level of carbohydrates for the general population is 50 per cent of daily energy intake (British Nutrition Foundation 1998). Wholegrains, vegetables, fruit and legumes are low-energy dense foods, promoting satiety and helping weight management. These are considered the most desirable carbohydrate sources as they are rich in fibre, essential nutrients and phytochemicals. Whole fruit is preferable to fruit juice due to the higher fibre content, which is beneficial to bowel health. Fibre from wholegrains also provides valuable nutrients that are not present in fibre supplements. In addition, wholegrains have numerous biological effects, positively influencing lipid metabolism and acting as antioxidant and weak hormones (Doyle *et al.* 2006). Less desirable carbohydrates include refined grains which have been milled to remove the bran and germ, such as white flour products including bread and pasta, and white rice. This process removes essential vitamins and minerals, making the grain of lower nutritional value. Sometimes these products are fortified with the micronutrients which have been lost, such as folic acid and B-vitamins; however, the valuable fibre and phytochemicals are not replaced.

Refined sugar is a high-energy, low-nutrient food, which affects the action of insulin to maintain blood sugar levels. Fluctuations in blood sugar result in cravings for more sugary foods, creating a cycle with the potential to lead to insulin resistance and eventually type-2 diabetes. Although honey is an unrefined form of sugar containing vitamins and minerals, it is also very concentrated and can be almost as problematic as refined sugar. Eating smaller, more frequent meals which include some protein helps regulate blood sugar levels.

The Glycaemic Index (GI) is an indication of the blood sugar response of the body to a standardised amount of carbohydrate in a food. The Glycaemic Load (GL) also takes into account the amount of food eaten. Low GL diets have been found to be useful in the control of blood sugar for conditions such as diabetes. Foods such as bread, rice, cereal and pasta can be rapidly converted to glucose resulting in stimulation of excess insulin. This interferes in essential fatty acid metabolism and directs excess calories to be synthesised into fat and cholesterol. Sugars (including honey, raw sugar, brown sugar, high-fructose corn syrup and molasses) and products that are major sources of these sugars (such as soft drinks) add substantial calories to the diet and thus can promote weight gain. In addition, most foods that are high in sugar do not contribute many nutrients to the diet and often replace more nutritious food choices. Therefore, limiting sugar consumption is recommended.

Fat

Fats form major structural components of cell membranes and provide a means of energy storage. Dietary fats also provide the fat-soluble vitamins A, D and E. The recommended level of total fat in the diet is less than 35 per cent of energy, with saturated fat intake limited to less than 10 per cent (British Nutrition Foundation 1998). There is no safe level attributed to intake of trans-fatty acids (found in margarines and foods containing partially hydrogenated oil) and these are best avoided.

The fatty acids Omega-6 (linoleic acid) and Omega-3 (alpha linolenic acid and its derivatives: EPA, DHA) are essential and must be provided through the diet. Foods that are rich in Omega-3 fatty acids such as oily fish, seeds and walnuts are considered beneficial, since increased Omega-3 is associated with reduced cardiovascular disease and overall mortality rate (WHO 2003; Ottoboni and Ottoboni 2004). While these essential fats are both required in the diet, the ratio between them is also relevant, with the ideal ratio of Omega-6 to 3 varying between 3/1 and 5/1 depending on the condition (Simopoulous 2002). Western diets tend to be far higher in Omega-6 (found in vegetable oil), with a ratio of around 15/1 – promoting cardiovascular disease, cancers and inflammatory conditions (Simopoulos 2002). It is noted that in areas where Omega-3 intake far exceeds Omega-6 (such as the Eskimo diet) cardiovascular problems are rare.

Protein

Proteins are a major functional and structural component of all cells and thus an adequate supply of protein is essential to maintain cellular integrity and function. They are required for the production of enzymes which control the body's digestive and metabolic processes, and the hormones which regulate them. An intake of 15 per cent of energy from protein is recommended for the general population (British Nutrition Foundation 1998). Adequate protein intake is essential during recovery from illness, and the best choices to meet protein needs are foods that are also low in saturated fat (e.g. fish, lean meat and poultry, eggs, yoghurt, nuts, seeds and legumes). Animal foods supply high levels of protein; however, a vegan diet, which excludes all animal foods and animal products, can meet protein needs if nuts, seeds, legumes and cereal-grain products are consumed in sufficient quantities, although supplemental vitamin B12 may be necessary. Legumes, nuts and seeds also supply essential fibre to the diet.

Vitamins, minerals and phytonutrients

The benefits of eating a variety of vegetables and fruits probably exceed the advantages of any individual constituents in these foods because the various vitamins, minerals and other phytochemicals in these whole foods act in synergy (Doyle *et al.* 2006). At least five portions a day of fruits and vegetables are recommended. One portion would be provided by:

- a small bowl of salad;
- two small fruit (e.g. plums, apricots);
- one medium fruit (e.g. apple, orange);
- a slice of a larger fruit (e.g. melon);
- two tablespoons of vegetables;
- a glass of fruit juice.

Fruits and vegetables are a rich source of antioxidants and are therefore a good defence against disease. Dark green, orange and red vegetables are particularly beneficial due to their higher proportion of phytochemicals. High intakes of sulphurophane containing cruciferous vegetables (broccoli, cauliflower, cabbage, brussels sprouts) are associated with longer survival time after diagnosis with ovarian cancer (Nagle *et al.* 2003).

Vitamins and minerals are labelled 'micronutrients' as they are required in small amounts. They are, however, immensely important and act as co-factors for the enzymes essential to all metabolic processes, including those required for healing and repair. They must be supplied through the diet and cannot be manufactured by the body. They are present in a wide range of foods and thus adequate supply must be obtained from consuming a varied diet. Even mild deficiency of single micronutrients such as zinc, selenium, iron, copper and vitamins A, C and E can result in altered immune responses (Chandra 1997).

Dietary supplements

These can supply vitamins, minerals, and also beneficial phytochemicals. There is a probable benefit in taking a standard multivitamin and mineral supplement containing approximately 100 per cent of the Reference Nutrient Intake (RNI) especially when chronically ill, as it may be difficult to eat a diet with adequate amounts of these micronutrients (Willett and Stampfer 2001; Fletcher and Fairfield 2002). The use of larger doses of vitamins, minerals and other dietary supplements may be beneficial but it is not recommended without professional advice and only after individual assessment by a nutritional practitioner. The Alpha-Tocopherol, Beta Carotene Cancer Prevention Study Group (1994) showed that high-dose beta-carotene *supplements* actually increased (not decreased) the rate of occurrence of lung cancer despite many observational epidemiologic studies suggesting that *dietary* beta-carotene was associated with lower risk for lung cancer. It has been hypothesised that individual antioxidant supplementation without adequate base-line levels of Vitamin C may be harmful. Since other vitamins and micronutrients at high doses have not been studied in large clinical trials, the study suggests caution in the use of high-dose nutritional supplements.

When considering supplementing vitamins and minerals to a chronically sick patient it may be necessary to first improve the patient's ability to digest and absorb nutrients. A nutritional practitioner may recommend other supplements such as probiotics and digestive enzymes to assist these processes, depending on an individual's needs.

Creating a balanced diet

General guidelines

A general guide for healthy eating is given by the Food Standards Agency in the form of the 'Eatwell Plate' (Food Standards Agency 2008). The plate is divided into sections to indicate the proportion of a meal that should come from each food group to ensure a balanced diet. It shows that about a quarter of the plate should contain protein foods (including dairy produce) with around one-third given to carbohydrates. Recall the negative aspects of refined carbohydrates such as white rice and pasta which are low in nutrients and fibre. These foods are commonly referred to as 'empty calories', since they do little other than to satisfy the appetite, representing a far lower nutritional value than their unrefined (complex) counterparts. A variety of fresh vegetables (excluding potatoes) should take up approximately one-third of the plate, to ensure a suitable intake of vitamins, minerals and phytonutrients, some of which are not found in any other food group. There is also a small allowance for high-fat and sugary foods; however, sugar should be minimised due to the negative health effects. Note that the recommendation to include fat does not take into account the difference between essential and harmful fats. Processed foods containing fat should be minimised, as they may contain harmful trans fats; however, other fats such as those found in fish, nuts and seeds are essential and known to be beneficial to health, as outlined above.

A similar model depicting a balanced diet is the Optimal Health Food Pyramid which shows that dairy products do not need to be included if a calcium supplement is taken (Murray *et al.* 2005). This suggests that so long as the calcium requirement is met, dairy foods are not necessary in the diet. Overreliance on dairy products should be avoided as some products such as cheese are high in saturated fat and low in fibre. Better still, the calcium requirement may be met without the

Table 10.1 Approximate calcium content of non-dairy foods per 100 g

Food	Calcium (mg/100 g)
Sardines (canned)	382 mg
Almonds (roasted)	291 mg
Spinach (boiled)	136 mg
Chinese cabbage (pak choi)	93 mg
Kale (boiled)	72 mg
Navy beans (boiled)	69 mg
Halibut (grilled)	60 mg
Oats	54 mg
Chickpeas (boiled)	49 mg
Broccoli (boiled)	40 mg
Tuna (skipjack, cooked)	37 mg

Source: figures calculated using data from U.S. Department of Agriculture (2007).

use of a supplement by using non-dairy food sources of calcium such as green leafy vegetables, sardines, tuna, halibut, almonds, oats, chickpeas and navy beans (U.S. Department of Agriculture 2007) (Table 10.1).

Food choices

In order to achieve maximum nutrient intake without increasing energy intake, it is recommended to choose nutrient-dense foods (whole and unprocessed) in preference to processed or refined items. Whole foods such as brown rice may be initially rejected by a person who is accustomed to a diet of largely refined foods. In this case brown and white rice may be mixed in a 50/50 ratio, then the amount of white rice gradually reduced.

Nutrients diminish over time, so freshly prepared fruit and vegetables are preferable to pre-prepared foods to ensure maximum nutrient density. There is inconclusive evidence as to whether organically grown produce has higher nutrient content than non-organic produce; however, it is worth buying organic if the budget allows, to avoid any toxic residues from pesticides that may be present in non-organic produce.

Cooking and preparation methods

Certain preparation methods within the home reduce the nutritional value of some foods – for example, crucial minerals and fibre are often discarded in vegetable peelings. In the case of potatoes, removing the skin reduces fibre by approximately 45 per cent, calcium by over 80 per cent and iron by as much as 95 per cent (U.S. Department of Agriculture 2007).

Cooking methods are also important, since the water-soluble vitamins B and C leach into cooking water and are often discarded. Spinach, for example, could lose as much as 64 per cent of its Vitamin C through cooking (Parker-Pope 2008). Other nutrients such as fats may be damaged at high temperatures and excessive heat creates harmful by-products, so it is preferable to choose relatively quick cooking methods using minimal oil such as steaming, poaching or stir frying with water, in preference to roasting, grilling or frying. Healthy fats such as olive oil can be added afterwards. If vegetables are boiled then it should be for the minimum amount of time to retain nutrients, and the cooking water reused, for example, in soups or beverages.

Consumption of raw fruit and vegetables may be an option for some people; however, others may lack the digestive capability to break down foods as efficiently as someone in optimal health, and pureeing or light steaming may be necessary. Light cooking of vegetables by methods that preserve nutrients such as steaming can increase the bio-availability of nutrients. For example, beta-carotene is better absorbed from cooked carrots and the antioxidant lycopene is better absorbed from cooked rather than raw tomatoes.

When cooking from fresh, it is useful to experiment with natural flavours such as garlic, lemon juice, ginger and coriander to create appetising meals. Many herbs and spices possess unique health benefits; for example, research has indicated that basil and bay have positive antioxidant activity (Hinneburg *et al.* 2006), and cinnamon may be used to reduce triglyceride and cholesterol levels in people with type 2 diabetes (Khan *et al.* 2003). Curcumin (found in turmeric) has also been indicated in the treatment of diabetes, with other benefits including anti-viral effects and the reduction of post-operative inflammation (Chattopadhyay *et al.* 2004).

Commercial processing

Commercial processing takes many forms and results in nutrient losses similar to those already outlined above. Data from the University of California show that the Vitamin C content of peas and carrots is reduced by over 85 per cent during the canning process (Parker-Pope 2008). In addition, commercial processing introduces undesirable substances such as salt, sugar and chemical preservatives to prolong shelf life or to enhance the flavour and palatability of food. Methods such as partial hydrogenation create harmful by-products and should be avoided for optimal health. The current recommendations from the World Cancer Research Fund (2007) indicate that intakes of processed meats (including smoked, cured and salted meats) should be minimised due to their association with cancer.

Water

Water in the body

Water is a key component of essential body fluids such as saliva, blood and lymph, providing lubrication around joints and the eyes, and aiding the removal of waste via stools and urine. It is estimated that water makes up 72 per cent of the body's fat-free weight (Garrow *et al.* 2000), with the percentage of total body weight ranging between 50 and 75 per cent, depending on age and sex (Seeley *et al.* 2006).

Water is present in all body tissues and provides a medium for cellular reactions to occur; thus adequate hydration is critical to all cellular and organ functions within the body. Water also helps to regulate metabolism and maintains the body temperature via perspiration. A small drop in body water causes signs of dehydration, including dry mouth, fatigue, difficulty focusing the eyes, confusion and poor concentration. Water intake should be monitored for all in long-term care; however, the older patient is at particular risk for dehydration because kidney function diminishes with age.

Constipation

A common cause of constipation is slow transit time through the gut, usually due to a combination of lack of fibre and inadequate water in the diet. Constipation appears to be more prevalent in the elderly population (Talley *et al.* 1996); however, it is not believed to be related to the actual ageing process, but is more likely linked to changes in diet, fluid intake and mobility of older people (Petticrew *et al.* 1997). Reduced mobility in those with long-term conditions could thus be expected to exacerbate any tendency towards constipation, regardless of the patient.

In a healthy individual, the large intestine absorbs water after digestion has been completed, creating solid matter ready for defecation. If the contraction of the colon muscle is sluggish, the stool remains longer in the colon and more water is absorbed, making the stool hard and dry. Straining to pass a hardened stool is associated with further complications, including the development of haemorrhoids, anal fissures, diverticulitis and hernias.

Liquids in the diet provide fluid to the colon, increasing the bulk and softness of the stools. Although fluid restriction has clearly been shown to be a major causative factor in constipation (Klauser *et al.* 1990), it is equally important to ensure that adequate dietary fibre is consumed in order to increase the actual stool volume and avoid water being lost in the urine. Note that chronic constipation can be a sign of more serious disorders and may require medical attention to avoid long-term complications.

Benefits of adequate water intake

Drinking eight glasses of water daily is generally advocated for good health; however, Maughan (2003) notes that the exact health risks associated with insufficient fluid intake are difficult to define. Some research has indicated links with various types of cancer (Shannon *et al.* 1996; Michaud *et al.* 1999), and adequate water intake is considered necessary for preventing the formation of kidney stones (Qiang 2004). Clinical observation has suggested that back and joint pain can be eased in up to 80 per cent of cases simply by drinking more water.

The human brain is estimated to comprise 85 to 95 per cent water, making it highly susceptible to changes in hydration. Research indicates that water restriction affects cognitive function (Grandjean and Grandjean 2007) and also contributes towards confusion in older people (Mentes *et al.* 1998). Depression has also been associated with inadequate fluid intake, and so maintaining hydration is especially important where this may be an issue.

Dehydration can be prevented by ensuring that the diet contains plenty of foods with high water content, such as soups, vegetables and fruit which help to hydrate the body in addition to any liquids consumed. It is advisable to avoid alcohol and caffeinated beverages, since these are known to have a diuretic effect. Diuretic drugs will have a more profound effect, and other medical drugs may also have a dehydrating effect on the body through side-effects such as diarrhoea. In cases of fever, diarrhoea or vomiting, a greater fluid intake will be required to replace lost water. Someone who is already severely dehydrated will have lost sugar and salts as well as water, and it is recommended to use rehydration solutions (available on advice from a pharmacist) instead of plain water, which can further dilute the salts and sugars in the body (NHS Direct 2008).

Appetite and motivating someone to eat

Long-term conditions may cause variations in appetite due to physical and psychoso-matic symptoms such as nausea and digestive discomfort, as well as food cravings for emotional comfort or perceived pain relief. Holistic care requires consideration of the body, mind and spirit, and there may be conflict between foods that meet emotional needs, and foods that best meet the body's nutritional needs. The motivation to eat nutritious foods needs to be maintained, and those suffering a long-term chronic illness may benefit from taking an active involvement in the management of symp-toms via the diet in order to help regain a sense of control over the condition.

Motivation (an inner drive or desire to perform an action) should be differentiated from compliance (the following of instructions). Motivation to eat is often low in chronic illness, and while spoon- or tube-feeding may result in compliance it does not achieve motivation. To improve motivation, Resnick (2001) recognises the important role of belief – saying that if a patient has the belief that eating can improve their health and well-being, their motivation to eat will increase. This means educating a someone regarding the benefits of foods specific to their condition, and in complex cases this may require the assistance of a nutritional practitioner. Setting challenging yet realistic goals is also an effective way to help motivate an adult, with appropriate goals being said to be those that are attainable in the near future (Bandura 1997). Giving social support, verbal encouragement and positive reinforcement for achieving these goals can further help to increase motivation (Resnick 2001).

There may be a number of reasons for low food intake not directly related to appe-tite, and understanding this is a step towards improving food intake. Mental disorders such as dementia may cause someone to forget the need to eat, while Parkinson's disease may affect the physical ability to prepare food. Stroke victims may experience limited movement, poor coordination and difficulty chewing and swallowing, along with psychological problems such as anxiety and fear of choking (Kumlien and Axels-son 2002). Those with dentures or missing teeth (less than 20 teeth) are also likely to experience difficulty in chewing (Budtz-Jorgensen *et al.* 2001). Depression and apathy can lead to rejection of food. If there are any signs of an eating disorder then profes-sional advice is essential.

If solid food is problematic then using soups or purees made from fresh ingredi-ents may provide a suitable solution. This renders food easier to digest and minimises problems with chewing for those with false teeth or coordination problems. All key food groups should be represented; vegetable soups, for example, could include lentils or other beans for protein. Potato or well-cooked brown rice may be used to thicken a soup and make it more substantial.

Eating should be a positive and enjoyable experience, so individual likes and dis-likes must be considered. The introduction of new, healthful foods is encouraged but may need to be introduced gradually into the existing diet to avoid undue stress at mealtimes. Where possible, the receiver of the food should take active involvement in choosing and preparing the meal. It is important not to become upset with a patient who refuses certain foods. Mealtimes should be made enjoyable, since stress reduces the production of digestive juices and nerves may cause nausea. A large plateful of food may be overwhelming if the appetite is poor, whereas smaller portions and healthy titbits such as a couple of oatcakes or a piece of fruit may be more palatable. Eating is a social activity and it may also be beneficial to share mealtimes with others.

Conclusion

A knowledge of nutritional requirements can assist the creation of balanced diets for the management of chronic conditions. However, since food does not simply fulfil physical needs but also plays a key role in the emotional and mental well-being of patients, nutritional knowledge alone is rarely enough. Other factors that need to be taken into consideration include understanding the emotional needs for certain foods, increasing the motivation to prepare and eat the right foods, enhancing digestive and absorptive processes, and not neglecting the social benefits of sharing meals.

In order to provide a nutritional programme for a specific condition, a professional assessment and a personalised treatment plan is necessary. A holistic nutritional practitioner will consider all aspects of a patient including emotional factors, lifestyle and personal preferences, and then a suitable dietary and supplementary programme may be given. However, even without the help of a practitioner, significant benefits can be made by making the right food choices.

Summary of key recommendations

- Eat whole, unprocessed foods for maximum nutrient density.
- Cook with fresh ingredients and avoid processed foods with high sugar, salt and other additives.
- Increase the consumption of Omega-3 fatty acids by including oily fish in the diet along with nuts and seeds.
- Avoid trans-fatty acids found in baked goods, biscuits, margarine and all products listing partially hydrogenated fats as an ingredient.
- Increase dietary fibre intake by including wholegrains, pulses, fruits and vegetables.
- Aim to drink eight glasses of water a day.
- Consume at least five portions of fruit and vegetables a day.
- Ensure that the diet is correctly balanced to represent all major food groups.
- Avoid sugar and refined carbohydrates which provide 'empty calories'.
- Consume smaller, more frequent meals and snacks to help keep blood sugar levels stable.
- Use a variety of herbs and spices to flavour food in preference to salt.
- Choose cooking and preparation methods to maximise nutritional content.
- Introduce new and unfamiliar foods gradually.
- View mealtimes as social occasions and share food with others.
- Aim to make mealtimes enjoyable, not stressful.
- Consider the emotional needs for food in addition to physical needs.
- A patient should be involved in the food preparation process if possible.

References

Bandura, A. (1997) *Self-efficacy: The Exercise of Control.* New York: W.H. Freeman.

Bates, C.J., Benton, H.K., Biesalski, H.B. *et al.* (2002) Nutrition and Aging: A Consensus Statement. *Journal of Nutrition, Health and Aging*, 6, 103–116.

Biernacki, C. and Barratt, J. (2001) Improving the Nutritional Status of People with Dementia. *British Journal of Nursing*, 10(17), 1104–1114.

British Nutrition Foundation (1998) *Nutritional Requirements.* Online. Available at: www.sstaffs. gov.uk/Docs/Nutritional%20Requirements.doc (accessed 16 May 2008).

Brooks, J.D., Ward, W.E., Lewis, J.E. *et al.* (2004) Supplementation with Flaxseed Alters Estrogen Metabolism in Postmenopausal Women to a Greater Extent than does Supplementation with an Equal Amount of soy. *American Journal of Clinical Nutrition,* 79, 318–325.

Budtz-Jorgensen, E., Chung, J.P. and Rapin, C.H. (2001) Nutrition and Oral Health. *Best Practice and Research Clinical Gastroenterology,* 15(6), 885–896.

Calle, E.E., Rodriguez, C., Walker-Thurmond, K. *et al.* (2003) Overweight, Obesity, and Mortality from Cancer in a Prospectively Studied Cohort of U.S. Adults. *New England Journal of Medicine,* 348, 1625–1638.

Chan, J.M., Holick, C.N., Leitzmann, M.F. *et al.* (2006) Diet after Diagnosis and the Risk of Prostate Cancer Progression, Recurrence, and Death (United States). *Cancer Causes Control,* 17, 199–208.

Chandra, R.J. (1997) Nutrition and the Immune System: An Introduction. *American Journal of Clinical Nutrition,* 99, 460S–463S.

Chattopadhyay, I., Biswas, K., Bandyopadhyay, U. and Banerjee, R.K. (2004) Turmeric and Cucurmin: Biological Actions and Medicinal Applications. *Current Science,* 87(1), 44–53.

Clifton, P.M., Noakes, M. and Keogh, J.B. (2004) Very Low-fat (12%) and High Monounsaturated Fat (35%) Diets Do Not Differentially Affect Abdominal Fat Loss in Overweight, Non-diabetic Women. *Journal of Nutrition,* 134, 1741–1745.

Doyle, C., Kushi, L.H., Byers, T. *et al.* (2006) Nutrition and Physical Activity During and After Cancer Treatment: An American Cancer Society Guide for Informed Choices. *CA: A Cancer Journal for Clinicians,* 56, 323–353.

Duncan, T.E. and McAuley, E. (1993) Social Support and Efficacy Cognitions in Exercise Adherence: A Latent Growth Curve Analysis. *Journal of Behavioral Medicine,* 16(2), 199–218.

Fletcher, R.H. and Fairfield, K.M. (2002) Vitamins for Chronic Disease Prevention in Adults: Clinical Applications. *JAMA,* 287, 3127–3129.

Food Standards Agency (2008) *Eat Well Be Well.* Online. Available at: www.eatwell.gov.uk/ healthydiet/eatwellplate/ (accessed 14 January 2009).

Garrow, J.S., James, W.P.T. and Ralph, A. (2000) *Human Nutrition and Dietetics* (10th edn). London: Churchill Livingstone.

Gil Gregorio, S.P. and Ramirez Diaz, J.M. (2003) Dementia and Nutrition. Intervention Study in Institutionalized Patients with Alzheimer disease. *Journal of Nutrition, Health and Aging,* 7(5), 304–308.

Grandjean, A. and Grandjean, N.R. (2007) Dehydration and Cognitive Performance. *Journal of the American College of Nutrition,* 26 (90005), 549S–554S.

Hinnerburg, I., Dorman, H. and Hitunen, R. (2006) Antioxidant Activities from Selected Culinary Herbs and Spices. *Food Chemistry,* 97(1), 122–129.

Joint WHO/FAO Expert Consultation on Diet, Nutrition and the Prevention of Chronic Diseases (2003) *Diet, Nutrition and the Prevention of Chronic Diseases: Report of a Joint WHO/FAO Expert Consultation.* Geneva, Switzerland: World Health Organisation.

Khan, A., Safdar, M., Khan, M.M.A. *et al.* (2003) Cinnamon Improves Glucose and Lipids of People with Type 2 Diabetes. *Diabetes Care,* 26(12), 3215–3218.

Klauser, A.G., Beck, A., Schindlbeck, N.E. *et al.* (1990) Low Fluid Intake Lowers Stool Output in Healthy Male Volunteers. *Z. Gastroenterology,* 28, 606–609.

Kumlien, S. and Axelsson, K. (2002) Stroke Patients in Nursing Homes: Eating, Feeding, Nutrition and Related Care. *Journal of Clinical Nursing,* 11, 498–509.

Maughan, R.J. (2003) Impact of Mild Dehydration on Wellness and on Exercise Performance. *European Journal of Clinical Nutrition,* 57 (Suppl. 2), S19–S23.

Mentes, J., Culp, K., Wakefield, B. *et al.* (1998) Dehydration as a Precipitating Factor in the Development of Acute Confusion in the Frail Elderly. In: Arnaud, M.J., Baumgartner, R., Morley, J.E., Rosenberg, I. and Toshikazu, S. (eds) *Hydration and Aging.* New York: Springer.

Michaud, D.S., Spiegelman, D., Clinton, S.K. *et al.* (1999) Fluid Intake and the Risk of Bladder Cancer in Men. *New England Journal of Medicine*, 340, 1390–1397.

Miller, D.K., Perry, H.M. and Morley, J.E. (1998) Relationship of Dehydration and Chronic Renal Insufficiency with Function and Cognitive Status in Older US Blacks. In: Vellas, B., Albarede, J.L. and Garry, P.J. (eds) *Hydration and Aging. Facts, Research, and Intervention in Geriatric Series.* New York: Serdi and Springer.

Murray, M., Pizzorno, J. and Pizzorno, L. (2005) *The Encyclopaedia of Healing Foods.* London: Time Warner Books.

Nagle, C.M., Purdie, D.M. and Webb, P.M. *et al.* (2003) Dietary Influences on Survival after Ovarian Cancer. *International Journal of Cancer*, 106, 264–269.

NHS Direct (2008) Dehydration. Online. Available at: NHSdirect.nhs.uk/help/a-z/index.aspx? letter D.

Nielsen, S.J. and Popkin, B.M. (2003) Patterns and Trends in Food Portion Sizes, 1977–1998. *JAMA*, 289, 450–453.

Nitenberg, G. and Raynard, B. (2000) Nutritional Support of the Cancer Patient: Issues and Dilemmas. *Critical Reviews on Oncology Hematology*, 34, 137–168.

O'Brien-Cousins, S. (1996) Exercise Cognition among Elderly Women. *Journal of Applied Sport Psychology*, 8, 131–145.

O'Brien-Cousins, S. (1997) Elderly Tomboys? Sources of Self-efficacy for Physical Activity in Late Life. *Journal of Aging and Physical Activity*, 5(2), 229–243.

Ottoboni, A. and Ottoboni, F. (2004) The Food Guide Pyramid: Will the Defects Be Corrected? *Journal of American Physicians and Surgeons*, 9(4), 109–113.

Parker-Pope, T. (2008) Finding the Best Way to Cook All Those Vegetables. *The New York Times*. The New York Times Company, 20 May.

Petticrew, M., Watt, I. and Sheldon, T. (1997) Systematic Review of the Effectiveness of Laxatives in the Elderly. *Health Technology Assessment*, 1(13), i–iv, 1–52.

Pirlich, M. and Lochs, H. (2001) Nutrition in the Elderly. *Best Practice and Research Clinical Gastroenterology*, 15(6), 869–884.

Qiang, W. and Ke, Z. (2004) Water for Preventing Urinary Calculi. *Cochrane Database of Systematic Reviews*, Issue 3.

Resnick, B. (2001) Weight Loss and Failure to Thrive: Evaluating and Motivating Older Adults Toward Recovery. *Annals of Long-term Care*, 9(7), 21–31.

Rock, C.L. (2005) Dietary Counselling is Beneficial for the Patient with Cancer. *Journal of Clinical Oncology*, 23, 1348–1349.

Rolls, B.J., Drewnowski, A. and Ledikwe, J.H. (2005) Changing the Energy Density of the Diet as a Strategy for Weight Management. *Journal of the American Dietary Association*, 105 (Suppl. 1), S98–S103.

Rolls, B.J., Morris, E.L. and Roe, L.S. (2002) Portion Size of Food Affects Energy Intake in Normal-weight and Overweight Men and Women. *American Journal of Clinical Nutrition*, 76, 1207–1213.

Schattner, M. and Shike, M. (2006) Nutrition Support of the Patient with Cancer, In: Shils, M.E., Shike, M. and Ross, A.C. (eds) *Modern Nutrition in Health and Disease. 10th edition.* Philadelphia, PA: Lippincott Williams and Wilkins.

Seeley, R.R., Stephens, T.D. and Tate, P. (2006) *Anatomy and Physiology, 7th edition.* Dubuque: McGraw-Hill.

Shannon, J., White, E., Shattuck, A.L. *et al.* (1996) Relationship of Food Groups and Water Intake in Colon Cancer Risk. *Cancer Epidemiology Biomarkers and Prevention*, 5, 495–502.

Simopoulos, A.P. (2002) The Importance of the Ratio of Omega-6/Omega-3 Essential Fatty Acids. *Biomedicine Pharmacotherapy*, 56(8), 365–379.

Slavin, J. (2003) Why Whole Grains are Protective: Biological Mechanisms. *Proceedings of the Nutrition Society*, 62, 129–134.

Talley, N.J., Fleming, K.C., Evans, J.M *et al.* (1996) Constipation in an Elderly Community: A Study of Prevalence and Potential Risk Factors. *American Journal of Gastroenterology*, 91, 19–25.

The Alpha-Tocopherol, Beta Carotene Cancer Prevention Study Group (1994) The Effect of Vitamin E and Beta Carotene on the Incidence of Lung Cancer and other Cancers in Male Smokers. *New England Journal of Medicine*, 330, 1029–1035.

U.S. Department of Agriculture, Agricultural Research Service (2007) *USDA National Nutrient Database for Standard Reference, Release 20. Nutrient Data Laboratory Home Page.* Online. Available at: www.ars.usda.gov/ba/bhnrc/ndl (accessed 12 January 2009).

Warren, J.L., Bacon, W.E., Harris, T. *et al.* (1994) The Burden and Outcomes Associated with Dehydration Among US Elderly. *American Journal of Public Health*, 84, 1265–1269.

Willett, W.C. and Stampfer, M.J. (2001) Clinical Practice. What Vitamins Should I Be Taking, Doctor? *New England Journal of Medicine*, 345, 1819–1824.

World Cancer Research Fund/American Institute for Cancer Research (2007) *Food, Nutrition, Physical Activity and the Prevention of Cancer: A Global Perspective.* Washington, DC: AICR.

World Health Organisation (2003) *Diet, Nutrition and the Prevention of Chronic Diseases: Report of a Joint WHO/FAO Expert Consultation.* Geneva: WHO.

11 Complementary and alternative medicine (CAM)

Nicola Robinson

Introduction

The use of complementary and alternative medicine (CAM) continues to increase worldwide and offers a wide choice for individuals, particularly for those with chronic health problems and long-term conditions (Boon *et al.* 2006). The World Health Organisation (WHO) has estimated that 80 per cent of the world's population rely on traditional forms of medicine particularly for their primary care (WHO 2003). While in China and India such traditional medicine is often an integral part of the healthcare system (Patwardhan *et al.* 2005), this is not the case in Western countries where there are different models of integrated healthcare (Halberstein 2005; Yesilada 2005; Robinson 2006). In the UK, CAM provision is varied and mostly provided by independent practitioners, some of whom work in conventional health-care. Users of CAM tend to present to CAM practitioners with chronic illnesses rather than acute self-limiting illnesses, and often when conventional medicine may have limited effectiveness (Cant 2005). Acupuncturists are often consulted by people with chronic pain, headache and migraine. Osteopaths and chiropractics are used for lower back pain. Other long-term conditions such as cancer, HIV/AIDS, diabetes, asthma, substance dependency, depression and anxiety are treated by a range of therapies.

In this chapter, CAM refers to the approaches to healthcare and treatment normally provided outside of conventional medical care. It outlines what is considered as CAM, who uses it and what for, and then explores in more detail the use of specific CAMs for various chronic health problems and long-term conditions by summarising some of the available evidence.

What is CAM?

Complementary and alternative medicine (CAM) as defined here includes a diversity of therapeutic practices and alternative healthcare approaches that fall outside the boundaries of conventional allopathic medicine (Hill 2003). It includes forms of treatment, diagnosis and/or preventive techniques that complement mainstream medicine and satisfying patient demand not met by conventional approaches. Complementary healthcare provision has, however, been increasing within conventional medical settings in the UK (Park 2006) when it may also be referred to as integrated care. In many cases this is just the availability of complementary medicine within conventional settings. However, it is important to be aware that this increased availability

Table 11.1 Categorising CAM

Category	Definition	Examples of CAM
Alternative medical systems	Built on a complete system of theory and practice	Traditional Chinese medicine, ayurveda, homoeopathy, naturopathy
Mind–body interventions	Techniques which enhance the mind's capacity to effect bodily function and symptoms	Meditation, mindfulness, autogenic training, prayer, art, music, dance
Biologically based therapies	Use of natural substances – scientifically unproven therapies	Herbs, foods, vitamins, dietary supplements
Manipulative and body-based methods	Based on manipulation and/or movement of one or more parts of the body	Chiropractic, osteopathy, massage
Energy therapies	Affecting or manipulation of energy fields surrounding and penetrating the human body	Qigong, reiki, therapeutic touch, electromagnetism

(due to increased numbers of complementary practitioners and over-the-counter preparations) is further influencing patients' choice and the development of new services.

CAM has different meanings for different people and this also creates assumptions and expectations about what CAM can offer in terms of treatment. It is perceived as either natural, traditional, holistic and/or as a way of altering body energy (Campbell 2002). CAM has been classified into five categories by the US National Centre for Complementary and Alternative Medicine (NCCAM). These categories and examples of CAM therapies are given in Table 11.1.

Who uses CAM ?

Most surveys on the use of CAM have focused on visits to CAM practitioners (Zoltman and Vickers 1999). This excludes other traditional and cultural practices which could also be considered as CAM which are self-administered such as the use of heating and cooling foods, specific herbs to treat illnesses, exercises such as yoga, Tai chi and Qigong, and religious rituals and practices (Robinson *et al.* 2008).

The number of people consulting a CAM practitioner trebled between 1981 and 1997 (Zollman and Vickers 1999) and continues to increase. A study in 1998 identified that 28 per cent of the population had used CAM in the previous year (Thomas *et al.* 2001). Up to 36 per cent of parents use CAM for their children; much of these are self-made home remedies (Robinson *et al.* 2008). Heightened public interest in the potential benefits of CAM continues to propel the growth of a multi-billion-dollar industry. Chinese herbal medicine increased from 33 per cent in 1990 to 42 per cent in 1997 in the USA (Eisenberg *et al.* 1998) and this trend has been noticed in most Western countries (Ernst 2000; Thomas *et al.* 2004, 2005). In 2004, approximately 10,000 tons of medicinal herbs were exported from China (Houghton 2004).

People's decision to use CAM is influenced by their age, gender, ethnicity, education and expectations and beliefs of health and illness, and whether they suffer from chronic conditions (Cant 2005; Ernst *et al.* 2006). The rise in the use of CAM is in part explained by the dissatisfaction and/or disappointment with allopathic medical treatment (Astin 1998), lack of trust in healthcare (Van den Brink-Muinen and Rijken 2006) and a lifestyle choice for individuals in search of a different experience (Giddens 1991).

Users of CAM generally pay for their treatment and are unlikely to tell their GP about their use (estimates range from 23 to 90 per cent) (Robinson and McGrail 2004). Ascertaining who is using CAM is, therefore, problematic. However, the majority of CAM use does not occur instead of conventional medical care, but in addition: people prepare home-made remedies and self-administer.

Patient care may be enhanced if doctors were educated about CAM as recommended by the House of Lords Report and the BMA (BMA 1993; HOL 2000). A recent article by Willison *et al.* (2007) suggested that disclosure of CAM use could be facilitated by paying greater attention to patient/client values, the use of an integrated community-based participatory approach or deploying it in public health initiatives. These strategies would act to enhance client-centred care and communication. Greater satisfaction with the CAM therapeutic encounter compared with GP consultations is often reported (Lee Treweek and Stone 2005).

CAM users may not be aware of the evidence of a particular therapy's effectiveness. The NHS National Library for Health, CAM specialist library has identified the major research evidence for CAM and is accessible to both public and professionals (www.library.nhs.uk/cam). The Cochrane Database of systematic reviews and other online databases such as PubMed are also useful for accessing information. Other CAM specific databases include: www.naturalstandard.com and http://naturaldatabase.com. The former, Natural Standard, includes evidence-based information covering herbs, supplements, therapies and specific conditions and is designed to aid clinical decision-making. The latter has an extensive database of scientific monographs on herbs and supplements and covers specific conditions.

CAM impacts upon healthcare delivery by creating individual choice and empowers individuals to seek other healthcare approaches. This is of particular importance in our rapidly ageing population where chronic disease and long-term conditions are and will become more prevalent. Health is not just a single goal to be universally achieved, it has degrees and levels. The UK government's commitment to self-care and the increasing use of complementary healthcare could therefore contribute and help to reduce demand on and cost to health services. The concept of well-being and good health, even for those living with a chronic disease, incorporates good nutrition, exercise, physical and mental health to improve quality of life.

Much of traditional self-care knowledge is acquired through family and peers and is not captured in the normal conventional medical consultation. This may have safety implications if there is a possibility for herbal preparations to interact with conventional medication.

CAM, chronic illness and long-term conditions

Any single model of healthcare is unlikely to be able to meet the range of needs for people with long-term, chronic and complex conditions; often more comprehensive health needs are required (Remsburg and Carson 2002). Funding mechanisms, healthcare systems and policies perpetuate this and much provision is based on what is 'medically necessary' (Dwyer 2004; Cronin-Wood 2007). The aim of care for those with such multiple needs must be the promotion of health and well-being, as well as the maintenance of independence and functional capacity, by keeping individuals healthy as long as possible through prevention, early detection and management of chronic disease.

People with chronic health problems report CAM use up to five times more than those without a chronic health problem (Van den Brink-Muinen and Rijken 2006). Research suggests that having more than one chronic disease is significantly and independently related to the use of CAM (McKenzie and Keller 2001; Egede *et al.* 2002; Al-Windi 2004; Burgmann *et al.* 2004). People with chronic illness and long-term problems are generally very knowledgeable about their condition and want to be included in any decision-making. A study by Cox *et al.* (2003) on women with endometriosis showed that those who used CAM were more likely to be assertive, take control and decide how to manage their illness.

Demand for CAM services is likely to increase with an ageing population (Van den Brink-Muinen and Rijken 2006; Dossey 1997). Where some CAM is being integrated into conventional medical settings, it is more likely where chronic disease cannot be treated by orthodox means, for example, cancer care and chronic pain (Aung 2006; Robinson *et al.* 2006). Public health solutions should include an integrated approach. Of key importance is that the ultimate goal for healthcare is to provide an effective approach, at reasonable cost and without harm.

The evidence for CAM use

The evidence tables in this chapter are, in part, based on the work of Ernst *et al.* (2006, 2008) and Spencer and Jacobs (2003). Much of the recent evidence for CAM use for a wide range of conditions has been synthesised and details of the key trials may be found in these publications. These are, however, just an indication of the topics that have been researched to date. Since 2000, several longitudinal studies have been funded in the USA by the National Centre for Complementary and Alternative Medicine (NCCAM), National Institutes of Health. These studies will in time produce evidence on specific CAM therapies (Zappa and Cassileth 2003). Please note: the number and quality of trials in CAM are increasing rapidly and readers must always look for new evidence systematically if they wish to have comprehensive knowledge on which to base any clinical decision-making. The details provided in the tables are on those CAMs which have been researched. Often studies have been methodologically poor. There are many CAMs and conditions which still remain to be investigated or well-controlled studies carried out. In the following tables CAM is identified as 'beneficial' if it has been shown to have demonstrable evidence of effectiveness. Those identified as 'likely to be beneficial' include studies where not all trials are of high quality, or they may either have only a small effect and therefore may not be clinically relevant, or may have preliminary encouraging data, or deserve further study, or there may be insufficient data available. Studies of 'unknown effectiveness' include some where preliminary evidence may be encouraging or evidence is either inconclusive or there are insufficient data, or data are contradictory or methodology is limited. Those studies identified as 'unlikely to be beneficial' include those where there is no evidence of effectiveness. For those 'likely to be ineffective or harmful', data are contradictory or benefit does not outweigh the risk, or there is no effect or the treatment is likely to be ineffective.

Chronic pain

Chronic pain affects many aspects of quality of life including daily, social and working activities. A survey of chronic pain of 46,394 patients in 15 European countries showed that prevalence varied between 12 and 30 per cent (Breivik *et al.* 2006). Of the 4839 people interviewed in depth, 59 per cent had constant pain and 69 per cent had used non-drug treatments. The most common non-drug treatments were: massage (30 per cent), physical therapy (21 per cent) and acupuncture 13 per cent, and 38 per cent found they had been extremely or very helpful. The therapies accessed varied depending on the country and local traditions of managing chronic pain. Back, knee, head, leg, shoulder, neck and hip pain accounted for 95 per cent of the pain reported. A summary identifying the use and evidence for specific CAMs for chronic pain is given in Table 11.2. A detailed review on evidence for CAM and pain may be found in Taylor *et al.* (2003).

Diabetes and cardiovascular disease

Various CAM therapies have been promoted as beneficial for the prevention and treatment of diabetes and cardiovascular disease. These include vegetarian diets, dietary supplementation, herbal remedies, stress reduction and relaxation (Haskell *et al.* 2003; McGrady and Kleshinski 2003). Whole systems approaches such as traditional Chinese medicine and Ayurveda have also claimed to be effective in prevention and treatment. In the case of diabetes, the basis of treatment is to lower blood glucose levels, maintain a healthy weight and avoid the development of complications. Evidence on the effectiveness for CAM is given in Table 11.3 and in two comprehensive reviews (Haskell *et al.* 2003; McGrady and Kleshinski 2003).

Mental health

Many people use CAM to alleviate symptoms of mental distress such as anxiety and depression as well as stress itself. Thomas *et al.* (2001) reported that 39 per cent of visits to UK CAM therapists were for stress and/or relaxation. CAM is also used for people with drug or alcohol dependence and have also been used for those with more severe conditions such as schizophrenia. CAM is also used by people who have not developed a specific health problem, but who want to find ways of improving mental health and general functioning. In this way CAM offers an integrated approach referred to as 'mind, body and spirit'. Conversely, some have argued that those with mental health problems are more easily persuaded to try other forms of care, are not psychologically strong and that the use of such treatments may identify such distressed patients (Sparber and Wootton 2002). Baron and Baron (2003) review the evidence to provide an overview of clinically significant CAM in psychiatry and people with mental health problems. Boucher *et al.* (2003) similarly reviewed the evidence for CAM in the treatment of alcohol and drugs. Table 11.4 details the levels of effectiveness for CAM and mental health problems, and drug and alcohol dependence.

Table 11.2 Evidence for CAM and chronic pain

	Back pain	Neck pain	Osteoarthritis	Rheumatoid arthritis
Beneficial	Acupuncture, osteopathy, relaxation, Alexander technique, herbal: capsacian, devil's claw, willow, massage	Acupuncture	Acupuncture, phytodolor	Omega-3 fatty acids, phytodolor (herbal mixture)
Likely to be beneficial	Autogenic training, massage, relaxation, yoga		Foods: avocado, soya bean Supplements: chondroitin, glucosamine, devil's claw, spa therapy	Relaxation, spa therapy, Tai chi
Unknown effectiveness*	Auriculotherapy, biofeedback, music therapy, yoga	Massage, relaxation	Arnica Herbs: capsaicin, comfrey, ginger, rose-hip, willowgreen lipped mussel, Chinese herb Duhuo Jisheng Wange, soy, music therapy, Tai chi, homoeopathy, magnets massage, yoga	Garlic glucosamine, green lipped mussels, homoeopathy, magnets, sativex, spiritual healing, Suogudan, tong luo kai bi (Chinese herbal)
Trade-off between benefits and harms	Black Cohosh (some association with liver damage)			Triptergium wilfordii
Unlikely to be beneficial			Eazmov (Ayurvedic)	Feverfew, probiotics, willow bark
Likely to be ineffective		Spinal manipulation	Bromelain, magnets, vitamin E	

Note
*Preliminary evidence encouraging or evidence either inconclusive or insufficient data.

Table 11.3 Evidence for CAM, diabetes and cardiovascular disease

	Diabetes	Hypertension	Angina
Beneficial	Guar gum, Psyllium (both reduce total and LDL cholesterol)	Biofeedback	Relaxation (as adjunct to conventional treatments, improves exercise tolerance and reduces pain)
Likely to be beneficial	Ayurveda (glucose-lowering effects of coccinia indica and gymmenia sylvestre, cinnamon, fish oil (lowers triglycerides), soy	Autogenic training, co-enzyme Q10, fish oils, hibiscus, Qigong, relaxation, Tai chi, yoga	Acupuncture (pain reduction)
Unknown effectiveness*	Biofeedback, blueberry leaf extract, some Chinese herbal products, chromium, co-enzyme Q10, fenugreek, French maritime pine, garlic, Panex ginseng, milk thistle, mulberry, red clover, reflexology, vitamin E, tea	Acupuncture, aromatherapy, Chinese herbal medicines, garlic, ginseng, green coffee bean extract, hawthorn, hypnotherapy, maritime pine, meditation, melatonin, pomegranate, probiotics, sesame, vitamins C and E	Abana (ayurvedic preparation), various Chinese herbal mixtures, homoeopathy, pomegranate, terminale arjuna
Unlikely to be beneficial	Breathing exercises (to lower blood pressure)	Breathing exercises, gingko, green algae, homoeopathy, olive leaf, red clover, soy	Chelation therapy
Likely to be ineffective	Glucosamine, magnesium, Xioke teazinc (no effects on HBA1c and glucose)	Chiropractic	Fish oil

Note
*Preliminary evidence encouraging or evidence either inconclusive or insufficient data.

Table 11.4 Evidence for CAM and mental health problems

	Depression	Anxiety	Drug/alcohol dependence	Schizophrenia
Beneficial	St John's Wort	Massage, music therapy, relaxation	Biofeedback (alcohol)	Music therapy
Likely to be beneficial	Autogenic training, massage, relaxation, yoga	Acupuncture, aromatherapy, guided imagery, hypnotherapy, meditation		
Unknown effectiveness*	Acupressure, acupuncture, aromatherapy, fish oil, guided imagery, hypnotherapy, lavender, mindfulness-based stress reduction, music therapy	Autogenic training, biofeedback, exercise Herbs: chamomile, gingko biloba, passion flower, lemon balm, reflexology, reiki, Tai chi, therapeutic touch	Acupressure, acupuncture (alcohol and heroin), therapeutic touch, yoga, some Chinese herbs, Qigong, relaxation	Acupuncture, art therapy, Chinese herbal medicine (combined with antipsychotics), gingko biloba, hypnosis, polysaturated fatty acids
Trade off between benefits and harms	Black Cohosh (some association with liver damage)			
Unlikely to be beneficial		Homoeopathy	Cranial electrostimulation gingko biloba (cocaine), hypnotherapy	
Likely to be ineffective		Valerian, chiropractic, flower remedies	Acupuncture (cocaine), relaxation (drug withdrawal)	

Note
*Preliminary evidence encouraging or evidence either inconclusive or insufficient data.

Table 11.5 Evidence for CAM and cancer

	Reducing cancer risk	Cancer treatment	Palliative care
Beneficial	Allium vegetables (garlic) (regular intake reduces risk of GI cancers) Exercise (reduces colon and breast cancer) Green tea (regular intake reduces risk of digestive tract and breast cancer) Tomato (lycopene) (regular intake reduces prostate cancer risk)		Aromatherapy (improves well-being and reduces anxiety) Exercise (reduces severity of adverse effects caused by conventional medicine) Massage (improves well-being)
Likely to be beneficial	Phytoestrogens (preliminary data suggest risk reduction, particularly prostate cancer)	Acupuncture (hot flushes, fatigue after chemotherapy)	Acupuncture (nausea, chemotherapy-related nausea and vomiting) Biofeedback, guided imagery Hypnotherapy (chemotherapy-related nausea and vomiting), relaxation (pain, improvement of anxiety, increase well-being) Music therapy (psychological problems)
Unknown effectiveness *	Antioxidants, calcium (colorectal cancer), dietary fibre, fish oil, Ginseng, vegetarianism	Traditional Asian herbal mixtures, beta glucan, essiac, gerson diet, macrobiotic diet, melatonin, mistletoe	Acupuncture (pain), Asian herbal mixtures Cannabinoids (pain control, appetite, quality of life) Co-enzyme Q10 (may reduce toxicity), fish oil, gingko, ginseng (fatigue and quality of life), homoeopathy, hypnotherapy (pain and fatigue), marigold (radiation-induced dermatitis), spiritual healing (reduce anxiety and increase well-being)
Unlikely to be beneficial	Breathing exercises (to lower blood pressure)		
Likely to be ineffective	Glucosamine, magnesium, xioke tea, zinc (no effects on HBA1c and glucose)	Di Bella therapy, Laetrile, shark cartilage, support group therapy, thymus gland extract	

Note
*Preliminary evidence encouraging or evidence either inconclusive or insufficient data.

Cancer and supportive palliative care

People treated with radiotherapy and chemotherapy for cancer undergo major life changes such as: they may be unable to work, their appearance changes, there are usually changes in their quality of life and they may feel ill as well as lacking in energy. This creates various psychological and emotional changes. In some situations CAM has been shown to help symptoms and improve quality of life and mood and reduce feelings of discomfort (Vaghela *et al.* 2007).

Research has demonstrated that people with cancer access CAM to a greater extent than those with other long-term conditions, and that this is increasing (Ernst 2000; Cassileth *et al.* 2001; Lewith *et al.* 2002). In a UK study, 32 per cent of people with cancer were found to have sought CAM treatment in a variety of settings (Lewith *et al.* 2002) as compared with Patterson *et al.*'s (2002) study which found that over 70 per cent of cancer patients had used at least one type of CAM and 17 per cent had seen a CAM practitioner. Other studies have shown that those with more physical discomfort and more progressive disease and those requiring palliative care had higher CAM use (Burstein *et al.* 1999; Baron and Baron 2003). CAM is often used by people with cancer in conjunction with conventional medicine.

A range of CAM treatments are used by people with cancer but the common ones are dietary treatments, herbs, homoeopathy, hypnotherapy, meditation, visualisation, relaxation, spiritual healing, aromatherapy and massage (Rees *et al.* 2000; Cassileth *et al.* 2001). Researchers suggest that cancer patients access CAM for three main reasons: symptom relief, to improve quality of life and to lengthen their lives (Oneschuk *et al.* 1998; Pan *et al.* 2000; Cassileth *et al.* 2001). CAM practitioners are also perceived as providing them with opportunities for a more caring therapeutic relationship, particularly in the case of palliative care. CAM is therefore sometimes used by people with cancer for emotional and psychological support.

Palliative care services are multidisciplinary and often include complementary therapists as an important part of their teams. There are similarities between palliative care and CAM in both their ethical and research approaches. Palliative care, like CAM, uses the term 'holistic and total care'. Many oncology units and hospices offer CAM for their patients and relatives, the aim being to offer care not cure (Kohn 1999). The curative potential of CAM therapies is unproven but they are generally less toxic. However, one of the main reasons why people with cancer use CAM is for symptom relief. Symptoms requiring relief are varied and include pain, nausea and vomiting, fatigue and breathlessness. It is, however, hard to separate out symptom relief and improved quality of life, since they are connected. For example, if pain is reduced, both mobility and sleep will improve. Scientific evidence for CAM for symptom management is still limited. A limited summary is given in Table 11.5, and further information may be found in Ernst *et al.* (2006, 2008), Heller *et al.* (2005) and Pham *et al.* (2003), and guidelines have been published which have acknowledged how CAM can enhance the quality of life for those with cancer and those requiring palliative care (Tavares 2003).

Conclusion

A central theme of CAM is promoting the body's capacity to self-heal. This may relate to how the user rather than the therapist brings about healing, their expectations, the strength of the therapeutic relationship and how an individual takes responsibility for their health. In the case of chronic disease, how the interaction occurs may depend on the individual's decision-making process and how and whether they can take responsibility for their health (Fouladbakhsh and Stommel 2008). Developing cooperation and trust between conventional and CAM practitioners will benefit the consumer and achieve a better-educated society whose members are equipped to manage their long-term health problems.

References

Al-Windi, A. (2004) Determinants of Complementary/Alternative Medicine (CAM) Use. *Complementary Therapy in Medicine*, 99(5), 889–893.

Astin, J.A. (1998) Why Patients Use Alternative Medicine: Results of a National Study. *Journal of American Medical Association*, 19, 1548–1553.

Aung, S.K.H. (2006) Bioethics and Complementary Medicine: An Overview and Personal Perspective. *Health Ethics Today*, 11(3), 9. Online. Available at: www.phen.ab.ca/materials/het/het11–03c.html (accessed 14 November 2008).

Baron, D.A. and Baron, A. (2003) Psychiatric Disorders. In: Spencer, J.W. and Jacobs, J.J. (eds), *Complementary and Alternative Medicine: An Evidence-based Approach*. St Louis: Mosby.

Boon, H.S., Verhoef, M.J., Vanderheyden, L.C. *et al.* (2006) Complementary and Alternative Medicine: A Rising Healthcare Issue. *Health Policy*, 1(3), 9–35.

Boucher, T.A., Culliton, P.D. and Bullock, M.L. (2003) Alcohol and Chemical Dependencies. In: Spencer, J.W. and Jacobs, J.J. (eds), *Complementary and Alternative Medicine: An Evidence-based Approach*. St Louis: Mosby.

Breivik, H., Collett, B., Ventafridda, V. *et al.* (2006) Survey of Chronic Pain in Europe: Prevalence, Impact on Daily Life, and Treatment. *European Journal of Pain*, 10(4), 287–333. Epub 10 August 2005.

British Medical Association (1993) *Complementary Medicine: New Approaches to Good Practice*. London: BMA.

Burgmann, T., Rawsthorne, P. and Bernstein, C.N. (2004) Predictors of Complementary and Alternative Medicine Use in Inflammatory Bowel Disease: Do Measures of Conventional Healthcare Utilization Relate to Use? *American Journal of Gastroenterology*, 99(5), 889–893.

Burstein, H.J., Gelber, S., Guadagnoli, E. *et al.* (1999) Use of Alternative Medicine by Women with Early-stage Breast Cancer. *New England Journal of Medicine*, 340, 1733–1739.

Campbell, A. (2002) *Complementary and Alternative Medicine: Some Basic Assumptions, in Alternative Medicine, Should we Swallow It?* London: Hodder & Stoughton.

Cant, S. (2005) Understanding Why People Use Complementary and Alternative Medicine. In: Heller, T., Lee-Treweek, G., Katz, J., Stone, J. and Spurr, S. (eds) *Perspectives on Complementary and Alternative Medicine*. London: Routledge.

Cassileth, B.R., Schraub, S., Robinson, E. *et al.* (2001). Alternative Medicine Use Worldwide: The International Union Against Cancer Survey. *Cancer*, 91(7), 1390–1393.

Cox, H., Henderson, L., Wood, R. *et al.* (2003) Learning to Take Charge: Women's Experiences of Endometriosis. *Complementary Therapies in Nursing and Midwifery*, 9(1), 62–68.

Cronin-Wood, K. (2007) Building Better Chronic Disease Prevention and Management Systems. *Hospital News*, Canada, May, pp. 8 and 16 (newspaper).

Dossey, B.M. (1997) Complementary and Alternative Therapies for our Ageing Society. *Journal of Gerontological Nursing*, 23(9), 45–51.

Dwyer, J.M. (2004) *Australian Health System Restructuring – What Problem is Being Solved? Australia and New Zealand Health Policy. Biomed Central*. Online. Available at: www.anzhealthpolicy.com/content/1/1/6) (accessed 17 November 2008).

Egede, L.E., Zheng Ye, X. and Silverstain, M.D. (2002) The Prevalence and Use of Complementary and Alternative Medicine Use in Individuals with Diabetes. *Diabetes Care*, 25(2), 324–329.

Eisenberg, D.M., Davis, R.B., Ettner, S.L. *et al.* (1998) Trends in Alternative Medicine Use in the United States. 1990–1997: Results of a Follow-up National Survey. *Journal of the American Medical Association*, 280, 1569–1575.

Ernst, E. (2000) Prevalence of Use of Complementary and Alternative Medicine: A Systematic Review. *Bulletin World Health Organisation*, 78, 252–257.

Ernst, E., Pittler, M.H. and Wider, B. (2006) *The Desktop Guide To Complementary and Alternative Medicine: An Evidence-based Approach* (2nd edn). St Louis: Mosby.

Ernst, E., Pittler, M.H., Wider, B. *et al.* (2008) *Oxford Handbook of Complementary Medicine.* Oxford: Oxford University Press.

Fouladbakhsh, J.M. and Stommel, M. (2008) Comparative Analysis of CAM Use in the US Cancer and Non Cancer Populations. *Journal of Complementary and Integrative Medicine*, 15(1), Article 19. Online. Available at: www.bepress.com/jcim/vol. 5/iss1/19/.

Giddens, A. (2000) *Modernity and Self Identity: Self and Society in the Late and Modern Age.* Cambridge: Polity Press.

Halberstein, R.A. (2005) *Medical Plants: Historical and Cross-cultural Usage Patterns. Annals of Epidemiology*, 15, 686–699.

Haskell, W.L., Luskin, F.M. and Marvasti, F.F. (2003) Atherosclerotic Vascular Disease. In: Spencer, J.W. and Jacobs, J.J. (eds) *Complementary and Alternative Medicine: An Evidence-based Approach.* St Louis: Mosby.

Hill, F.J. (2003) Complementary and Alternative Medicine: The Next Generation of Health Promotion? *Health Promotion International*, 18(3), 265–271.

Houghton, P. (2004) UK Needs Greater Expertise in TCM. *Pharmaceutical Journal*, 273, 125.

House of Lords (2000) *Select Committee on Science and Technology – Sixth Report on Complementary and Alternative Medicine (CAM).* Online. Available at: www.publications.parliament.uk/pa/ld199900/ldselect/ldsctech/123/12301.htm (accessed 16 October 2008).

Katz, J. (2005) CAM in Supportive and Palliative Cancer Care. In: Heller, T., Lee-Treweek, G., Katz, J., Stone, J. and Spurr, S. (eds) *Perspectives on Complementary and Alternative Medicine.* London: Routledge.

Kohn, M. (1999) *Complementary Therapies in Cancer Care.* London: Macmillan Cancer Relief.

Lee-Treweek, G. and Stone, J. (2005) Critical Issues in the Therapeutic Relationship. In: Heller, T., Lee-Treweek, G., Katz, J., Stone, J. and Spurr, S. (eds) *Perspectives on Complementary and Alternative Medicine.* London: Routledge.

Lewith, G.T., Broomfield, J. and Prescott, P. (2002) Complementary Cancer Care in Southampton: A Survey of Staff and Patients. *Complementary Therapies in Medicine*, 1092, 100–106.

McGrady, A. and Kleshinski, J.F. (2003) Diabetes Mellitus. In: Spencer, J.W. and Jacobs, J.J. (eds) *Complementary and Alternative Medicine: An Evidence-based Approach.* St Louis: Mosby.

McKenzie, J. and Keller, H.H. (2001) Vitamin-mineral Supplementation and Use of Herbal Preparations Among Community-living Older Adults. *Canadian Journal of Public Health*, 92(4), 286–290.

Oneschuk, D., Fennell, L., Hanson, J. *et al.* (1998) The Use of Complementary Medications in Cancer Patients Attending an Outpatient and Symptom Clinic. *Journal of Palliative Care*, 14(4), 21–26.

Paltiel, O., Avitzour, M., Preretz, T. *et al.* (2001) Determinants of the Use of Complementary Therapies by Patients with Cancer. *Oncology*, 19(9), 2439–2448.

Pan, C.X., Morrison, R.S., Ness, J. *et al.* (2000) Complementary and Alternative Medicine in the Management of Pain, Dyspnea, and Nausea and Vomiting Near the End of Life: A Systematic Review. *Journal of Pain and Symptom Management*, 20(5), 374–387.

Park, J. (2006) In Praise of Integrated Health. *Complementary Therapies in Medicine*, 14(3), 173–174.

Patterson, R.E., Neuhouser, M.L., Hedderson, M.M. *et al.* (2002) Types of Alternative Medicine Used by Patients with Breast, Colon, or Prostate Cancer: Predictors, Motives, and Costs. *Journal of Alternative and Complementary Medicine*, 8(4), 477–485.

Patwardhan, B., Warude, D., Pushpangadan, P. *et al.* (2005) Ayurveda and Traditional Chinese Medicine: A Comparative Overview. *eCAM* 2(4), 465–473.

Pham, P.T.K. and Primack, A. (2003) Cancer. In: Spencer, J.W. and Jacobs, J.J. (eds) *Complementary and Alternative Medicine: An Evidence-based Approach*. St Louis: Mosby.

Rees, R.W., Feigel, I., Vickers, A. *et al.* (2000) Prevalence of Complementary Therapy Use by Women with Breast Cancer: A Population Survey. *European Journal of Cancer*, 36, 1359–1364.

Remsburg, R.E. and Carson, B. (2002) Rehabilitation. In: Lubkin, I.M. and Larson, P.D. (eds) *Chronic Illness – Impact and Interventions* (5th edn). Toronto/London/Singapore/Boston: Jones and Bartlett.

Robinson, A. and McGrail, M.R. (2004) Disclosure of CAM Use to Medical Practitioners: A Review of Qualitative and Quantitative Studies. *Complementary Therapies in Medicine*, 12, 90–98.

Robinson, N. (2006) Integrated Chinese Medicine. *Complementary Therapies in Clinical Practice*, 12, 132–140.

Robinson, N., Donaldson, J. and Watt, H. (2006) Auditing Outcomes and Costs of Integrated Complementary Medicine Provision – The Importance of Length of Follow up. *Complementary Therapies in Clinical Practice*, 12(4), 249–257.

Robinson, N., Blair, M., Lorenc, A. *et al.* (2008) Complementary Medicine Use in Multi-ethnic Paediatric Outpatients. *Complementary Therapies in Clinical Practice*, 14, 17–24.

Sparber, A. and Wootton, J. (2002) Surveys of Complementary Medicine: Part V. Use of Alternative and Complementary Therapies for Psychiatric and Neurological Diseases. *Journal of Alternative and Complementary Medicine*, 8(1), 93–96.

Spencer, J.W. and Jacobs, J.J. (eds) (2003) *Complementary and Alternative Medicine: An Evidence-based Approach*. St Louis: Mosby.

Tavares, M. (2003) *National Guidelines for the Use of Complementary Therapies in Supportive and Palliative Care*. London: NCHSPCS/FIH.

Taylor, A.G., Galper, D.I., D'Huyvetter, K. *et al.* (2003) Pain. In: Spencer, J.W. and Jacobs, J.J. (eds) *Complementary and Alternative Medicine: An Evidence-based Approach*. St Louis: Mosby.

Thomas, K.J. and Coleman, P. (2004) Use of Complementary or Alternative Medicine in a General Population in Great Britain. Results from the National Omnibus Survey. *Journal of Public Health*, 26(2), 152–157.

Thomas, K., Nicholl, J. and Coleman, P. (2001) Use and Expenditure on Complementary Medicine in England: A Population Based Study. *Complementary Therapies in Medicine*, 9, 2–11.

Thomas, K.J., Coleman, P. and Nicholl, J.P. (2005) Trends in Access to Complementary Medicines via Primary Care in England 1995–2001. Results from a Follow-up National Survey. *Family Practitioner*, 20(5), 575–577.

US National Centre for Complementary and Alternative Medicine (NCCAM) (n.d.) *What is Complementary and Alternative Medicine?* Online. Available at: http://nccam.nih.gov/health/whatiscam. (accessed 19 August 2008).

Vaghela, C., Robinson, N., Gore, J. *et al.* (2007) Evaluating Healing for Cancer in a Community Setting from the Perspective of Clients and Healers: A Pilot Study. *Complementary Therapies in Clinical Practice*, 13(4), 240–249.

Van den Brink-Muinen, A.A. and Rijken, M.P. (2006) Does Trust in Health Care Influence the Use of Complementary and Alternative Medicine by Chronically Ill People? *BMC Public Health*, 691,012. Online. Available at: http://www.biomedcentral.com/1471–2458/6/188 (accessed 15 September 2008).

Willison, K.D., Williams, P. and Andrews, G.J. (2007) Enhancing Chronic Disease Management: A Review of Key Issues and Strategies. *Complementary Therapies in Clinical Practice*, 13, 232–239.

World Health Organisation (2003) *WHO Traditional Medicine Strategy 2002–2003, World Health Organisation Document, WHO/EDM/TRM/2002.1*. Geneva: World Health Organisation.

Yesilada, E. (2005) Past and Future Contributions to Traditional Medicine in the Health Care System of the Middle East. *Journal of Ethnopharmacology*, 100, 135–137.

Yuan, J., Kerr, D., Park, J. *et al.* (2008) Treatment Regimens of Acupuncture for Low Back Pain – A Systematic Review. *Complementary Therapies in Medicine*, 16(5), 295–304.

Zapper, S. and Cassileth, B. (2003) Complementary Approaches to Palliative Oncological Care. *Journal of Nursing Care Quality*, 8, 22–26.

Zollman, C. and Vickers, A. (1999) ABC of Complementary Medicine: Users and Practitioners of Complementary Medicine. *British Medical Journal*, 319, 836–838.

12 Caring for the spirit

The Reverend Fr. Alan Brown

Introduction

Spirituality is a relatively easy topic to discuss. It is, however, immensely difficult to define. Indeed it may be impossible to define, but perhaps can be better described. Swinton and Pattison (2001, 25) describe it thus:

> Spirituality can be understood as that aspect of human existence which relates to structures of significance that give meaning and direction to a person's life and helps them deal with the vicissitudes of existence. It is associated with the human quest for meaning, purpose, self transcending knowledge, meaningful relationships, love and a sense of the holy. It may or may not, be associated with a specific religious system.

For Coyte *et al.* (2007, 23):

> It can refer to the essence of human beings as unique individuals 'what makes me, me and you, you'. So it is with the power, energy and hopefulness within a person. It is life at its best, growth and creativity, freedom and love. It is what is deepest in us – what gives us direction, motivation. It is what enables a person to survive bad times, to overcome difficulties, to become themselves.

The reflections by Swinton and Pattison, and Coyte *et al.* provide an excellent start to the understanding of what spirituality might mean for people. Not everyone is the same, of course. No two people have absolutely the same life experiences and outlook, although sets of experiences and like-mindedness may at times bring people together. This is perhaps why organisations which support people who live with particular illnesses or disabilities tend to be relatively successful. The sharing of experiences is one way of gaining greater understanding of how things are for oneself and for others. Having said this, the above reflections are written in a positive way. It would, of course, be wonderful if we could all feel as positive about life, as these reflections imply.

The journey of life

In Chapter 2 of this book, Carl Margereson describes the trajectory and impact of long-term conditions, which include the development and impact of symptoms;

experiencing loss; changes in self-concept and subsequent loss of self-esteem; the problem of social stigma, where both the person and others around them now see themselves differently; changes in social networks and levels of support; finding new ways of coping and adjustment; the power of perceived control and the experience of chronic stress. When brought together, simple as this list of variables may seem, it provides a stark backdrop to the patient/client experience.

Unfortunately, we are human and fragile beings; who can be knocked about on the journey of life more easily than we think. Where a person's journey brings major changes in expectations – physical ability, psychological ability, employment prospects, marriage prospects – the possibility of an early death, questions about the meaning of life, which we wouldn't perhaps think about at other times, become more important. Conversations with patients about such issues don't usually start out with opening gambits such as 'Now let's talk about your spirituality'. But this is precisely what we are talking about, even though the term 'spirituality' might never be used, since this list of variables equates to the vicissitudes of life which Swinton and Pattison are talking about above.

None of these stages need occur in a linear fashion of course. Indeed, an individual may become stuck at a particular point of the trajectory, never really getting away from the sick role. A young friend of mine who has a long-term condition, never fails to remind me, when challenged to do something outside of their perceived 'safe activity state', that they have a long-term condition and need to take care of their health. Well, this is so, but in reality they could do more than they do, but they have somehow been overtaken by the sick role, in a way which has almost devoured them. This is not to underestimate, though, quite how disastrously life can change for people. Facing the 'never again to' is very tough: never to breathe properly, never to walk; never to have sex in the way it was known before. As professionals and ministers we inevitably talk of these issues with a certain detachment, for no matter how close we might get to the person, it is only they who can understand their own situation from within. Individuals may work through the trajectory and somehow come out of it at the other end, being stronger and more fully human; on the other hand they might go round and round parts of the cycle like a merry-go-round and never seem to reach a level of fulfilment. Williams (2006, 13) talks well of zig-zag journeying where:

> we pick up bits and pieces of our true selves. We begin to discover who and what we really are. Our freedom to travel is most importantly the freedom to travel inwards to our own depths. Inwards and downwards is the most vital of all the directions we go. This is not an alternative through the zig-zag. It is the same journey better understood and more fully appreciated.

This all takes time, of course. We may not always recognise the journey that we are on as a journey. Such travels can be painful; arrival, if we ever really arrive, can be even more painful, or can bring us to some sort of resolution. The journey is an individual one for each person, no two people are alike and the effects of a serious illness or an accident, while common enough in symptomatology and diagnosis, are unique to the individual in the ways in which they affect their lives. An example of this, in the world of spinal injuries, would be the psychological and spiritual effects of dealing with a revised body image and sexual function. Here, loss isn't simply loss, it is the lack of movement and sensation, often replaced by tremendously severe neuropathic pain. It is dealing with having to move about in a wheelchair all the time, not just once a day, but all day, every day. It is dealing with not being able to walk, always having to look for ramps instead of being able to negotiate kerbs; of using hand controls to drive a car instead of pedals; of using condoms and catheters to urinate; of being incontinent of faeces when the bowel is upset; of wanting to have children of your own and not being able to father them yourself; of not being able to feel more than half of your partner beside you in bed in the way that you used to; in being forever wrapped in a wheelchair instead of standing to full height.

While I recognise the danger of over-emphasis here, none of us can know how we would react to any of these things. We would all do so differently, facing the challenges in different ways. Some people would feel totally overcome by this type of situation, others will face it head-on and build a new life, as Williams says, 'the journey better understood and more fully appreciated'. But such journeys can take a very long time. Again, this young friend of mine, when faced with a possible sexual encounter some seven years after having a spinal injury, had to come face to face with the realities of how he was going to feel, or indeed, in some parts of his body, not feel, during his relationship with his first girlfriend since the accident. There was a new awakening, a new drilling-down into self.

A life of changes

It isn't simply the physical things of life which make a difference. Again this young friend of mine had been training for a professional career. Through one difficulty or another, including an absolute lack of money, it took him five years to resume his studies. He had, previously, always come top of the class. On the resumption of his studies, when he received the feedback for his first assignment which had been marked as a very clear pass, he broke down and cried. It had taken him five years to know that although he cannot walk, his brain is still what it was and that he can still compete with others in the classroom.

It isn't simply the person who has to deal with the changes which occur when affected by a long-term condition. As noted in the trajectory, relatives and friends are affected also. In his book *Looking Up* (2008), Tim Rushby-Smith discusses the effects of spinal injury on himself and also on his wife, who was pregnant at the time of his accident. Rushby-Smith muses on how he will cope with assisting to look after a newborn baby and assisting his wife, and in another part of the book his wife comments that she wishes he wasn't paralysed. While Tim and his wife set about rebuilding their lives, his wife was clearly mourning for the days they had together when he could walk, didn't have immense pain and could do the things they enjoyed doing together which are now curtailed, at least to some extent. It could be said, therefore, that we travel alone and yet in community with others, be they family, friends, professionals and anyone else whom we meet along the way who have significance for us, either in the long or short term.

These stories about my young friend and Tim Rushby-Smith, above, point to the need for life experience alongside the support which others can give. The receiving of the mark from the teacher did more good than a hundred conversations about how well my friend would do if he would but allow himself a chance and 'give it a go'. Tim only knew what life would be like in relation to having a child when his child was born. What are such experiences about? They are about lifting the spirits; of finding a new spirituality; the journeying on to a new path of enlightenment about the self and the world in which we are engaged; the continued search for meaning.

Searching for meaning

Spirituality and the consideration of religious beliefs in relation to healthcare is often one of the last, if not the last issue, to be considered by health professionals as the patient or client journeys on through their health experience. As I begin to write this chapter it is Ash Wednesday. In the Christian calendar, it is the start of Lent, a period of 40 days when Christians have time to reflect on their own spiritual and religious well-being, their place in the Church and in society, and to consider, in general, what life means for them.

Such reflections take time and effort. If anything meaningful is to be gained from the activity, those undertaking the reflection have to plumb the depths of their innermost being. This is neither comfortable, nor to be embarked upon lightly. It would be a mistake though to think that only those with a religious belief need, at some point in their lives, to plumb such depths and to try to make sense of that which is around them.

When Simon Robinson and I published a book on *Spirituality and the Practice of Healthcare* (Robinson *et al.* 2003) we began with an extract from a book by Hugo Gryn. Gryn was born in Czechoslovakia in 1930, the son of a prosperous Jewish family. In 1944 the Gryn family were deported to Auschwitz. Hugo and his mother survived but his brother and father died while in the camp. After the war Gryn emigrated to the United States where he trained as a rabbi. He later moved to England where he was a rabbi in a London synagogue for 32 years, becoming a regular radio broadcaster, for many years on BBC's Radio 4's *The Moral Maze*. I make no apology for using it again here, for it provides a very clear scenario of the helplessness and futility of life which can overcome us.

> When we arrived at Auschwitz, it was a bright, sunny day and a series of jet streams appeared in the sky. They may have been experimental V2 bombs, but I had not seen such a sight before, and for a while, I believed that God himself would intervene.... Hope was to believe that evil would be destroyed, even though it looked invincible, with no evidence whatsoever of forces for good.... And there was faith. That God knew what was happening. That he let it happen and that it had a purpose. Most of the time this was difficult. Too difficult.
>
> I knew then, and I know now, that my survival had nothing to do with being different or better or more deserving. And one of my burdens, indeed an irrational sense of guilt ever since, has been precisely that I do not know why I survived. In all sorts of ways much of what I have tried to do and tried to be ever since has been to give some sense of meaning to that survival.
>
> (Gryn 2000, 248)

Gryn was talking about a very particular situation in Auschwitz. He could not comprehend this particular situation at the time. Indeed the meaning of it eluded him for more than half a century. It is clear from his writing that although it remained incomprehensible, this did not stop him continuing to work at finding meaning and purpose from the experience. So it is with people who have long-term conditions, or at least it can be. It is a reasonable question to ask 'Why me?' in many different situations. The question in the end is unanswerable in an absolute form, but it is part of the human psyche that we return to this question time and time again, during our lives, in many different situations. Some of these situations will be positive ones and we will be jubilant. In the context of this chapter, it is more likely that the question is being asked in a more searching, perplexed way.

People with long-term conditions can find themselves in an ever-changing set of circumstances as their condition develops, or complications occur. They are, in a sense, in a permanent dialogue with it and with themselves. During this dialogue the person may encounter a series of hopes, joys and deaths. These may include the hope of becoming fully well, to be restored to that level of health which they had before, or to be even better; joy isn't simply being happy all of the time, but it is the recognition that even small things can bring a sense of fulfilment or well-being, whether caused by finding new ways to do something, or recognising that we are still worthwhile human beings. Death is the final act, yet in truth we live through a series of deaths and rebirths throughout the whole of our lives. Becoming disabled or losing one's job is a form of death and we have to find ways of being reborn; that renewal which makes us feel human, loved and able to love.

When things are going well in our lives, we don't often truly think about how things are, for we take many things for granted. When we are faced with a long-term condition, we are brought up sharply into the realities of life and we may well realise that we are far from perfect. None of us are perfect. We only need to look in the mirror to see that. Given this recognition, a key to keeping going can be the real sense of hope for the future. Not the hope of a miracle, although somehow some people seem to experience these, but a way of finding a settlement with how things are and finding a way forward which accommodates the illness or physical problem and allows us to move on.

Hope isn't simply something of the mind, it is mixed with the personal experiences which we have, physical, psychological, social and emotional. In terms of the physical, it can be in the loving touch of another. Love in this context is not that in which we are in a sexual encounter with someone. Rather, it can be the touch of a professional who recognises us for the person who we are. In recent years, we have become much more mechanistic in our medical treatments and have perhaps lost the notion of therapeutic touch which conveys to another that they are valued. Psychological hope is the will to regain the balance of momentum which enables us to keep going through the thick and thin of life. Social hope is to do with relationships in the wider social context, of being part of the community in which we live and have our being; to becoming fulfilled members of society, however this fulfilment is attained. Emotional hope is the reliance on others, be it a partner, relative, a series of friends or indeed God or some other 'higher being' depending upon the person's faith structure and experience. As will be recognised, this emotional hope is not supported by any one of these elements alone, but by the whole physical, social and psychological constructs which make our lives unique.

Prayer and music can be just as beneficial to people as medication. In the zig-zag of life, we can find that we have a lot of space inside us to fill. At times, illness or injury can drag us down and we can begin to feel empty inside. We will all have known, at some point or another, that sense of an open cavern in our hearts. Somehow, the void has to be filled. As Fisher (2009, 61) says, 'silent prayer, over time, has the ability to unclutter our heart and mind and to give us interior room to breathe'. This has something to do with knowing just where we are. Music can do the same, for through music we can sometimes begin to reach the depths of our soul and, odd as it may seem, to be in paradise at the same time. To be taken on to a different plane.

Within this search for meaning is the constant fear of failure: failure to be well, failure to do things right, failure to make amends. Professionals also encounter the fear of failure: failure to do the right thing – which isn't necessarily the same thing as doing things right, failure to do your best. This is simply another part of our human fragility. But unless we can allow ourselves to be released from the paralysis of fear, whether as patient/client or professional, we will not learn to fly and to be the person that we have been born to be. We sometimes have to let go of the past to enable the future. The search for meaning can at times make life look even more confused, but unless we enter into this search, we become stifled and fail to grow.

Affirmation has a significant part to play in our spiritual well-being. In this context, affirmation isn't simply the need for the professional to affirm the worth of the patient/client. Affirmation works both ways round. It is based on trust and on the recognition that we all need to be told that it is 'OK' to be who we are and where we are, and for us to know that there are people alongside us upon whom we can rely. While we might question whether a young person with motor neurone disease can feel good about dying, there is something about knowing, as we approach death, that we have done what we could, while we could, to the best of our ability and for someone to be able to tell us so. Such conversations, which are made up of honesty and compassion, are not easy, but they are necessary. They are, to use a rather old-fashioned-sounding phrase, the intensive care of charity, to give oneself to the other as entirely as possible.

Relevance of spirituality in a changing world

The world is in change and we have, where possible, to move with the times. This doesn't always come easily. When I trained as a nurse in the late 1960s, it was common for prayers to be led by the Ward Sister at the nurse's station at the beginning of the day. Contrast this with a report in the *Guardian* in February 2009, where a nurse who had been suspended for offering to pray for a patient while fixing her dressings had been allowed to return to work on the understanding that she asks patients in advance if they have any spiritual needs (*Guardian* 2009b). It would have been good practice if the nurse had done this in the first place, as the patient had been taken aback by the nurse's offer and had reported her because it was thought that others might be equally offended. It is clear from this scenario that we have seen spirituality and prayer move from being, at least in some places, at the heart of the NHS service 40 years ago, to the margins of provision.

If we believe what much of the media tells us, it would be easy to believe that we live in a totally secular society. This is not true, or at least it is not totally true. Dr Rowan Williams, the Archbishop of Canterbury, recently commented that, 'Britain is not a secular country, but it is uncomfortably haunted by the memory of religion and doesn't quite know what to do with it ... a society which is religiously plural and

Table 12.1 Belonging to a religion in Great Britain

	1996 (%)	2006 (%)
Christian		
Church of England/Anglican	29.3	22.2
Christian – no denomination	4.7	9.6
Roman Catholic	8.9	9.0
Presbyterian/Free Presbyterian/Church of Scotland	3.8	2.5
Baptist/Methodist	3.0	2.4
United Reformed Church (URC)/Congregational	0.8	0.1
Brethren	0.1	–
Other Protestant/other Christian	2.2	1.7
Non-Christian		
Islam/Muslim	1.8	3.3
Hindu	0.6	1.4
Jewish	0.3	0.5
Sikh	0.2	0.2
Buddhist	0.5	0.2
Other non-Christian	0.4	0.4
No religion	42.6	45.8
Refusal/not answered/didn't know	0.8	0.6

Source: British Social Attitude Surveys. Reproduced with permission.

confused and therefore not necessarily hostile' (*Guardian* 2009c, 5). The statistics given in Table 12.1 provided by British Social Attitude Surveys and published in *Religion or Belief: A Practical Guide for the NHS* (DoH 2009) shows that although there has been a general trend downward during the past ten years in the number of people who purport to belong to one of the major world faiths, the reduction has not been as dramatic as many would have us believe. It is important therefore that when we are caring for people with long-term conditions, we take account of their particular religious needs, if any, and their spiritual needs.

Religion and spirituality

Religion and spirituality are not the same, although many people see them as being synonymous with each other. It is quite possible to have a sense of spirituality without any formal attachment to a particular religion. Religions vary as to what is held to be good practice. For the Muslim it will be praying five times a day and attending Friday prayers. For the Christian it will be attending church on days of Obligation, such as Ash Wednesday, Easter and so on. As noted in *Religion or Belief* (DoH 2009, 11), many religions recognise a power or powers that exist outside the laws of nature yet are in relationship with, and have an influence on, natural reality. This power or powers may, depending upon the situation and the experience of the person, be perceived to be either good or bad. As has been said earlier, it is not unusual for people to ask the 'Why me?' question when faced with the challenges of a long-term condition. This type of question is only one of a myriad questions which a person might ask. Others include: 'What have I done to deserve this, it must be something bad?' 'Is this God's retribution?' 'How do I make sense of this?' 'If God is good, how come this has happened?' Personally, I have a belief in a loving God who has no wish to incur any form of retribution on anyone. Not everyone has the same view. I recall being taken up very short when the young friend of mine with a spinal injury related to me that in his own country, Kosovo, there was a very deep religious suspicion that he had done something terribly wrong in his past and that the spinal injury had been inflicted upon him because of this. He went on to say that in his country, many people would not even look at him or touch his wheelchair, because it was thought that he was less than human. Such experiences are exceptionally hard for people to bear, and stem from ignorance, fear and an unjust set of superstitions held by those around them.

The Bible talks, in one or two places, of demonic possession. Some people who have a mental illness feel that they are possessed by demons. Evangelical Christians firmly believe in a deliverance ministry, where, at the extreme, exorcism has a place. Who is to say whether this is right or wrong? There is much in the world that we cannot understand. It would seem to me though that where people do talk of God, it should be in a supportive and loving way and not in a way where demonic notions are given sway. A truly holistic view of the human condition should involve a balanced approach, taking into account the spiritual, psychological, social and physical dimensions of the situation in which the person finds themselves. This is not to say that religious identity should be set aside, far from it, but it should be contextualised in a meaningful way.

Spirituality and learning difficulties

During the writing of this chapter, I learned of the death, at the age of 43, of Christopher Nolan. Christopher, born with cerebral palsy, became a world-renowned writer. He could neither speak nor control his hands but typed using an ingenious system which enabled words to bubble out of him. His first book, *Damburst of Dreams*, which was published when he was 16, was hailed as a 'jubilant lawless debut' (*Guardian* 2009a, 23), in which Christopher had 'plummeted into language like an avalanche, as if it were his one escape route from death – which of course it was'.

Christopher's life is a wonderful example of how the spirits can be lifted when the person is given the opportunity to be creative and human. While Christopher would no doubt have loved to have been able to speak, to control his hands, to be able to walk, his writings took him far beyond that state which many of us who are untroubled by any form of long-term condition can envisage. The simple message here is that no matter with whom we are in contact, we have a duty of care to enable them, as best we can, to reach the goals which they can either set for themselves, or we, as professionals, along with their carers and with the person themselves, can bring about with a sense of mutuality and love.

Spirituality and mental health

Common symptoms of mental ill-health include: sleep problems 29 per cent, fatigue 28 per cent, irritability 22 per cent, worry 20 per cent, depression 12 per cent, concentration and forgetfulness 10 per cent, depressive ideas 10 per cent, anxiety 9 per cent, somatic symptoms 7 per cent, worry about physical health 7 per cent, obsessions 6 per cent, phobias 5 per cent, compulsions 3 per cent and panic 2 per cent. From these statistics we can discern that a considerable number of the population live their lives affected, to some degree, by mental stress. This may or may not be experienced long term, but the effects are nevertheless burdensome when they occur. It would be wrong, too, to see this catalogue of mental health problems as being independent from those which are experienced by those with a long-term condition where often psychological distress and mental health problems can develop. All those with a long-term condition are likely to worry to some degree about their physical health. Some will become depressed, and a minority, though no less important for that, will consider the final act of suicide.

It is important therefore that the state of the person's mental health is not forgotten when considering how they are coping with their long-term condition, be it an impaired physical state or psychiatric illness, as this will affect their spirituality.

End of life: death and dying

None of us really likes to contemplate the end of our lives. Or do we? It has become clear in recent years that some people prefer to end their lives by means of assisted suicide, rather than carry on in an ever-demeaning state of physical and mental anguish. To assist someone to do this in the United Kingdom is against the law and so we have seen an increase, in the past few years, of people taking their last journey into parts of Europe where they are able to follow this course of action. There has been much publicity in recent months about whether the parents of a young rugby player who suffered a cervical spine injury should be taken to court, for assisting him, not to take his own life, but for accompanying him on his last journey to where this act would take place. In the end, the Crown Prosecution Service decided that there would be no advantage in taking any further action.

This scenario brings home to us the reality of illness and death. Some people, as in this case, whether rightly or wrongly, choose the time of their passing. Others continue to the end of their life, with a mixture of hope, fear, sadness, loss and grief. Not everyone, even towards the very end, wishes to leave this world a sadder place because of their death. I am reminded of a woman who asked a music therapist in a hospice if she could go to the music room with him. Once there, she pulled from her dressing-gown pocket the words of the song 'My Way'. Suffering from chronic lung disease, singing was almost impossible and yet, with the help of some oxygen off she set accompanied by the music therapist, and she sang the song the whole way through. Her song had been recorded and was played at her funeral a week later. Her singing was her way of saying goodbye to the people whom she loved and it was a recognition of a life lived.

Other people will prefer to die quietly and alone. Yet others will ask for reconciliation (known in the past as confession) and the laying-on of hands of a priest, something which I have been privileged to undertake on numerous occasions. What has always struck me is the way in which people want to come to the end of their life in an honest and settled way. To somehow be in charge of themselves, and to look back on their life openly and with a sense of having travelled. We return again to the zig-zag of life about which Williams talked earlier.

In order to help people towards this honest and settled death, we have, as professionals, to be willing to talk about the subject of death and not to shy away from it. It is self-evident that only those who have experienced death fully know about it. As a clergyman, in the preparation for someone approaching their death, I do my best to make sense of the unknown and unknowable. I can only do this through my own faith and belief system, through my interpretation of the scriptures and other writings and through my own experiences. And yet, in discussion with many people who have been approaching the end of their life, I have realised that the only thing I could give them, in absolute terms, was faithful friendship, mixed with my own belief of a loving God who would somehow be there for them in whatever the next world had to bring. It never quite seems to be enough, but reality is reality and sometimes we have to be satisfied with that.

The role of the chaplain

Hospital chaplains are often brought into healthcare situations towards the end of a person's life. This need not be the case. The chaplain is able to be included, with the patient's agreement, at any stage of the person's illness or long-term condition. Inevitably, if the person is in hospital for a long time, the chaplain has the opportunity to get to know them very well. One of the things which chaplains often have and other health professionals do not is time to spend with the patient. People often like to tell their stories, to plan the time they have left, be it long or short, and the chaplain is able to give the person space to have a conversation.

Chaplains are able to assess what sort of spiritual care a person might need. This assessment may take the form of a number of questions made up from the following framework (Cobb 2005, 46–47):

- An understanding of the person's spiritual orientation in relation to their life context.
- Identifying any practical consequences this may involve in the provision of care.
- Establishing beliefs or practices that facilitate coping and factors that may hinder spiritual well-being.
- Recognising the significance of beliefs in the experience of injury or illness and making healthcare decisions.
- Determining any support or resources needed.

The types of questions which can be helpful include:

- 'Is your faith/spirituality/religion helpful to you?'
- 'Do you have any spiritual or religious beliefs, can you tell me about them?'
- 'Are there things which we need to know about your faith/spirituality/religious beliefs that would help us in caring for you?'
- 'Can we provide anything for you to support you in your faith/spirituality/ religion?'
- 'Would you like to talk with someone about these matters?'
- 'Would you like us to arrange for a member of your faith community to visit you?'

These questions can equally well be asked by nurses and other healthcare professionals. Spiritual care assessments rely on the sensitivity and discernment of staff as well as the trust which has developed between the staff and the patient/client. This should be underpinned by a systematic approach to the assessment of spiritual care.

Therefore both staff and patients/clients should be aware that the assessment of spiritual well-being is part of healthcare and provides an opportunity for any spiritual care needs to be expressed.

Chaplains can also provide very good links to local communities, worship centres, mosques, churches and so on, and are equally there for relatives and friends of the patient/client and their carers, including professional staff.

Conclusion

As may be seen, the topic of spirituality isn't only something which is of interest to ministers of religion. Nurses are expected to undertake a spiritual assessment alongside a multitude of other more tangible assessments. Apart from ascertaining an individual's religion, which is only one variable to be considered, questions, as noted above, can be asked to enable the person to provide an insight into their spiritual needs and distress. Unfortunately, nurses are notoriously bad at this, but it isn't at all impossible for them to do, if the right approach is taken. Such assessments are a two-way proposition and require time for conversation.

People who have long-term conditions of whatever age face isolation, resulting in an inner loneliness. The importance of affirming the worth of an individual and finding ways in which life can be lived to the full, celebrating the past, present and what is to come, cannot be underestimated. Confirmation of who we are through the expression of a narrative which is clearly listened to and valued is vital. Occasionally there has to be a reconciliation of time, place and situation, and an acknowledgement of past hurts and current fears. Such reconciliation is a skilled process, requiring the helper to be clear about who they are and the ways in which such reconciliation might take place. New ways of looking at the world, even though in some contexts it may seem to be coming to an end, are as important as life itself.

References

Cobb, M. (2005) *The Hospital Chaplains Handbook.* Norwich: Canterbury Press.

Coyte, M.H., Gilbert, P. and Nicholls, V. (eds) (2007) *Spirituality, Values and Mental Health: Jewels for the Journey.* London: Jessica Kingsley.

Department of Health (DoH) (2009) *Religion or Belief: A Practical Guide for the NHS.* London: Department of Health.

Fisher, P. (2009) *Outside Eden, Finding Hope in an Imperfect World.* London: SPCK.

Gryn, H. (2000) *Closing Shadows.* London: Viking.

Guardian (2009a) Christopher Nolan: Writer With Cerebral Palsy Who Won the Whitbread with *Under the Eye of the Clock. Guardian*, 23 February, 35.

Guardian (2009b) Nurse Suspended over Prayers Goes Back to Work. *Guardian*, 24 February, 14.

Guardian (2009c) *UK Haunted by Religion, Says Archbishop. Guardian*, 23 March, 5.

Robinson, S., Kendrick, K. and Brown, A. (2003) *Spirituality and the Practice of Healthcare.* Basingstoke: Palgrave Macmillan.

Rushby-Smith, T. (2008) *Looking Up.* London: Virgin Books.

Swinton, J. and Pattison, S. (2009) Come All Ye Faithful. *Health Service Journal,* 20 December, 24–25.

Williams, H.A. (2006) *Living Free.* London: Continuum UK.

Part IV

Specific conditions

Introduction

Part IV outlines a range of long-term conditions which have been the subject of National Service Frameworks. The overall aim of this section is to outline, in a direct and comprehensible way, the aetiology, trajectory, evidence-based treatment and holistic care for each condition. In so doing, the authors of each chapter, specialists in their own field, describe how services can respond effectively to the overall health and well-being of people with a range of chronic health problems.

Individuals with long-term conditions are cared for in many different settings. For example, those with asthma are not cared for solely in respiratory wards, or those following a stroke on a specialist stroke unit, or those with heart failure on a cardiology unit. Neither are individuals with severe mental health problems only cared for by specialist secondary or tertiary health services. Nor is it not uncommon for individuals diagnosed with a malignant neoplasm to also have other chronic health problems (such as COPD and coronary artery disease) and to also experience mental distress.

The majority of individuals with long-term disorders are either at home or being cared for in non-specialist care settings with their principal carer likely to be a loved one who may have no formal medical or nursing training. However, even professional carers may lack an understanding of other long-term conditions as there is a tendency for expert knowledge to focus in particular specialist areas. The lines of demarcation that are clearly drawn between health and social care services often also extend to separate specialist staff from the wider health and social community. As such, the individual with multiple or complex needs, and their carers, may not receive appropriate treatment or may experience fragmented care which may impact on the trajectory of their illness and undermine their overall quality of life and well-being.

It is hoped that non-professional and professional carers and specialists alike may find much in these chapters to enhance the care and treatment they provide to people with other co-morbid health conditions and assist in the promotion of the biological, psychological, emotional, social and spiritual health and functioning of individuals.

13 Long-term neurological conditions

Sue Thomas

Introduction

Improving the care of people with long-term conditions is a key government target and the *National Service Framework for Long Term Neurological Conditions* (NSFLTnC) published in March 2005 has a ten-year implementation plan to achieve this priority (DoH 2005). With our ageing population there has been an increase in the incidence and prevalence of neurological disability overall and this trend is likely to continue owing to increased life expectancy and improvements in medical care. Currently there are approximately ten million people across the United Kingdom with a long-term neurological condition (LTnC). These individuals account for 20 per cent of acute hospital admissions and are the third most common reason for people seeing their GP. It is estimated that 350,000 people in the UK need help with daily living activities owing to a neurological condition and 850,000 people extend care to this user group (DoH 2005).

Neurological conditions have a considerable impact upon health and overall well-being. Individuals who have neurological problems may experience a wide range of complex physical, sensory, cognitive, psychological, emotional, behavioural and social difficulties and will have a broad range of needs that impinge not only on their own lifestyle but on that of their family and carers. Access to a wide range of health, social and voluntary care services throughout the duration of the illness is required, as a direct or indirect consequence of the condition or of its complications. These support services need to be planned, coordinated and well managed in order to be both timely and accessible. There is accumulating evidence that properly planned, accessible and integrated multidisciplinary services, delivered by skilled, multidisciplinary teams can improve, not only the care given to individuals with a LTnC, but also the quality of their lives and that of their carers (NHS Modernisation Agency 2005).

The NSFLTnC is aiming to transform the way health and social care services are supporting people, encouraging the concept that appropriate team-working and improved disease management and self-care strategies can deliver better care by preventing or solving many of the problems that neurological conditions may cause. Specifically this chapter will outline how the NSFLTnC aims to raise standards of care for people with neurological problems. It will provide a brief overview of the more common neurological conditions and their effects, and how neurological conditions should be managed by health and social care services throughout the whole patient pathway.

Overview of long-term neurological conditions

A long-term neurological condition results from disease or injury to the body's nervous system; for example, to the brain, spinal cord or the peripheral nerves. There are a range of neurological conditions which are classified into the following categories by the NSFLTnC:

- Sudden-onset conditions, for example, acquired brain injury or spinal cord injury followed by a partial recovery.
- Intermittent and unpredictable conditions, for example, epilepsy or early multiple sclerosis where relapses and remissions lead to variations in the care that is required.
- Progressive conditions like Parkinson's disease, later stages of MS and motor neurone disease (which can be rapidly progressive).
- Stable neurological conditions that have changing needs owing to the ageing process, for example, cerebral palsy in adults.

While it is outside the scope of this chapter to review every neurological condition, it is important to highlight some of the most common. Parkinson's disease (PD), for example, is a common progressive neurological disorder caused by a loss of the dopamine-producing nerve cells in the part of the brain that controls movement (substantia nigra) (NICE 2006). There is no cure for the disease which predominantly affects movement. The risk of developing PD increases with age, and more men than women are affected. The symptoms include tremors, speech problems, muscle stiffness, trembling of limbs that may cause slowness and shuffling gait, loss of facial expression and loss of voice. In later stages of PD, some patients develop impaired cognitive ability and dementia. Other impairments that develop include swallowing difficulties, depression and bladder and bowel problems (NICE 2006). Symptomatic treatment may include speech therapy, functional assessment of work and self-care activities with rehabilitation, and physiotherapy for gait re-education. There is no single drug of choice in the initial pharmacotherapy of early PD; however, NICE (2006) suggests that the drugs levodopa (which is converted into dopamine in the brain) and dopamine agonists may be most effective in symptom control for people with early PD. Anticholinergic medication may be used for young people with early PD but there are side-effects of such drugs which may exacerbate the symptoms, such as agitation and confusion. Levodopa therapy will be needed for people with later PD and surgery (deep brain stimulation) may be beneficial for some.

Multiple sclerosis (MS) is the most common neurological condition in young adults and is most often diagnosed between the ages of 20 and 40. It is an inflammatory, autoimmune disease in which the body's own immune system attacks itself. In MS the target is cells in the brain and spinal cord. Symptoms vary depending on which part of the nervous system is affected and can include (NICE 2003):

- fatigue;
- changes in skin sensation (e.g. numbness);
- muscle spasms, weakness and stiffness;
- bladder problems (including incontinence and urinary tract infections);
- bowel problems (including constipation);

- mobility problems (including reduced movement in joints);
- psychological problems (including emotional outbursts, depression and anxiety, problems with memory and thought processes);
- pain;
- sexual problems;
- eye problems (including blindness);
- swallowing difficulties;
- speech difficulties.

MS is a highly complex variable condition which can have significant physiological and psychosocial impacts. Eighty-five per cent of people will have 'relapsing remitting MS' (RRMS) where an individual has relapses (or exacerbations) which can last for days or weeks, where any of the above symptoms may be experienced followed by remissions. Half of people with RRMS will develop the secondary progressive form of MS (SPMS) within ten years of diagnosis. This form is characterised by a gradual worsening of symptoms and less remission. Ten to 15 per cent of people are diagnosed with 'primary progressive MS' (PPMS) in which there are few if any remissions and symptoms develop and worsen. Some treatments are available and specialist care can help people to manage conditions. Medication includes high doses of the steroid methylprednisolone to reduce inflammation and some people with RRMS and SPMS (who are experiencing relapses) may benefit from beta interferon or glatiramer acetate (NICE 2003). In 2007, NICE approved natalizumab (tysabri) as a treatment for rapidly evolving, severe RRMS. Between 50 per cent and 75 per cent of people with MS have tried complementary and alternative therapies (CAM) (MS Society 2006) and NICE (2003) tentatively suggests that a 'multi-modal therapy' which includes reflexology, massage, magnetic field therapy and fish oils may be helpful for people with MS in terms of their general sense of well-being.

Epilepsy is the most common neurological disorder characterised by recurrent unprovoked seizures (Blume *et al.* 2001). A seizure is caused by a sudden burst of excess electrical activity in the brain. Around 50 million people worldwide have epilepsy with almost 90 per cent of these people living in developing countries (WHO 2009). Epilepsy is more likely to occur in young children or over the age of 65, but it can occur at any time (National Society for Epilepsy 2009) and there are over 40 different types of seizure (NSA 2009). Common types include the following:

- Generalised tonic-clonic seizures (previously called grand mal) where there is loss of consciousness, the person falls down and their body stiffens and starts to jerk uncontrollably.
- Generalised absence (previously called petit mal) where there is a brief loss of consciousness but the person does not fall down, there are usually no abnormal movements and the person appears as though they are daydreaming.
- Simple partial where the person is fully aware of the seizure and there is an abnormal twitching movement of part of the body, for example, head, eyes, hand or arm, or a tingling sensation. The person may sense odd smells, sounds or tastes.
- Complex partial where the person experiences odd tastes or smells or *déjà vu*; a dream-like state follows. During an attack, lip smacking, grimacing or fidgeting may occur which can be followed by generalised seizure.

It is not possible to prevent epilepsy from developing but for those with the condition there are numerous anti-epileptic drugs (AED) available and the medication treatment strategy should be individualised according to the seizure type, the type of epilepsy the person suffers from, other medications the person takes and co-existing health problems, the individual's lifestyle, and personal preferences (NICE 2004). Psychological interventions (such as relaxation, cognitive behaviour therapy and biofeedback) may be beneficial adjunctive therapies to improve quality of life, as is knowledge of how to avoid seizures occurring from triggers such as alcohol, stress, strobe lighting and lack of sleep.

The Department of Health has recognised the importance of developing better stroke services by including specific milestones, targets and actions in the *NSF for Older People* (DoH 200b) and through the *National Stroke Strategy* (DoH 2007a), so stroke is not one of the specific conditions covered in the NSFLTnC (see Chapter 19).

National Service Framework for Long Term Neurological Conditions

The NSFLTnC was developed in an effort to raise the standard of care for people with neurological conditions such as PD, MS and epilepsy. These conditions are used as examples throughout the NSFLTnC text. The key themes of this policy are to promote independent living, care planned around the needs and choices of the individual, easier, timely access to services and joint working across all the agencies and disciplines concerned in care provision and delivery.

At the centre of the NSF are 11 quality requirements (QRs) designed to provide services that are supportive and appropriate at every stage of the disease from diagnosis until the end of life. The QRs in this NSF are more qualitative than measures used in previous NSFs as they include a new 'user-friendly' typology to systematically assess the evidence supporting the QRs. This typology reflects the value placed on the opinions of service users and carers and their families/carers as well as the views of professionals when assessing the evidence base (DoH 2005). This reinforces the fact that users' and carers' opinions and choices should be central to care provision in health and social care, and although this NSF focuses on neurological conditions much of this policy is equally applicable to all LTCs.

Many LTnCs have also benefited from the development of National Clinical Guidelines in recent years which outline the evidence-based care and treatment required from a national perspective. These guidelines are developed by the National Institute for Health and Clinical Excellence (NICE) with advice from expert clinicians, nurses, therapists and service users, such as epilepsy (NICE 2004) and multiple sclerosis (NICE 2003). Underpinning all of the quality requirements in the NSF is the delivery of 'a person-centred service'. People with LTnC can have very complex needs that can affect physical, emotional and mental functioning. The condition can impact on differing aspects of their lives including family and carers, education, housing, employment and finance. A person-centred service requires all aspects of an individual's life to be taken into account when assessing needs. Neurological disorders are also lifelong once a diagnosis has been established so it is important that individuals are allowed to make informed choices about how to manage their lives in living with the condition that they have.

An effective person-centred service needs:

- good coordination;
- services planned in an integrated way around the needs of the person;
- an understanding of the skills of different professionals and the role of different agencies;
- an integrated assessment of health and social care needs;
- up-to-date information given at the appropriate time along the patient pathway;
- involvement of the patient and carer in the decision-making process;
- access to both generalist and specialist advice;
- support to help individuals self-care;
- encouragement to the individual to join support groups relating to their condition.

In other words, seeing the right person at the right time in the right setting with the right information to help make informed choices (Modernisation Agency 2005).

There are a number of key stages in the process of providing person-centred care and these hinge on successful care planning. Figure 13.1 details a LTC care planning model devised for the NHS Modernisation Agency and is useful in understanding the pathway to person-centred care.

Entry into the system

At diagnosis individuals, family and carers will need to cope with the diagnosis and there will be initial information needs. Information on neurological conditions is widely available through the Internet and World Wide Web (see 'Further Information'), patient organisations, magazines and journals, and in shops and libraries. Too much information can be overwhelming, however, so it is important that individuals are directed to appropriate sources of information from the outset. The pathway shown in Figure 13.2 suggests a route for providing information.

The author suggests that professional healthcare workers involved in an individual's care can often suggest the most reliable information sources. Patient charities are also a good starting point for information, and the majority of these charities will produce information leaflets. Information prescriptions are also a relatively new and useful way for individuals with LTC and contain a series of links or signposts to guide people to sources of information about conditions and treatments, care services, benefits advice and support groups (see 'Further Information').

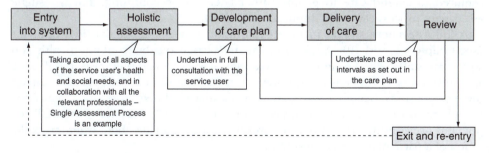

Figure 13.1 Care Planning Stages Model (source: NHS Modernisation Agency (2005). Reproduced by permission).

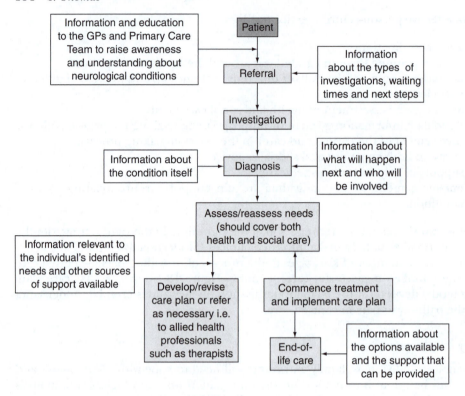

Figure 13.2 Pathway outlining key points for information giving (source: NHS Modernisation Agency (2005). Reproduced by permission).

Holistic assessment

A holistic assessment of need is the next key stage in the pathway of living with a LTC. *The NHS Plan* (DoH 2000) proposes a single assessment process (SAP) across health and social care. This single assessment process was initially highlighted in the *NSF for Older People* (DoH 2001b) and it is also valuable for people with LTnC, as it helps build a framework for identifying need and streamlining the care-planning process. Individuals should be invited to play as full a part as possible in the assessment process including elements of self-assessment. The wide range of professionals required to extend care to people with LTnC can be confusing, and the single assessment process can avoid duplication of effort.

A full assessment should include exploration of a set of standardised domains (see Chapters 5 and 19). Assessment can be carried out by front-line health and social care staff such as community nurses, social workers and therapists, but if more specialist assessment needs to be undertaken (e.g. assessments of cognitive impairment or pensions/benefit advice), an appropriately qualified professional may additionally need to be involved. What is important in a full assessment is that all the domains are considered and that no presumptions are made about whether exploration of a particular area is important.

The White Paper *Our Health, Our Care, Our Say* (DoH 2006) included a commitment to develop a common assessment framework (CAF) (DoH 2009b) for adults which would improve outcomes for adults by ensuring a personalised and holistic assessment of need focused on delivering individual outcomes, support joint working between health and social care services and increase efficiency through better information sharing. The CAF is not intended to be another assessment tool or rigid structure to be followed but something that builds on the SAP and care programme approach (CPA), and encourages information sharing between all those involved in supporting individuals and carers living with a LTnC (see 'Further Information').

Development of the care plan

Once the assessment has been completed care planning can be undertaken, taking into consideration the factors that are important to the individual and their family and carer.

The Generic Choice Model for LTC (DoH 2007a) (Figure 13.3) illustrates the important areas to consider in this process through two stages. The key issues in stage 1, at diagnosis and for immediate care post diagnosis, are:

- what matters to the individual and their carer;
- having access to expert support, advice and information;
- that all decisions are genuinely shared between the individual and their health professional.

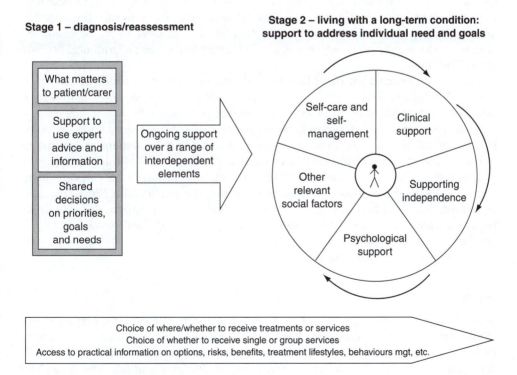

Figure 13.3 Generic Choice Model for LTC (source: DoH (2007). Reproduced by permission).

For stage 2, 'Living with a LTC', the specific elements that need to be considered are:

- self-care and care management;
- clinical support;
- psychological support;
- relevant social factors.

In theory the NHS Choice agenda (DoH 2007b) should enable a person with a LTnC to assemble, with the help of their healthcare professional, information about their life, available care and treatment options which will in turn enable a personalised package of treatment and care to be developed. The assessment and care-planning process allows the identification of specific needs and desired outcomes and encourages the design of support services that can best help maintain independence.

All individuals with a LTnC should have a care plan. There are a number of potential benefits to implementing successful care planning, including continuity of care, managing risks and helping individuals to control and manage their condition. Ideally care plans may be seen as a dynamic route map (Matrix Research and Consultancy 2005), which will be held by that individual and regularly evaluated and reviewed with them by their clinical team. Reviews should be based on clinical need which includes self-assessment. Arrangements should also be in place so that all people with a LTnC have a named point of contact for advice and information – this might be through a care manager or key worker scheme. This person would then be responsible for coordinating the input from all relevant agencies and producing the care plan. The care assessment and planning process ensures that appropriate services are available to provide support to enable the individual to receive continuity of care through the differing stages of the disease as well as if they need to transfer from, for example, children and younger persons' services to adult services or across geographical boundaries if they move.

Local arrangements for providing information to the person with a LTnC must ensure that information is quality assured, culturally appropriate information in a range of formats on all relevant aspects of service provision – how to manage their condition and wider social inclusion issues, for example, employment and transport. People should also be able to access education and self-management programmes that are tailored to their individual needs and at differing stages of their condition.

Personalised care planning should be a continuous process with the care plan regularly reviewed. All those involved in planning, the person with the LTnC and professionals should have an equal say in the discussion, negotiation, decision-making and review of the plan. The process needs to be led by the individual and based on their goals, aspirations and lifestyle wishes (Matrix Research and Consultancy 2005) (see 'Further Information').

Self-care

Self-care is increasingly recognised as an important component of the management of all LTnCs, and has been highlighted as a government health priority in England. Patients are known to obtain information from a wide range of sources, although little systematic research has been carried out on the factors which inform healthcare-seeking decisions. Concepts that have been developed for patient empowerment include telephone contact and support such as Own Health (Pfizer 2007), lay-led self-care support programmes such as the *Expert Patient Programme* (EPP) (DoH 2001a) and the Working in Partnership Programme (www.wipp.nhs.uk). WIPP was established as part of the General Medical Services contract in 2004 to provide support for primary care on developing self-care programmes. WIPP is now housed at self-care connect, an online resource for both professionals and people with LTCs (www.selfcareconnect.co.uk).

The EPP is an opportunity for people with LTnCs to come together with others and develop more skills to help them cope with the difficulties of long-term health problems. The programme is a course comprising six sessions of two and a half hours on consecutive weeks. Each week, participants are introduced to cognitive skills, that is, ways to build upon how they already deal with their conditions from day to day. This training offers course participants the opportunity to add to the skills they already use to:

- deal with problems like fatigue, pain, isolation, fear, frustration;
- manage their symptoms;
- access appropriate exercise for maintaining and improving their strength, flexibility and endurance;
- understand nutrition and the importance of this to their condition;
- communicate with family, friends and healthcare professionals;
- learn how to evaluate new health information.

EPP is led by people who have personal experience of living with a long-term condition. Evaluation of outcomes from the original research by Kate Lorig (Lorig *et al.* 1993) and cited by the Department of Health (DoH 2001a) indicates that patients who have participated in the EPP demonstrate:

- 9 per cent reduction in visits to GPs;
- 6 per cent reduction in visits to A&E;
- 9 per cent reduction in outpatient visits;
- 15 per cent increase in visits to pharmacists.

and

- reduced severity of symptoms;
- significant decrease in pain;
- improved life control and activity;
- improved resourcefulness and life satisfaction.

As with any skill, self-management needs to be learned and practised. This course aims to develop healthy lifestyle habits. These will complement any current or imminent medical or surgical treatment. The goal is for people to achieve the greatest possible physical capability and pleasure from life, despite living with their LTnC.

Self-management courses for people with long-term conditions are not new. They have been used and carefully researched in several countries, including the UK. Research has found that many benefits come from attending a course (Lorig *et al.* 1993). It can lead to:

- better symptom control;
- greater understanding of how to cope with the day-to-day problems listed above, including effective use of limited energy;
- a more active lifestyle;
- raised self-esteem and confidence;
- fewer visits to hospital and shorter stays;
- developing a partnership of care with healthcare professionals;
- more effective use of resources;
- increase in quality of life.

The importance of lay health workers has in the past been underestimated. Lay volunteers who have experience of certain illnesses are being used successfully to support and coach patients facing similar challenges.

Compliance and adherence to healthcare has come under increasing criticism in recent years and it has been suggested that interactions with patients should not be used as opportunities to reinforce instructions around treatment: rather, they should be seen as opportunities for the expertise of patients and health professionals to be shared in order to arrive at mutually agreed goals.

Emphasis on a 'doctor-centred' model of healthcare can lead to problems resulting in non-concordance and respect for the patient's agenda is fundamental in healthcare and is achieved more readily with lay health workers who have experienced similar health problems themselves. It is widely agreed that healthcare professionals need better to understand patients' constructions of symptoms and illnesses, and also their needs and expectations of healthcare, particularly in different cultural contexts. There is also a need to have a better understanding of the best ways of providing information to enable people to deal with their health concerns themselves, and of ways to help them to use services most effectively and efficiently.

Delivery of care

With the complexity of neurological conditions it will be essential that there is a multidisciplinary multi-agency approach to care and that this care is coordinated. In terms of care delivery consideration needs to be given to individuals at differing stages of their disease because the support given at diagnosis may be insufficient to support that person throughout the continuum of the disease. Individuals particularly need support at diagnosis to help understand the disease and its likely effects so that they can take an active role in the management of their own condition. As the disease progresses advice is needed to assist the person to remain healthy, to avoid complications and to prevent and manage crises.

Living with Parkinson's disease (PD)

To help understand the delivery of care across the time course of a disease an example of PD is used as an illustration. To aid understanding of the needs of people who have PD the disease was classified into four stages through a series of workshops which explored the disease process. The consultation surrounding this 'model for care' was undertaken following the World Health Organisation Declaration on PD (WHO 1997). A working group was formed which consisted of professionals and people living with

PD who reached consensus agreement on the stages of the disease. This was later published and has been the basis for educational training for professionals in PD ever since (MacMahon and Thomas 1998). The identified stages were: diagnosis; maintenance; complex; and palliative care (see Table 13.1). To see how long individuals would spend in each of the identified stages an audit of those living with the disease was undertaken in Cornwall using retrospective case note analysis (MacMahon *et al.* 1999). This has shown that typically someone will spend around one and a half years in a diagnostic phase, almost five to six years in a maintenance (fairly stable) stage, four and a half to almost five years in the complex stage and just over two years in a stage where palliative care is likely to be required (MacMahon and Thomas 1998).

Using this four-stage approach the aims, assessment needs, care management and outcomes required for someone living with PD were developed by a separate consensus group which included patients and carers, GPs, consultant neurologists and geriatricians, therapists and specialist and generalist nurses (PDS Primary Care Task Force 1998). The model depicts the different pathways followed in each stage of the disease.

Pathways visually illustrate and aid understanding of the range of support that each stage of PD requires. All LTnCs could be illustrated using a similar model and be of benefit to the professionals involved in care and to those living with the diseases, and are potentially useful as a lingua franca to case delivery.

Handling complications

Due to the longevity of neurological conditions many patients will maintain their lifestyle without accessing health and social care on a regular basis. Many may cope with problems that may be easily solved with expert advice which is why it is important to ensure that regular review is undertaken and that individuals are taught how to use health and social care services properly so that they can seek advice before any problem turns into a crisis. There has always been a culture of blaming anything and everything on the underlying diagnosis, often making individuals unsure of whether to speak to their doctor or nurse about problems that may arise.

Bakheit (2006) outlined the atypical presentations of acute illness in individuals with a LTnC which may increase the severity of a previously stable condition. Unexplained deterioration in mobility in a previously mobile person is commonly described or the need for increased assistance from others to cope with daily living activities which may indicate that an acute illness is developing. The most common causes of illness are urinary tract and respiratory infections. Other causes include accidental falls, dehydration and adverse drug effects. A deterioration from 'normal' in the individual's functional or mental abilities should not be attributed to the underlying neurological disorder until inter-current illness has been excluded and it is useful for individuals living with LTnCs to recognise the presenting signs of inter-current illness (see Table 13.2).

Rehabilitation

One of the main priorities of the NSFLTnC is that all people with neurological conditions remain as independent as possible and receive access to community rehabilitation services in order that they can achieve their maximum potential. This means flexible individualised programmes of rehabilitation and support that focus on goals beyond basic daily living activities so that the individual can participate fully in a range of life roles. Rehabilitation should be multidisciplinary and include the availability of specialist neurological expertise like neuropsychology to address the range of challenges that often present with neurological problems, for example, behavioural problems post brain injury. Good community rehabilitation has a great deal in common with good social care support and interventions will need to focus on wider social participation such as leisure and recreational activities including those provided by the voluntary sector.

Research has demonstrated that multidisciplinary/multi-agency community rehabilitation that is centred on a person's home can provide cost-effective services to help people reintegrate into the community. Increased independence can mean lower overall costs for supporting someone with a neurological impairment. This in turn reduces the burden on carers and reliance on health and social care services, and can lead to substantial cost savings in the longer term through maintaining independence and enabling social participation.

Existing good practice and evidence suggests that fully integrated rehabilitation includes:

Table 13.1 Care pathways for Parkinson's disease

Diagnosis stage	*Maintenance stage*

Aims
• Development of disease awareness
• Reductions in symptoms and distress
• Facilitate acceptance and understanding of diagnosis
	Aims
	• Morbidity relief
	• Maintenance of function and self-care
	• Promotion of normal activities
	• Reassessment
	• Avoid unnecessary medical dependency
	• Reduce symptoms
	• Avoid side-effects
	• Alert for complications:
	  • constipation
	  • postural hypotension

Assessment • To ascertain accurate diagnosis • Evaluate disability • Assess support available • Estimate patient understanding	

Management
• Develop care plan
• Consider multidisciplinary referral:
  • nurse specialist
  • physiotherapist
  • occupational therapist
  • speech and language therapist
  • dietician
• Ensure regular access to rehabilitation interventions
• Provide patient information on employment, driving, finances
	Management
	• Review care plan
	• Provide patient/carer education (consider expert patient programme)
	• Assistance and advice with medication
	• Drug therapy
	• Ensure regular access to rehabilitation interventions and regular review meetings with therapists:
	  • nurse specialist
	  • physiotherapist
	  • occupational therapist
	  • speech and language therapist
	  • dietician

Stage outcomes • Reduction in patient distress • Effective patient control	*Stage outcomes* • Symptom reduction • Treatment concordance • Maintenance and promotion of normal activities

Table 13.1 continued

Complex	Palliative
Aims	*Aims*
• Morbidity relief • Maintenance of function and self-care despite advancing disease • Assistance and adaptation of environment to promote daily living activities • Reassessment because of increasing disability and complexity • Symptom control	• Relief of symptoms and distress for patients and carers • Reassessment • Morbidity relief • Maintenance of dignity and function despite advancing disease • Avoidance of treatment-related problems • Symptom control • Re-evaluation of goals of therapy
Management	*Management*
• Support and explore areas of uncertainty • Advice on practical problems, management of non-motor symptoms and prevention of complications • Referral/liaison as in prior stages may be required + psychiatrist/community psychiatric nurse • Neurosurgery • Carer support	• Consider referral to specialist palliative care team • Advice on administration of medication • Progressive dopaminergic drug withdrawal • Analgesia • Sedation • Support and exploration of patient and carer uncertainties • Counselling/psychology/psychiatry • Communication and realistic planning • Realistic goals/forward planning • Bereavement issues • Prevention of complications • Urinary incontinence • Constipation • Motor fluctuations
Outcomes	
• Optimum symptom control • Minimalisation of disability • Treatment concordance • Reassess goals of therapy/care	
Non-motor symptoms	*Outcomes*
• Balance • Sleep disturbance • Anxiety • Urinary problems • Bowel problems • Dribbling saliva • Speech difficulties • Memory failure and confusional episodes	• Absence of distress • Maintenance of dignity • Symptom control

Source: MacMahon and Thomas (1998).

- providing appropriate information and education about the condition including practical advice, support and skills training for the person, family and carer;
- access to family counselling and sexual counselling if required;
- coordinated health and social care resources to support people in specially designed programmes to prevent them from developing secondary complications and help them maintain skills and abilities;
- providing adequate and appropriate social care support in and outside of the home that takes account of cognitive or behavioural problems that may affect a person's ability to care for themselves;
- interventions that focus on leisure and recreation;
- enabling individuals to do practical problem-solving and increasing their involvement in the local community to develop local support networks and access to housing-related support services.

In north Hampshire a Rehabilitation Action Plan was designed for people with acquired brain injury by a team that included individuals from the neurological

Table 13.2 Changes that suggest an acute illness in individuals with LTnC

Unexplained functional deterioration
- Reduced mobility falls
- Increased dependency on carers when previously independent

Increase in neurological impairment
- Increase in muscle spasticity and/or muscle spasms
- Reduction in muscle strength of a partially weak limb
- Worsening of dysphagia or dysarthria
- Increase in epileptic seizures

Change in cognitive function or behaviour
- Confusion states
- Sudden deterioration in pre-existing dementia
- Agitation, irritability, aggressive behaviour
- Hallucinations (in some conditions like Parkinson's disease)

Non-specific symptoms
- Sudden changes in blood pressure/heart rate
- Excessive fatigue, lethargy and sleepiness
- Urinary incontinence

Source: Bakheit (2006).

rehabilitation team, the national brain injury association Headway, Social Services, the Acute Trust and carers. The plan is an assessment record that focuses on goals for the brain-injured person, accessible by all agencies involved in care. It uses 13 functions of daily living to assess how the client is able to perform in these areas and, in conjunction with a key worker, the client and carer can together agree future goals for development. Functions of living include aspects such as ability to maintain a safe environment, communicating, eating and drinking, washing and dressing, mobilisation, working and playing, and expressing sexuality. The model for activities of daily living builds on work originally done by Nancy Roper in 1976 (Roper *et al.* 1980, 2000). These functions for living are reviewed on a regular basis. The plan is held by the patient so that anyone involved in care can have immediate access to the assessment and can see what the goals are and what progress has been made. The plan contains a record sheet of all professional contacts; action on this was considered essential by both the client and the carer (NHS Modernisation Agency 2005).

Personal health budgets in care delivery

As part of the Lord Darzi NHS Next Stage Review (DoH 2008), the government is piloting personal health budgets as a way of giving patients greater control over their own care delivery (DoH 2009a). This means that individuals will be able to decide which services they receive and the providers from which they receive those services. Personal budgets sit in a spectrum of policies of personalisation, which also includes choice and care planning. The main aim of introducing these budgets is to create a more personalised NHS. It may be that only a relatively small number of individuals with LTnCs would find that their needs lend themselves to a personal health budget, but their impact on the way care is delivered may be much wider for us in the future because this will take individuals away from care traditionally delivered by health and social care professionals. Personal budgets are really an extension of care planning.

The key differences are that the patient is aware of the resource implications for that care planning and will therefore have much greater control over how the budget for their care is spent. Potentially this could make a real difference to patients' lives by giving greater independence and control. Take, for example, the patient with multiple sclerosis (MS) who wants to go shopping or to work but has to wait at home for community services to get her up each day. With her personal budget she could purchase private support or a personal assistant who could do this for her. Some patients are already doing this, of course, but such personal budgets will empower people with LTnCs to have increasing degrees of user control over resources.

Family and carers in LTnC

Family and carers often play a huge role in supporting people with a LTnC. A survey carried out in Great Britain in 1995 and published by the Office for National Statistics (ONS 1998) has shown that there are 5.7 million carers in the UK providing unpaid care to an ill, frail or disabled family member, friend or partner. For some neurological conditions that typically affect younger people (MS or spinal cord injury) there is often a near-normal life expectancy post diagnosis so caring needs could easily span 40 to 50 years, which is a huge commitment. Carers often manage despite remarkably difficult circumstances but their caring role is undoubtedly at a huge cost to themselves. Family relationships and roles change in caring and cause severe financial and psychological pressure, particularly where there are cognitive, emotional and behavioural problems. The past two decades have seen increasing focus on the needs of carers but there are still many carers who may not be able to make informed choices about their own health and are frequently only identified as the result of a crisis occurring which results in their being no longer able or willing to continue caring.

Many carers take on the role willingly but it is vitally important that they are supported so that the caring relationship does not break down. The Carers Equal Opportunities Act 2004 (implemented from April 2005) has placed duty on councils to inform carers of their right to an assessment of their own needs. This should take account of their needs in respect of their caring role, wishes to undertake paid employment, and participation in training or leisure activities. All carers should have their own integrated health and social care assessment at diagnosis, and then throughout the course of the disease – for example, when the caring situation changes as the individual moves into a different stage of the disease. Carers should also have their own written care plan.

The support that is available to carers should be flexible and responsive, and be able to respond to issues such as emergency situations, where highly dependent support is required at short notice. There should also be appropriate support for children in the family and opportunities for respite breaks across a range of settings. Children who extend care should also be given special consideration.

Conclusion

This chapter has outlined some of the key elements to consider throughout the pathway of living with an LTnC. Many of the problems experienced by individuals, families and carers throughout the course of diseases can be overcome by the use of modern treatments and therapies, and by an understanding of the organisation and

Table 13.3 Useful contacts (including helpline support)

Epilepsy Action
Member-led epilepsy association raising awareness of epilepsy and providing support, advice and information to people living with the condition

www.epilepsyaction.org.uk
Helpline: Freephone 0808 8005050
Email: helpline@epilepsy.org.uk
Txt msg: 0779 780 5390 info

Parkinson's Disease Society
Charity funding research focusing on transforming lives. Nurses and specialist advisers on the helpline can offer support and advice. Also offer a wide range of information sheets, booklets and DVDs

www.parkinsons.org.uk
PDS National Office
215 Vauxhall Bridge Road
London SW1V 1EJ

Tel: 020 7931 8080
Helpline: 0808 8000303
Email: enquiries@parkinsons.org.uk

Multiple Sclerosis Society
UK charity for people affected by multiple sclerosis offering information and support. Over 350 local branches

www.mssociety.org.uk
MS Society
MS National Centre
372 Edgware Road
London NW2 6ND

Tel: 020 8438 0700

Motor Neurone Disease Association
UK charity working to help people with MND secure the care and support they need. Promote research into causes, treatment and a cure

www.mndassociation.org
Motor Neurone Disease Association
PO Box 246
Northampton NN1 2PR

Tel: 01604 250505
Email: enquiries@mndassociation.org

The Stroke Association
UK-wide charity funding research into prevention, treatment and better rehabilitation. Helps those following stroke and their families directly through its rehabilitation and support services

www.stroke.org.uk
Stroke Information Service
The Stroke Association
240 City Road
London EC1V 2PR

Tel: 0845 3033 100
E-mail: info@stroke.org.uk

Information Prescriptions (NHS)
Professionals, patients, service users or carers can access national information on a number of long-term conditions and create their own information prescriptions at NHS Choices

www.informationprescription.info
Rachel Porter
Project Manager – Information Prescriptions
Patient and Public Empowerment
Department of Health

Email: Rachel.Porter@dh.gsi.gov.uk
Tel: 0113 254 6503
NHS Choices
www.nhs.uk/yourhealth/pages/informationprescriptions.aspx

Centre for Policy and Ageing
Single Assessment Process
Common Assessment Framework

www.cpa.org.uk/sap/caf_more_about.html
Centre for Policy and Ageing
25–31 Ironmonger Row
London EC1V 3QP

Tel: 0207 5536500
Email: cpa@cpa.org.uk

NHS Choices
Individuals with an LTnC can get help and guidance with the care planning process and making their own care plan at NHS Choices

www.nhs.uk/YourHealth/Pages/CarePlans.aspx

management in local health, social and voluntary services. A multidisciplinary team in which a care manager or key worker plays a pivotal role in the areas of clinical management coordination, liaison and education will facilitate better care and is a key requirement for effective care, and for the individual and carer living with the LTnC nothing is more powerful than the right information, given at the right time in the right setting. The key principles contained in this chapter should guide these processes.

References

Bakheit, A.M.O. (2006) Recognition of Acute Illness in People with Chronic Neurological Disability. *Postgraduate Medical Journal*, 82, 267–269.

Blume, W., Luders, H., Mizrahi, E. *et al.* (2001) Glossary of Descriptive Terminology for Ictal Seminology: Report of the ILAE Task Force on Classification and Terminology. *Epilepsia*, 42(9), 121–208.

Office for National Statistics (1998) *Informal Carers in 1995*. London: ONS. Online. Available at: www.statistics.gov.uk/pdfdir/980514–1.htm (accessed 10 March 2009).

Department of Health (DoH) (2000) *The NHS Plan: A Plan for Investment, Plan for Reform*. London: The Stationery Office.

Department of Health (DoH) (2001a) *The Expert Patient Programme: A New Approach to Chronic Disease Management for the 21st Century*. London: Department of Health.

Department of Health (DoH) (2001b) *National Service Framework for Older People*. London: Department of Health.

Department of Health (DoH) (2005) *National Service Framework for Long Term Neurological Conditions*. London: Department of Health.

Department of Health (DoH) (2006) *Our Health, Our Care, Our Say: A New Direction for Community Services*. London: Department of Health.

Department of Health (DoH) (2007a) *National Stroke Strategy*. London: Department of Health.

Department of Health (DoH) (2007b) *Generic Choice Model for Long Term Conditions*. London: Department of Health.

Department of Health (DoH) (2007c) *Our NHS, Our Future – NHS Next Stage Review*. London: Department of Health.

Department of Health (DoH) (2008) *Information Prescriptions Evaluation. Final Report Recommendations and DH Responses. Gateway Reference 10316*. Online. Available at: www.dh.gov.uk/en/Healthcare/PatientChoice/BetterInformationChoicesHealth/Informationprescriptions/index.htm (accessed 5 March 2009).

Department of Health (DoH) (2009a) *High Quality Care for all Primary Care and Community Services. Personal Health Budgets: First Steps*. London: Department of Health.

Department of Health (DoH) (2009b) *Common Assessment Framework for Adults. A Consultation on Proposals to Improve Information Sharing Around Multi-disciplinary Assessment and Care Planning*. London: Department of Health.

Department of Health (DoH) (2009c) *Supporting People with Long Term Conditions: Commissioning Personalized Care Planning*. London: Department of Health.

Lorgi, K.R., Mazonson, P.D. and Holman, H.R. (1993) Evidence Suggesting that Health Education for Self Management in Patients with Chronic Arthritis has Sustained Health Benefits While Reducing Health Care Costs. *Arthritis and Rheumatism*, 36(4), 439–446.

MacMahon, D.G. and Thomas, S. (1998) Practical Approach to Quality of Life in Parkinson's Disease. *Journal of Neurology*, 245 (Suppl. 1), S19–S22.

MacMahon, D.G., Thomas, S. and Campbell, S. (1999) Validation of Pathways Paradigm for the Management of Parkinson's Disease. *Parkinsonism and Related Disorders*, 5, S53.

Matrix Research and Consultancy (2005) *NHS Modernisation Agency: Good Care Planning for People with Long Term Conditions: Updated Version.* London: Department of Health.

Multiple Sclerosis (MS) Society (2006) *MS Essentials 18: Complementary and Alternative Medicine.* Online. Available at: www.mssociety.org.uk/support_and_services/free_publications/ms_essentials_18.html (accessed 6 March 2009).

National Collaborating Centre for Chronic Conditions (2006) *Parkinson's Disease National Clinical Guideline for Diagnosis and Management in Primary and Secondary Care.* London: Royal College of Physicians.

National Institute for Health and Clinical Excellence (NICE) (2003) *Multiple Sclerosis. Management of Multiple Sclerosis in Primary and Secondary Care.* London: NICE.

National Institute for Health and Clinical Excellence (NICE) (2004) *The Epilepsies: The Diagnosis and Management of the Epilepsies in Adults and Children in Primary and Secondary Care.* London: NICE.

National Institute for Health and Clinical Excellence (NICE) (2006) *Parkinson's Disease: Diagnosis and Management in Primary and Secondary Care.* Online. Available at: www.nice.org.uk/CG035 (accessed 6 March 2009).

National Society for Epilepsy (2009) *What is Epilepsy?* Online. Available at: www.epilepsynse.org.uk/AboutEpilepsy/Whatisepilepsy (accessed 6 March 2009).

NHS Choices website (2009) *Your Guide to Long Term Conditions and Self Care.* Online. Available at: www.nhs.uk/yourhealth/Pages/Homepage.aspx (accessed 5 March 2009).

NHS Modernisation Agency (2005) *Action on Neurology. Improving Neurology Services – A Practical Guide.* London: Department of Health.

Office of National Statistics Health Statistics Quarterly (2001) *Winter 2001 Stroke Incidence and Risk Factors in a Population Based Cohort Study.* London: ONS.

Parkinson's Disease Society Primary Care Task Force (1998) *Parkinson's Aware in Primary Care. A Guide for Primary Care Teams Developed by the Primary Care Task Force for PDS (UK).* London: PDS.

Pfizer Limited (2007a) Own Health ® Birmingham: Successes and Learning from the First Year. Online. Available at: www.politics.co.uk/opinion-formers/press-releases/health/nhs-direct-joins-forces-with-pfizer-health-solutions-and-humana-europe-$1227918$366373.htm (accessed 10 March 2009).

Pfizer Limited (2007b) The Effect of a Telehealth Service on Patient Outcomes in the UK. Online. Available at: www.politics.co.uk/opinion-formers/press-releases/health/nhs-direct-joins-forces-with-pfizer-health-solutions-and-humana-europe-$1227918$366373.htm (accessed 10 March 2009).

Professor The Lord Darzi of Denham (2008a) *High Quality Care for All: NHS Next Stage Review Final Report.* London: HMSO.

Roper, N., Logan, W.W. and Tierney, A.J. (1980) *The Elements of Nursing.* Churchill Livingstone.

Roper, N., Logan, W.W. and Tierney, A.J. (2000) *The Roper–Logan–Tierney Model of Nursing: Based on Activities of Living.* Edinburgh: Elsevier Health Sciences.

Working in Partnership Programme (2009) *Self Care.* Online. Available at: www.wipp.nhs.uk/self-care (accessed 10 March 2009).

World Health Organisation (1997) Global Declaration of PD. Online. Available at: www.epda.eu.com/globalDeclaration/ (accessed 10 March 2009).

World Health Organisation (2009) *Epilepsy Aetiology Epidemiology and Prognosis Fact Sheet 999.* Geneva: WHO. Online. Available at: www.who.int/mediacentre/factsheets/fs999/en/index.html (accessed 10 March 2009).

14 Diabetes

Helen Robson and Zoë Berry

Introduction

Diabetes is a condition arising from a reduction in activity or secretion of insulin resulting in raised blood glucose. Persistently high blood glucose levels increase individual risk of vascular problems arising, including coronary artery disease, and eye and kidney damage (NICE 2004a). Owing to the potentially devastating impact of diabetes on individuals and their families (DoH 2001), standard one of the *National Service Framework for Diabetes* (NSFD) (DoH 2001) requires that health services have strategies in place to reduce the risk of the population developing type 2 diabetes, to reduce associated inequalities and to improve the diagnosis of diabetes. This chapter focuses on those people who have already received a diagnosis and for whom diabetes is a long-term condition.

Epidemiology

In the UK, diabetes affects approximately two million adults with another possible half a million people with undiagnosed diabetes, and these numbers are rising (DoH 2001). By far the most common form of diabetes is type 2 (between 85 per cent and 90 per cent of all people with diabetes) (DoH 2001; NICE 2004a, 2004b). Type 2 diabetes is most commonly diagnosed in people over the age of 40, but is increasingly being seen in younger people, reflecting the effects of sedentary life-style as part of the trend towards increasing globalisation and industrialisation affecting all societies (DoH 2001; Song 2008). The UK has one of the highest rates of type 1 diabetes in the world which also appears to be increasing, and it is estimated that over 12 per cent of all deaths in the 20- to 79-year age bracket are as a result of diabetes (DoH 2008).The incidence of diabetes rises with age with 5 per cent of people over the age of 65 in the UK having diabetes, and the rate in people over the age of 85 years is 20 per cent (DoH 2001). While more men are diagnosed with diabetes in England, more women die from the condition (DoH 2001).

In a recent study examining the prevalence and incidence of diabetes in the UK, Massó-González *et al.* (2009) found a rise of 74 per cent in new cases from 1997 to 2003. The study also found that the prevalence of diabetes in the UK population almost doubled between 1996 (2.8 per cent) and 2005 (4.3 per cent). While the rise in new cases remained similar over this period for type 1 diabetes, the vast majority of new cases were of type 2 diabetes, which is often associated with obesity. Indeed, between 1996 and 2005, the proportion of individuals newly diagnosed with type 2 diabetes who were obese increased from 46 per cent to 56 per cent. The risk of developing diabetes is around 20 times greater in the very obese (those with a body mass index of over 35) than in people with a body mass index of between 18 and 25 (DoH 2008).

People from black and minority ethnic groups and those from less affluent and socially excluded groups are particularly prone to develop type 2 diabetes and to suffer the consequences arising from complications (DoH 2001). The incidence, prevalence and progression of type 2 diabetes also vary by ethnic group (Erens *et al.* 1999). It has been recognised that in particular South Asians, Black Caribbeans and West Africans residing in the UK are at a higher risk of developing the disease (Riste *et al.* 2001). Death from complications is three and a half times higher among the poorest people in the UK than among the richest and socially excluded communities, including prisoners, refugees and asylum seekers, and people with learning disabilities or mental health problems may receive poorer quality and less timely care (DoH 2001).

Aetiology

Glucose is required by the body's cells for energy, especially the muscles. Insulin is secreted by special islets of beta cells in the pancreas and helps to transport glucose from the blood and maintains blood glucose levels within normal limits. All food carbohydrates are eventually changed into glucose and so carbohydrate metabolism will be affected by reduced sensitivity to insulin of cells or reduction in or lack of insulin secretion. The causes of disordered carbohydrate metabolism in type 1 and type 2 are not the same and each will be reviewed. The stages of diabetes range from individuals who maintain normal blood glucose levels on diet alone to those requiring insulin for survival. However, there is an age-related decline in glucose tolerance with fasting blood glucose levels increasing in older people (Reaven and Reaven 1980; Chen *et al.* 1985).

Type 1 diabetes

Type 1 accounts for between 5 and 15 per cent of all cases of diabetes, is due to the islet cells not secreting insulin and usually occurs in younger people with onset before age 40. It is now known that there is an auto-immune response that destroys the beta cells of the pancreas and can occur years before the onset of any symptoms (Eisenbarth 1986). It is not possible to prevent or reverse type 1 diabetes and there is a strong genetic susceptibility with increased risk where other family members have the disease. There is still little known about the possible triggers that activate the complex auto-immune responses leading to type 1 diabetes. Sometimes type 1 diabetes can develop later in life and can be difficult to differentiate from type 2 diabetes. However, in the onset of type 1 diabetes after childhood there is often weight loss and hyperglycaemia (high blood glucose) which is not affected by diet or tablets and leads to rapid progression to insulin therapy.

Type 2 diabetes

In this type of diabetes either the cells become less sensitive to insulin (insulin resistance) or the pancreas is not secreting enough (ß-cell dysfunction). An insulin-resistance syndrome (also called the metabolic syndrome) has been identified and is characterised by abdominal obesity, raised fasting glucose, raised blood pressure, and deranged lipid profile. This syndrome, not characteristic of type 1 diabetes, is believed to be triggered by both genetic and environmental factors such as excess calorie intake and reduced levels of physical activity, and is also associated with an inflammatory process in the body (Daniels *et al.* 2005; Donath *et al.* 2008).

Assessment and diagnoses

Standard two of the NSFD requires that services will develop, implement and monitor strategies to identify people who do not know they have diabetes. This can be achieved through an increased awareness of the signs and symptoms of diabetes and testing of those individuals who have not developed symptoms but who fall within one of the high-risk groups. Those experiencing symptoms such as passing large amounts of urine, increase in thirst due to fluid loss and possible weight loss should be assessed by a healthcare professional.

In type 1 diabetes, particularly in younger people, symptoms can develop very quickly, and a serious condition called diabetic ketoacidosis (DKA) may result in life-threatening coma. In type 2 diabetes the onset may be slower and symptoms such as tiredness, visual difficulties and recurrent yeast (Candida) infections in the mouth and genitals may present for many months before diagnosis. As the disease progresses, more serious complications can develop including staphylococcal infections (e.g. boils), weakness and numbness in hands and feet, impotence and circulatory problems (Kumar and Clark 2002).

Because the symptoms of diabetes may be easily missed or ignored, patients who are not diagnosed within five to ten years of the onset of the disease may present with symptoms of subsequent complications such as eye damage or problems with the peripheral circulation of the feet and legs. Diagnosis may be delayed if problems are attributed to increasing age or are misinterpreted. In some, diabetes may be discovered on routine screening although diagnosis is never made on the basis of urine testing ('dipstick') or a stick reading of a finger-prick blood glucose test alone.

Diagnosis of diabetes needs to be confirmed by an appropriately qualified healthcare professional. Blood glucose testing must be through accredited laboratory services, in line with World Health Organisation diagnostic criteria (WHO 1999, 2006) and diagnosis confirmed if classic symptoms are associated with:

- a random venous plasma glucose concentration ≥11.1 mmol/l
- a fasting plasma glucose concentration ≥7.0 mmol/l (whole blood ≥6.1 mmol/l)
- two-hour plasma glucose concentration ≥11.1 mmol/l two hours after 75 g anhydrous glucose in an oral glucose tolerance test (OGTT).

Where there are no symptoms, additional testing is needed with at least one additional glucose test result on another day with a value in the diabetic range essential for diagnosis, either fasting, from a random sample or from the two-hour post-glucose load. If the fasting or random values are not diagnostic the two-hour value should be used (Diabetes UK 2008).

Following testing, people may be identified as having either impaired glucose tolerance (IGT) or impaired fasting glycaemia (IFG) where there is difficulty maintaining blood glucose levels within the normal range but where levels are below the diabetic range. Impaired glucose tolerance is often associated with the metabolic syndrome. These individuals, however, do not have diabetes but are at increased risk of developing the disease as well as cardiovascular problems (DoH 2001). They should therefore be alerted to the symptoms of diabetes and screened regularly for early diagnosis and to assess risk of cardiovascular disease.

Clinical care

General care principles

The general principle of diabetes management will be to maintain optimal control of blood glucose levels. The views and preferences of individuals with diabetes should be integrated into their healthcare as the management of diabetes typically involves a considerable element of self-care. People with diabetes should have the opportunity to make informed decisions about their care and treatment in partnership with healthcare professionals (NICE 2004a, 2008a). An individual care plan should be developed and reviewed annually, modified according to changes in wishes, circumstances and medical findings (NICE 2004a), and should address:

- diabetes education including nutritional and dietary advice;
- insulin therapy and oral glucose control therapy as appropriate;
- self-monitoring;
- arterial risk factor surveillance and management;
- late complications surveillance and management;
- means and frequency of communication with the professional care team;
- follow-up consultations including next annual review.

Glucose control and therapy

Diabetes cannot be cured but treatment can be very successful. Good control of blood glucose and blood pressure can increase life expectancy and improve quality of life for people with both type 1 and type 2 diabetes (DoH 2001) by avoiding many of the complications explored later. In type 1 there is an absolute loss of insulin production and insulin therapy will be required by injections every day. In type 2 diabetes lifestyle changes including a healthier diet, weight loss and increased physical activity may help improve glucose levels significantly, but tablets and/or insulin may be necessary where good control is not achieved.

Insulin therapy

Although animal insulin from pigs and cows was used in the past, in the West manufactured biosynthetic human insulin is used. Analogue insulin, for example, has been modified by genetic engineering to give an altered form of natural insulin, but which has the same effect in the body in terms of glucose control. There are a variety of different preparations with some having a very rapid onset and short duration, and others having a much slower rate of absorption with longer action, and these are outlined in Table 14.1.

Because the liver normally releases glucose at a fairly steady rate there is a corresponding release of insulin to maintain normal blood glucose levels. At mealtimes there is an additional release or bolus of insulin for up to two hours after food is eaten to ensure that glucose in the bloodstream can be taken up into the cells of the body. For people with type 1 diabetes there may be multiple insulin injection (basal bolus) regimens or twice-daily pre-mixed or isophane insulin injections. For those with type 2 diabetes who require insulin this may also include a basal insulin regimen with oral hypoglycaemic agents.

Pre-filled insulin pens

Although special plastic insulin syringes are available, pre-filled injection pens offer a discreet and convenient method of delivering insulin, and cartridges are available for most varieties of insulin. Injection is usually into fat on the abdomen or thigh with accidental intramuscular injection leading to possible erratic blood glucose control. If there is little subcutaneous fat, then by 'pinching up' the skin at the injection site, using a short needle and inserting it at a 45-degree angle, problems can usually be avoided. Injections should be rotated within sites but not between sites for insulin given at one time of day and sites should be monitored regularly for problems (NICE 2004a). Needles should be disposed of carefully with sharp containers made available and local policy followed.

Continuous subcutaneous insulin infusion (CSII)

CSII (also called 'pump therapy') is recommended as a treatment option for adults and children 12 years and older with type I diabetes who meet specific criteria (NICE 2008b). Equipment utilises a small pump reservoir which is battery operated and where a computer chip allows the exact dose of insulin to be delivered with

Table 14.1 Different insulins used in treatment of diabetes

Type	Examples	Action
Short acting Used for mealtime glucose control	Rapid-acting insulin (analogues): • aspart (Novorapid) • lispro (Humalog) • glulisine (Apidra)	Onset 15 minutes Peak 1 hour Duration 3 to 4 hours
	Soluble (Unmodified) insulin (Actrapid)	Onset 30 minutes Peak 2 to 3 hours Duration 8 hours
Intermediate acting	Isophane (neutral protamine Hagedorn or NPH)	Onset – 2 to 4 hours Peak 6 to 7 hours Duration 20 hours
Long acting	Insulin analogues: • detemir insulin • glargine insulin	Onset 1 to 3 hours Duration 20 to 24 hours
Biphasic	Mix of rapid/short acting with intermediate	Available in different proportions

booster amounts possible to cover mealtimes. The pump is attached to a thin plastic tube which has a needle at the end allowing continuous insulin to be delivered under the skin 24 hours a day. Devices are becoming popular and increasingly user-friendly, allowing more flexible lifestyles while achieving good glucose control. However, while an insulin pump may offer better control with fewer hypoglycaemic episodes, where control is achieved with multiple daily injections there may be no additional benefit (Pickup and Renard 2008).

Anti-diabetic drugs in type 2 diabetes

In type 2 diabetes where diet and lifestyle change do not achieve effective blood glucose control, antidiabetic tablets will be prescribed (Table 14.2). Their action is to either increase insulin output by the pancreas, increase sensitivity of the cells to insulin or decrease absorption of carbohydrate from the intestine. Metformin is often the first-line drug for type 2 diabetes, particularly for overweight individuals, and offers some cardiovascular protection (NICE 2008a). A sulfonylurea may be another option where overweight is not a problem. Side-effects from the commonly used metformin or sulfonylureas are rare and often reduce after a while but where side-effects continue and are troublesome, treatment should be reviewed by a specialist health professional. The thiazolidinediones (glitazones) may cause significant fluid retention and are not suitable for people with heart failure. Sometimes tablets and insulin are required in type 2 diabetes but evidence suggests that the best option may be to commence insulin alone rather than in combination (Massi-Benedetti and Orsini-Federici 2008).

An alternative therapy for those with type 2 diabetes is *Exenatide* which increases insulin secretion, suppresses glucose production and slows gastric emptying. It may be useful in people with type 2 diabetes for whom tablets are failing to achieve good control particularly those who are obese, and it is associated with the prevention of weight gain. It is not administered via a traditional needle and syringe but is delivered subcutaneously in a pre-filled pen and may be an acceptable option where there is a needle phobia. It is required twice a day usually before meals. It is not suitable for those with type 1 diabetes as an alternative to insulin. Common side-effects are nausea, vomiting and diarrhoea which may subside over time and, when used with tablets, there may be increased risk of hypoglycaemia.

Table 14.2 Anti-diabetic drugs for type 2 diabetes

Drug group and action	Examples
Sulfonylureas – improve insulin secretion in pancreas	Tolbutamide, glipizide, gliclazide, glimepiride
Meglitinides – improve insulin secretion but very rapid action	Repaglinide, nateglinide
Biguanides – increase glucose transport across cell membrane	Metformin
Thiazolidinediones (glitazones) – increase sensitivity of cells to insulin	Pioglitazone, rosiglitazone
Alpha glucosidase inhibitors – decrease absorption of glucose from intestine	Acarbose

Non-concordance rates with therapy are high where, for example, there is weight gain with a specific drug or interference with daily routines and in many cases treatment is often suboptimal with poor monitoring following initial prescribing (Calvert *et al.* 2007).

Hypoglycaemia

Occasionally individuals with diabetes on drug or insulin therapy may experience periods when blood glucose levels fall below the normal level of between 4–7 mmols/l. Hypoglycaemia is one of the most feared complications of diabetes and understanding the physiological responses induced by hypoglycaemia and monitoring glycaemic therapy can help reduce its occurrence (Cryer 2004; Briscoe and Davis 2006). In hypoglycaemia a sequence of physiological events is triggered in the body and a number of anti-insulin hormones released to protect the brain, resulting in shakiness, anxiety, nervousness, palpitations, sweating, dry mouth, pallor, pupil dilation and tingling. Glucose deficiency to the brain may result in irritability, confusion, speech difficulty, headaches, fits, coma and even death (McAulay *et al.* 2001). Those with diabetes and their carers need to be made aware of the signs and symptoms and prompt management of hypoglycaemic attacks.

Supporting self-care

Education concerning self-monitoring of blood glucose, diet, physiological insulin replacement, medication and lifestyle are important to maintain good glycaemic control, avoid hypoglycaemia and prevent long-term complications (Briscoe and Davis 2006). Supporting self-care is an important strategy in the management of diabetes and the development of a collaborative working relationship can empower individuals with diabetes (DoH 2001). There are a number of elements which are important in supporting self-care. Adults with diabetes should be offered up-to-date information on the existence and means of contacting diabetes support groups (local and national), and the benefits of membership (NICE 2004a). Culturally appropriate, flexible education programmes and advice should be offered to all adults with diabetes and to those who may share responsibilities for caring.

The Year of Care programme is a project led by Diabetes UK and the National Diabetes Support Team (NHS Diabetes) in partnership with the Health Foundation and the Department of Health (Diabetes UK 2008). The Year of Care outlines the ongoing support that individuals can expect to receive in a year, and a major aim of the programme is to develop an infrastructure supporting self-management and collaborative care. Useful information on this programme is available online (Diabetes UK 2008; National Diabetes Support Team 2008).

Regular monitoring of blood glucose levels is critical for those on insulin therapy but may only be required on occasion for those on diet only or on tablets. Self-monitoring skills should be taught close to the time of diagnosis and initiation of insulin therapy. Structured assessment of self-monitoring skills, the quality and use made of the results obtained and the equipment used should be made annually. Self-monitoring skills should be reviewed as part of an annual review, or more frequently according to need, and reinforced where appropriate. Self-monitoring should be performed using meters and strips chosen by adults with diabetes to suit their needs, and usually with low blood requirements, fast analysis times and integral memories. Monitoring using sites other than the fingertips (often the forearm, using meters that require small volumes of blood and devices to obtain those small volumes) cannot be recommended as a routine alternative to conventional self-blood glucose monitoring (NICE 2004a).

Non-pharmacological management of diabetes

Nutritional information sensitive to individual needs and culture should be offered from the time of diagnosis of diabetes, and delivered by professionals with specific and approved training (NICE 2004a, 2008a). This may be complicated if the person is obese or underweight; has an eating disorder; has raised blood pressure or renal failure. Examples of structured programmes of education available are the DESMOND Collaborative 2005 for people with type 2 diabetes and the DAFNE evidenced-based structured education programme for those with type 1 diabetes (NICE 2003).

Emphasis should be placed on eating a healthy, balanced diet that is applicable to the general population and in particular high-fibre, low-glycaemic-index sources of carbohydrate in the diet, such as fruit, vegetables, wholegrains and pulses; include low-fat dairy products and oily fish; and control the intake of foods containing saturated and trans-fatty acids. The glycaemic index is a ranking of foods according to their direct effect on blood glucose levels (Jenkins *et al.* 1981). Dietary advice should be integrated with a personalised diabetes management plan, including other aspects of lifestyle modification, such as increasing physical activity and losing weight. Substitution of sucrose-containing foods for other carbohydrates in the meal plan is allowable, but care should be taken to avoid excess energy intake. Foods marketed specifically for people with diabetes are to be discouraged (NICE 2008a).

Adults with type 1 diabetes should be advised that physical activity can reduce their enhanced arterial risk in the medium and longer term (NICE 2004a). Those who choose to integrate increased physical activity into a healthier lifestyle should be offered information about appropriate intensity and frequency of physical activity and the possible effect of activity on blood glucose levels, namely that they are likely to fall over. As such, appropriate adjustments of insulin dosage and/or nutritional intake for exercise and post-exercise periods, and the next 24 hours, may be required.

Identification and management of complications

Standard 10 and 11 of the NSFD require local services to improve detection and management of long-term complications. Health services must develop, implement and monitor agreed protocols and systems of care to ensure that all people who develop long-term complications of diabetes receive timely, appropriate and effective investigation and treatment to reduce risk of disability and premature death. This involves carrying out risk assessment of the possibility of short-term complications such as diabetic ketoacidosis and hyperosmolar non-ketotic acidosis (HONK) and screening for long-term complications relating to the eyes (retinopathy), renal system (nephropathy), the feet and lower limbs, problems with the nervous system (neuropathy), cardiovascular issues and risks associated with the diabetic patient who is pregnant. We will now explore these issues.

Diabetic ketoacidosis (DKA)

DKA is a potentially life-threatening complication of diabetes affecting some people with type 1 and type 2 diabetes on insulin. Caused by a severe deficiency of insulin, consistently high blood glucose levels result, and because glucose cannot enter the cells the body breaks down fat leaving ketones (acid) as a waste product. Blood acidity is harmful to the body and may lead to shock, kidney failure, multiple organ failure and death if not promptly treated (NICE 2004a). DKA can develop during illness or infection (such as pneumonia), or following an event such as trauma or surgery where insulin requirement is usually increased, and advice from a health professional is important particularly where dietary intake is poor.

Early signs of DKA include thirst and passing large volumes of urine as the body attempts to flush the ketones out. Nausea and vomiting may follow with rapid, deep breathing (hyperventilation), confusion, drowsiness and possible coma. Deterioration can be rapid and treatment usually requires hospitalisation so that intravenous insulin can be given and salt and water losses replenished, together with treatment of any predisposing cause.

Hyperosmolar non-ketotic syndrome (HONK)

This is a serious condition with a death rate of 58 per cent affecting mainly older people with type 2 diabetes, and may be the first sign that they have diabetes. HONK may occur when blood glucose becomes very high (>40 mmols) and can develop over several weeks. Symptoms include passing urine frequently, increased thirst, confusion which may develop into drowsiness and possible coma as severe dehydration results (DoH 2001). Ketones are not usually present in the urine, hence the name, because there may still be some insulin production. Admission to hospital is required for fluid replacement and administration of insulin. Regular screening for diabetes in high-risk groups and awareness of this complication is therefore essential.

Retinopathy

Changes to small blood vessels in the eye can lead to a condition called diabetic retinopathy, a leading cause of blindness in people under the age of 60 years in industrialised countries (NICE 2003). Often there are no symptoms in the early stages or any pain, so screening is crucial. Eye screening performed at diagnosis needs to be repeated annually with any change in vision reported immediately for further investigation. Diabetic retinopathy can be treated with laser therapy but eye care includes good control of blood glucose levels and blood pressure. In 2003 the Diabetes National Service Framework Delivery Strategy set a target that by the end of 2007 100 per cent of people with diabetes would be offered screening for retinopathy (DoH 2003). However, screening attendance rates are significantly lower in younger people, in those with type 1 diabetes and in areas with the highest levels of deprivation (Millett and Dodhia 2006).

Nephropathy

Morbidity and mortality from kidney disease are important complications of diabetes. A higher proportion of individuals with type 1 diabetes compared with type 2 progress to nephropathy, primarily because death in the latter from cardiovascular causes is more common than death from renal failure (Dinneen and Gerstein 1997; Molitch 1997). High glucose levels affect the filtering ability of the kidneys, allowing albumin to pass through, and the presence of small amounts of albumin in the urine (microalbuminuria) is a signal of relatively early nephropathy and an independent risk factor for cardiovascular disease (Lin *et al.* 2008). In the early stages treatment such as the use of ACE inhibitors can prevent kidney disease from becoming worse.

Additional symptoms of renal impairment may include fatigue, sleep difficulties, poor appetite, gastric problems and poor concentration, and eventual renal failure may require dialysis and transplantation. Annual specialist monitoring is recommended so that early detection of kidney problems can be identified. Early referral to a nephrologist is required if progressive renal impairment is evident, particularly if hypertension is poorly controlled (see Chapter 20).

Neuropathy

Neuropathy is damage to nerves and in the case of diabetes can arise from long periods of uncontrolled high blood sugar. This may cause tingling or burning sensations in the extremities, with numbness potentially leading to skin damage and ulceration, possibly necessitating amputation. Autonomic neuropathy is a dysfunction of the involuntary nervous system which controls, for example, the bladder, digestive system, cardiovascular system and genitals. This can result in a variety of problems such as gastroparesis which can result in bloating and vomiting, and erratic blood glucose control as normal transit and digestion of food is affected. Some people may experience a loss of the warning signs of hypoglycaemia with potentially serious results.

Although poor blood sugar regulation can cause damage to the autonomic nervous system, it is important to remember that other causes may explain symptoms. Autonomic neuropathy may also be an underlying cause of bladder-emptying problems (NICE 2004a) and in men with diabetes erectile dysfunction (impotence) is a common problem with an increase in incidence with age. The causes are complex and the problem may occur, despite a normal level of desire for sex and normal levels of male hormones. Most antihypertensive medications commonly used for people with diabetes are associated with this problem as well as obesity, smoking and lack of exercise. Following normal outcomes for physical examination and biochemical investigation, drug treatment may be prescribed. Medication may be effective but timely referral to a urologist or psychologist may be necessary so that other possible management interventions may be considered.

Davies *et al.* (2006) estimates that in the UK 500,000 people have painful diabetic peripheral neuropathy with 80 per cent of these having moderate to severe pain which has been found to have a significant effect on quality of life (Benbow *et al.* 1998).

While NICE (2004a) recommends the initial use of simple analgesics (paracetamol, aspirin), in many instances of neuropathic pain these are ineffective and other treatments may need to be considered (see Chapter 6).

Foot care

Because diabetic neuropathy causes reduced sensation it may not always be possible to feel pain following injury to the lower limbs, and this can be particularly problematic if there are circulatory problems owing to delayed healing and increased risk of infection. Carers should encourage care of feet and nails through education and instruction, and local policy should be followed regarding foot care and chiropody services. Toe-nails should be carefully trimmed and, avoiding the cuticles, any sharp edges carefully filed. Feet should be kept clean using a mild soap and dried thoroughly. Regular inspection of the feet should be carried out for cracks and wounds, particularly where these may be hidden, and on no account should blisters be opened or the skin damaged in any way. Appropriate well-fitting footwear is important together with non-abrasive loose-fitting cotton socks that are changed daily. Special footwear such as insoles and shoe inserts may be required if there is a deformity, corns or previous ulcers (NICE 2004b).

Inspection of feet by carers on a daily basis is particularly important where individuals have physical disability, visual and cognitive impairment. Healthcare professionals should carefully screen for foot complications during visits and at least one-year intervals (NICE 2004b), noting:

- skin condition;
- shape and deformity of feet;
- appropriateness of shoes;
- impaired sensory nerve function;
- vascular supply (including peripheral pulses).

Where there is high risk of foot complications, further education and specific assessment of other contributory risk factors is important, and where there is ulceration, specialist podiatry care and antibiotics may be needed (NICE 2004b). In extreme cases, amputation of heavily ulcerated or ischaemic lower limbs may be necessary (DoH 2001).

Cardiovascular and arterial risk

Atherosclerosis is a major threat to the microvasculature for people with and without diabetes (Dokken 2008) and this process involves the build-up of lipids (fats) in the blood vessel walls. In diabetes, although microvascular diseases give rise to retinopathy and nephropathy in particular, the major macrovascular complications are coronary heart disease, stroke and peripheral vascular disease, all of which are grouped together as cardiovascular disease (Gostling 2006). For people with diabetes it is suggested that there is a two- to fourfold increase in risk for cardiovascular disease compared to those with normal glucose tolerance (Wood *et al.* 2005).

In diabetes elevated glucose levels contribute to a number of complex physiological changes leading to inflammatory changes in the walls of blood vessels. Indeed, diabetes has long been considered a state of chronic, low-level inflammation (Pickup *et al.* 1997). However, in type 2 diabetes the picture is more complicated as risk is further increased by the presence of the metabolic syndrome where there is obesity, impaired fasting glucose, hypertension, low high-density lipoprotein (HDL) cholesterol and elevated triglycerides (Meigs *et al.* 2007). HDL cholesterol offers some protection by helping to remove low-density lipoprotein (LDL) cholesterol from the circulation. Diabetes is also associated with an increase in clotting factors in the blood so that clot formation can contribute to myocardial infarction (heart attack) and cerebrovascular accident (stroke) (Dokken 2008).

Individual risk assessment in terms of possible cardiovascular complications is crucial in those with diabetes. Effective blood glucose control is essential and it has been shown that where type 2 diabetes is intensively managed (compared, for example, with diet alone), there is significant risk reduction for microvascular complications and some risk reduction for myocardial infarction (UKPDS (1998)).

Blood pressure monitoring will be required and treatment for hypertension commenced where there are sustained readings over 140/90 mmHg (Williams *et al.* 2004) to achieve a target of less than 130/80 mmHg in instances of kidney, eye or cerebrovascular damage and less than 140/80 mmHg in others (NICE 2008a). Review should be every six months where there is hypertension, otherwise annually. It is important to remember that in the presence of autonomic neuropathy postural hypotension may occur where there is a sudden fall in pressure on standing, possibly resulting in falls.

As abnormal lipid levels also predict risk of cardiovascular disease, these need to measured and cholesterol-lowering statins (e.g. simvastin) may be prescribed. To reduce the risk of clotting episodes an anti-thrombotic (anti-clotting) agent may be considered in those aged 50 years and over with a blood pressure greater than 145/90 mmHg, or in those under 50 years who have other significant cardiovascular risk factors. In such cases a daily low dose of aspirin (75 mg) or clopidogrel (if aspirin intolerance) may be offered (NICE 2008a).

Time should be taken to review lifestyle so that appropriate assistance can be given in helping individuals to address issues such as smoking cessation, weight reduction, diet modification and physical exercise.

Pregnancy and diabetes

Hormonal and metabolic changes occur as a natural part of pregnancy but where there is pre-existing diabetes mellitus these changes further complicate the regulation of glucose metabolism. In the non-diabetic woman, pregnancy stimulates an increased production of insulin to maintain normal glycaemic levels and an increase in pancreatic cells to meet demand. During the first three months of pregnancy an increase in fat stores enables fat to be released later to support the increased demands of the foetus for glucose and amino acids. Placental hormones exert an influence over the metabolic status of the woman and create a resistance to the effects of insulin for the duration of her pregnancy.

Reabsorption of glucose which occurs in the kidney may be compromised even when blood glucose levels are within normal limits, causing glycosuria (excess sugar in the urine), which in the non-pregnant state would be prevented by adequate insulin production. Consequently, urinalysis as an assessment of diabetic status during pregnancy is inadequate. In diabetes raised levels of blood sugar cause glucose to be irreversibly bound to haemoglobin, which at a high level is known to be associated with congenital abnormalities. The rate of congenital abnormalities in pregnancies of women with diabetes was found to be four to ten times higher than that of women without diabetes (Kapoor *et al.* 2007).

It is unsurprising therefore that given the above changes during pregnancy, the phenomenon of gestational diabetes exists. This is a diabetic state which occurs for the period of pregnancy only and resolves itself following delivery. However, as this is a time-limited condition, in that it exists for the gestational period only, rather than a long-term condition, the information here relates more specifically to those women who have a pre-existing diabetic state.

Maternal complications

In a woman with diabetes who is pregnant the levels of insulin required to maintain a healthy blood glucose level can be up to four times that of her usual dose. Women who have type 2 diabetes often require insulin at this time in their life, although requirements return to normal immediately following delivery. Type 1 diabetes generally becomes more unstable during pregnancy, with increased levels of insulin required as the pregnancy advances. The instability of the diabetic control can lead to increased risk of glycosuria and greater risk of urinary tract infections, and increased risk of ketoacidosis can lead to nausea and vomiting. Nausea and vomiting are often associated with symptoms of pregnancy independently of any diabetic concerns, but these 'natural' symptoms of raised hormone levels can severely hinder a woman's ability to maintain a stable glycaemic control, at a time when this is essential for her own and her foetus's health. Alongside this the relative instability of her diabetes would inevitably carry the increased risks associated with the complications of diabetes generally.

In 2007 the Confidential Enquiry into Maternal and Child Health (CEMACH) produced a report outlining the poorer outcomes associated with pregnancy and childbirth for those women who have diabetes mellitus (CEMACH 2007). As well as increased risk of congenital abnormalities, the report outlines a four to seven times greater risk of perinatal mortality, a fivefold increase in stillbirth and identifies that these babies were three times more likely to die within their first three months of life. Given these significant risks it is of particular concern that this same report found that fewer than 20 per cent of NHS Trusts in the UK had any multi-disciplinary pre-conception services.

Other complications associated with diabetes and pregnancy include increased risk of an excess of amniotic fluid (polyhydramnios) which is present in around 18 per cent of pregnancies in women with diabetes. This can lead to a premature rupture of the membranes due to over-distension of the uterus and subsequent increased risk of infection (Gilbert 2007). Pre-eclampsia is also more common in women with diabetes, and has been found to be two times the usual incidence, particularly where there has been poor diabetic control during the pregnancy and there also exists evidence of renal compromise (Howarth *et al.* 2007). Miscarriage and pre-term labour are more common in this group of women, and diabetic retinopathy can be severely exacerbated as a consequence of the pregnancy.

Where there has been poor diabetic control and maternal blood sugars have remained high, the foetal response is to produce insulin which causes increased protein and fat deposits. This leads to the development of a large baby (macrosomic) which has a much higher birth weight and increases the risk of birth trauma, obstructed labour and the need for health professionals to intervene providing an assisted delivery. This may lead the medical team and the mother towards the decision to undergo an elective Caesarean section at around 38 weeks in order to minimise this risk and the associated trauma to the mother, and this decision must be balanced against the increased risks of prematurity and respiratory distress syndrome. These complications are also found to be more prevalent in babies produced by women with diabetes, as it is believed that hyperglycaemia and hyperinsulinaemia cause a delay in the foetal lung maturity (Walkinshaw 2004). Where the diagnosis of a macrosomic foetus is made (i.e. birthweight over 4000 g) by ultrasound scanning, the woman should be informed of the risks and benefits of a vaginal birth, induced labour and Caesarean section, and encouraged to consider her options with her healthcare team. If a vaginal delivery is considered to be the most appropriate method, the woman's blood glucose levels will be closely monitored and controlled throughout the process, often utilising intravenous dextrose and an insulin infusion to aid the closely controlled levels.

In intrauterine life, the foetus will produce higher levels of insulin in response to the high maternal blood sugar levels. Following delivery the baby's pancreas continues to produce excess insulin initially, causing the baby to become hypoglycaemic. Early feeding within two hours of the birth is therefore essential to prevent hypoglycaemia, and the baby's blood sugar levels should be routinely monitored to assist early detection of any such difficulties.

Overall, a woman who has diabetes should be made aware that this will affect her maternity care from the outset. It will inevitably limit her ability to choose her own maternity care and direct her own birth plan, and there should be greater contact with health professionals and more rigorous antenatal care and treatment. Her concordance and partnership in this endeavour is the key to a successful outcome and therefore much care and thought must be given to collaboration which will result in increased perceived control over her choices and care generally.

A woman who has diabetes mellitus should be encouraged to plan a pregnancy and to ensure that she takes great care of her diabetic control in preparation for this. Foetal abnormalities can occur due to poor diabetic control in the very early days of the pregnancy, before the woman is aware that she has conceived. Care for the woman should be offered on a collaborative basis including midwives, obstetricians, dieticians and medics, but it is imperative that the woman herself is fully involved in her care and understands the condition in terms of monitoring of blood glucose levels, administration of insulin and in relation to diet. Treatment and care must take into account individual needs and preferences, and women should be encouraged to make informed decisions in partnership with healthcare professionals (NICE 2008c).

Partners and/or other family members should also be included in the educational aspects of caring for the woman's diabetic control during the pregnancy, to support her during periods of physical or emotional stress, or diabetic crisis, where it may be imperative that they take on the management of her blood sugar monitoring and controls. During the postnatal period again, the support and education of the woman and her partner or other family member is essential to minimise the risks associated with the transition of glycaemic control back to the non-pregnant status, and the considerations necessary where the woman chooses to breastfeed.

Mental ill-health and diabetes

There is evidence that people with mental health problems have elevated rates of diabetes (Gough and Peveler 2004). The prevalence of diabetes among people with schizophrenia, for example, is believed to be two to four times higher than the general population and elevated rates are also found among those with depression. The relationship between mental health problems and hyperglycaemia was first noted early in the twentieth century (Kohen 2004). Since that time successive studies have continued to identify that those with serious mental illness are one of the highest risk categories of the population for developing diabetes, although the mechanisms involved are complex.

Having diabetes doubles the risk of developing a depressive-type illness compared with that of the general population (Anderson *et al.* 2000) and this occurs commonly around the time of diagnosis and latterly as diabetic complications become apparent. However, despite depression being a relatively common health problem, it often goes undiagnosed and therefore untreated by health professionals (Panzarino 1998) (see Chapter 15). Symptoms of depression, for example, poor self-esteem, reduced motivation and energy levels and impaired cognitive functioning, can further compound the diabetes as the depressed person becomes less motivated, and less able to cope with diet and treatment which are integral to good control. The co-existence of depression and diabetes has been associated with poorer glycaemic control and an increase in complications associated with diabetes. There is a also a link with the generally poorer quality of lifestyles in those experiencing mental health problems and the increased risk of smoking and lack of exercise (Harris and Baraclough 1998). This, in turn, decreases quality of life and leads to both increased disability and use of healthcare services, leading ultimately towards an increased risk of mortality in this group (Egede *et al.* 2005). In short, the co-existence of diabetes and depression potentially creates the downward spiral effect of the diabetes being less well managed, complications becoming more pronounced, and this, in turn, has an adverse impact on the depressive illness (Ciechanowski *et al.* 2000).

Studies also suggest that depressive illness can adversely affect recovery from the physical complications associated with diabetes, such as infection, or myocardial infarction secondary to cardiovascular disease. Co-existence of physical and mental health problems results in worse prognosis and has a severe effect on quality of life generally. Health services responsible for the care of people with diabetes need to consider the mental state of those they treat which should be included in routine assessments. Where people with diabetes have underlying depression, the impact of their mental health status may be under-assessed or neglected by professionals in favour of pursuing assessment and questioning around their physical health (Wright 2006). Yet treatment for depression, in the form of antidepressant medication or psychological therapy, can have a beneficial outcome in regulating glycaemic control longer term, and therefore improve the prognosis and quality of life for this client group (Goldney *et al.* 2004).

Interaction between diabetes and schizophrenia is compounded by multiple risk factors. There are significantly high rates of first-degree relatives of people with schizophrenia with type 2 diabetes which suggests that diabetes and schizophrenia may have a genetic association (Mukherjee *et al.* 1989) with schizophrenia itself possibly being an independent risk factor for diabetes (Kohen 2004). This genetic predisposition in people with schizophrenia appears to be compounded by unhealthy lifestyles (Disability Rights Commission (DRC) 2006). For example, people with schizophrenia have a higher incidence of heavy smoking: 68 per cent of people with schizophrenia smoke more than 25 cigarettes a day compared with 11 per cent of the general population (Kelly and McCreadie 1999). Sedentary lifestyles and poor nutrition have also been found to be contributing factors to ill-health generally in those with a serious mental illness (DRC 2006) and are identified as risk factors associated with developing type 2 diabetes. McCreadie *et al.* (1998) found that people with schizophrenia are more likely to consume a diet which is higher in saturated fat and sugar, and low in fibre. This diet profile is also known to promote metabolic diseases in the general population, as well as adversely affecting the longer term health outcomes in schizophrenia (Peet 2004).

Psychiatric medication is often associated with weight gain, specifically antipsychotic medication, mood stabilisers and antidepressants (Robson and Gray 2009). Treatments for psychiatric symptoms may also increase risk of diabetes as there is evidence that antipsychotic medication has a clear association with impaired glucose metabolism, which is considered to be a pre-diabetic state. The implication of antipsychotic medication in the development of diabetes is, however, not a phenomenon specific to newer medications. Within a year of the introduction of chlorpromazine, the first wave of antipsychotic medication, in the 1950s, there was evidence that this drug had an adverse impact on glucose metabolism. In recent years, the newer, atypical antipsychotics have been implicated in the increase of diabetes among those with serious mental illness, particularly clozapine and olanzapine. This is, in part, due to the weight gain associated with these drugs, but also as a consequence of their effects on glucose regulation. Expert consensus, however, suggests that treatment with antipsychotic medication remains essential to stabilise the psychiatric condition prior to working with the client to stabilise their diabetic status.

Poorer diet is compounded by a lack of regular exercise in people with serious mental health problems and increases risk of obesity and therefore type 2 diabetes. The sedentary lifestyle of those in this group is often linked with the sedating effects of prescribed medication as well as aspects of depression or schizophrenia which can affect individual motivation to get active and lose weight. However, evidence from studies carried out by Faulkner and Sparkes (1999) demonstrated that where exercise was used as a therapeutic activity for people specifically with schizophrenia, over a ten-week period the benefits were truly holistic, improving aspects of social, physical and psychological health in the participants.

Therefore, where risk of diabetes is increased in those with schizophrenia, health promotion, advice and extra support will be needed if risk is to be reduced. In particular, a healthier eating plan should be encouraged, including specifically reducing fat and sugar content, and increasing intake of fruit, vegetables and foods with higher fibre content (DoH 2001). Smoking cessation advice should also be offered. Furthermore, active screening for diabetes and impaired glucose tolerance has found that 30 per cent of people with schizophrenia have one of these two conditions, although they were not aware of it. This often leads to people only seeking medical advice once complications of diabetes have become established and symptoms develop.

The clinical goal should be to identify diabetes in those with mental health problems as early as possible, preferably in the pre-diabetic stage, with a view to early intervention, thus slowing disease progression and avoiding complications (NICE 2002; Sainsbury Centre for Mental Health 2003). However, within the population of those with serious mental health problems there is evidence that although they have more frequent contact with health services, they were found to be less likely to report physical healthcare symptoms spontaneously, and some of their symptoms of mental illness, such as cognitive impairment, social isolation and suspicion, may contribute to their not seeking care or adhering to treatment (Phelan *et al.* 2001).

Table 14.3 Useful contacts (including helpline support)

Diabetes UK Organisation for people with diabetes, funding research, campaigning and helping people live with the condition Local support groups available	www.diabetes.org.uk/ Diabetes UK Central Office Macleod House, 10 Parkway, London NW1 7AA Tel: 020 7424 1000 Email: info@diabetes.org.uk
NHS Diabetes Works with and supports communities helping to design, commission and deliver safe, high-quality and personalised diabetes services	www.diabetes.nhs.uk/ NHS Diabetes 3rd Floor, St John's House 30 East Street Leicester LE1 6NB Tel: 0116 295 2045/2080 Email: enquiries@diabetes.nhs.uk
Insulin Dependent Diabetes Trust (IDDT) Charity organisation offering advice and support for people living with diabetes	www.iddtinternational.org Insulin Dependent Diabetes Trust PO Box 294 Northampton NN1 4XS Tel: 01604 622837 Email: enquiries@iddtinternational.org
Diabetes Research and Wellness Foundation A charity offering support, advice and education to people living with diabetes and the general public	www.drwf.org.uk/default.aspx Diabetes Research and Wellness Foundation 101–102 Northney Marina Hayling Island Hampshire PO11 0NH Tel: 023 92 637 808 Email:enquiries@drwf.org.uk
Juvenile Diabetes Research Foundation Charity which funds type 1 diabetes research. Provides information for families affected by diabetes.	www.jdrf.org.uk/default.asp?section=2&sectionTitle=Home Juvenile Diabetes Research Foundation 19 Angel Gate City Road London EC1V 2PT Tel: 020 7713 2030 Email:info@jdrf.org.uk

Conclusion

A recurring theme throughout this book is the empowerment of individuals with long-term conditions who are the real experts in care. In a number of areas professional and support groups interested in diabetes care have led the way in terms of developing appropriate strategies so that self-management becomes a reality. Effective glycaemic control and reduction in all risk factors contributing to both micro- and macrovascular complications is crucial. If this is to be achieved then individuals with diabetes need the skills, knowledge and motivation so that they are at the centre of all care activities and fully involved in decision-making. Carers need to be aware of the increased risk of diabetes in some groups and, with many different professionals involved in care, effective communication is important, with partnership and collaboration the central tenets in the care planning process.

References

Anderson, R.J., Lustman, P.J., Clouse, R.E. *et al.* (2000) Prevalence of Depression in Adults with Diabetes; A Systematic Review. *Diabetes,* 49 (suppl. 1), A64.

Benbow, S.J., Wallymahmed, M.E. and MacFarlane, I.A. (1998) Diabetic Peripheral Neuropathy and Quality of Life. *Quarterly Journal of Medicine,* 91, 733–737.

Briscoe, V.J. and Davis, S.N. (2006) Hypoglycemia in Type 1 and Type 2 Diabetes: Physiology, Pathophysiology, and Management. *Clinical Diabetes,* 24, 115–121.

Calvert, M.J., McManus, R.J. and Freemantle, N. (2007) The Management of People with Type 2 Diabetes with Hypoglycaemic Agents in Primary Care: Retrospective Cohort Study. *Family Practice,* 24, 224–229.

Chen, M., Bergman, R.N., Pacini, G. *et al.* (1985) Pathogenesis of Age-related Glucose Intolerance in Man: Insulin Resistance and Decreased Beta-cell Function. *Journal of Clinical Endocrinologial Metabolism,* 60, 13–20.

Ciechanowski, P.S., Katon, W.J. and Russo, J.E. (2000) Depression and Diabetes: Impact of Depressive Symptoms on Adherence, Function and Costs. *Archives of Internal Medicine,* 160 (21), 3278–3285.

Confidential Enquiry into Maternal and Child Health (CEMACH) (2007) Diabetes in Pregnancy: Are we Providing the Best Possible Care? Findings of a National Enquiry. Online. Available at: www.cemach.org.uk. (accessed 10 March 2009).

Cryer, P.E. (2004) Current Concepts: Diverse Causes of Hypoglycemia-associated Autonomic Failure in Diabetes. *New England Journal of Medicine,* 350, 2272–2279.

Daniels, S.R., Arnett, D.K., Eckel, R.H. *et al.* (2005) Overweight in Children and Adolescents: Pathophysiology, Consequences, Prevention, and Treatment. *Circulation,* 111, 1999–2012.

Davies, M., Brophy, S., Williams, R. *et al.* (2006) The Prevalence, Severity, and Impact of Painful Diabetic Peripheral Neuropathy in Type 2 Diabetes. *Diabetes Care,* 29, 1518–1522.

Department of Health (DoH) (2001) *National Service Framework for Diabetes: Standards.* Online. Available at: www.dh.gov.uk/en/Publicationsandstatistics/Publications/PublicationsPolicyAndGuidance/DH_4002951 (accessed 26 February 2009).

Department of Health (DoH) (2003) National Service Framework for Diabetes: Delivery Strategy. Online. Available at: www.dh.gov.uk/en/Publicationsandstatistics/Publications/PublicationsPolicyAndGuidance/DH_4003246 (accessed 4 April 2009).

Department of Health (DoH) (2008) Five Years On: Delivering the Diabetes National Service Framework. Online. Available at: www.dh.gov.uk/en/Publicationsandstatistics/Publications/PublicationsPolicyAndGuidance/DH_087123 (accessed 4 April 2009).

Diabetes UK (2008a) *Getting to Grips with the Year of Care: A Practical Guide.* London. Diabetes UK. Online. Available at: www.diabetes.org.uk/upload/Professionals/Year%20of%20Care/

Getting%20to%20Grips%20with%20the%20Year%20of%20Care%20A%20Practical%20 Guide.pdf (accessed 2 April 2009).

Diabetes UK (2008b) Care Recommendations. New Diagnostic Criteria for Diabetes. Online. Available at: www.diabetes.org.uk/en/About_us/Our_Views/Care_recommendations/New_ diagnostic_criteria_for_diabetes_/ (accessed 28 February 2009).

Dinneen, S.F. and Gerstein, H.C. (1997) The Association of Micro Albuminuria and Mortality in Non-insulin-dependent Diabetes Mellitus. *Archives of Internal Medicine*, 157, 1413–1418.

Disability Rights Commission (DRC) (2006) Equal Treatment: Closing the Gap. Interim Report. Online. Available at: http://83.137.212.42/sitearchive/DRC/PDF/mainreportpdf- healthFIpart1.pdf (accessed 4 March 2009).

Dokken, B. (2008) The Pathophysiology of Cardiovascular Disease and Diabetes: Beyond Blood Pressure and Lipids. *Diabetes Spectrum*, 21(3), 160–165.

Donath, M.Y., Schumann, D.M., Faulenbach, M. *et al.* (2008) Islet Inflammation in Type 2 Diabetes: From Metabolic Stress to Therapy. *Diabetes Care*, 31, S161–S164.

Egede, L.E., Nietert, P.J. and Zheng, D. (2005) Depression and All Cause and Coronary Heart Disease Mortality among Adults With and Without Diabetes. *Diabetes Care* 28(6), 1339–1345.

Eisenbarth, G.S. (1986) Type I Diabetes Mellitus: A Chronic Autoimmune Disease. *New England Journal of Medicine*, 314, 1360–1368.

Erens, B., Primatesta, P. and Prior, G. (eds) (1999) *Health Survey for England: The Health of Ethnic Minority Groups*. London: HMSO.

Faulkner, G. and Sparkes, A. (1999) Exercise Therapy for Schizophrenia: An Ethnographic Study. *Journal of Sport and Exercise*, 21, 39–51.

Gilbert, E. (2007) *Manual of High Risk Pregnancy and Delivery* (4th edn). Missouri: Mosby.

Goldney, R.D., Phillips, P.J. and Fisher, L.J. *et al.* (2004) Diabetes, Depression and Quality of Life: A Population Study. *Diabetes Care*, 27(5), 1066–1070.

Gostling, C. (2006) Diabetes as a Cardiovascular Disease: Addressing the Risk. *British Journal of Cardiac Nursing*, 1(3), 117–125.

Gough, S. and Peveler, R. (2004) Diabetes and its Prevention: Pragmatic Solutions for People with Schizophrenia. *British Journal of Psychiatry*, 184 (suppl. 47), s106–s111.

Harris, E. and Barraclough, B. (1998) Excess Mortality of Mental Disorder. *British Journal of Psychiatry*, 173, 11–53.

Howarth, C., Gazis, A. and James, D. (2007) Associations of Type 1 Diabetes Mellitus, Mater- nal Vascular Disease and Complications of Pregnancy. *Diabetic Medicine*, 24, 1229–1234.

Jenkins, D.J.A., Baldwin, J.M., Barker, H. *et al.* (1981) Glycaemic Index of Foods. A Physiologi- cal Basis for Carbohydrate Exchange. *American Journal of Clinical Nutrition*, 34, 362–366.

Kapoor, N., Sankaran, S., Hyer, S. *et al.* (2007) Diabetes in Pregnancy: A Review of the Current Evidence. *Current Opinion in Obstetrics and Gynaecology*, 19, 586–590.

Kelly, C. and McCreadie, R.G. (1999) Smoking Habits, Current Symptoms and Premorbid Characteristics of Schizophrenia Patients in Nithsdale, Scotland. *American Journal of Psychia- try*, 156, 1751–1757.

Kohen, D. (2004) Diabetes Mellitus and Schizophrenia: Historical Perspective. *British Journal of Psychiatry*, 184 (suppl. 47), s64–s66.

Kumar, P. and Clark, M. (2002) Diabetes Mellitus and Other Disorders of Metabolism. In *Clin- ical Medicine* (5th edn, pp. 1069–1121). London: W.B. Saunders.

Lin, J., Glynn, R.J., Rifai, N. *et al.* (2008) Inflammation and Progressive Nephropathy in Type 1 Diabetes in the Diabetes Control and Complications Trial. *Diabetes Care*, 31, 2338–2343.

Massi-Benedetti, M. and Orsini-Federici, M. (2008) Treatment of Type 2 Diabetes with Com- bined Therapy: What are the Pros and Cons? *Diabetes Care*, 31, S131–S135.

Massó-González, E., Johansson, S., Wallander, M. *et al.* (2009) Trends in the Prevalence and Incidence of Diabetes in the UK – 1996 to 2005. *Journal of Epidemiological Community Health*, 63, 332–336.

McAulay, V., Deary, I.J. and Frier, B.M. (2001) Symptoms of Hypoglycaemia in People with Diabetes. *Diabetic Medicine*, 18, 690–705.

McCreadie, R., McDonald, E., Blacklock, C. *et al.* (1998) Dietary Intake of Schizophrenic Patients in Nithsdale, Scotland: A Case Control Study. *British Medical Journal*, 317, 784–785.

Meigs, J.B., Rutter, M.K., Sullivan, L.M. *et al.* (2007) Impact of Insulin Resistance on Risk of Type 2 Diabetes and Cardiovascular Disease in People with Metabolic Syndrome. *Diabetes Care*, 30, 1219–1225.

Millett, C. and Dodhia, H. (2006) Diabetes Retinopathy Screening: Audit of Equity in Participation and Selected Outcomes in South East London. *Journal of Medical Screening*, 13, 152–155.

Molitch, M.E. (1997) Management of Early Diabetic Nephropathy. *American Journal of Medicine*, 102, 392–398.

Mukherjee, S., Schnur, D.B. and Reddy, R. (1989) Family History of Type 2 Diabetes in Schizophrenic Patients. *Lancet*, I, 495.

National Diabetes Support Team (2008) Partners in Care: A Guide to Implement a Care Planning Approach to Diabetes Care. NHS Diabetes. Online. Available at: www.diabetes.nhs.uk/news-1/Partners%20in%20Care.pdf (accessed 4 April 2009).

National Institute for Health and Clinical Excellence (NICE) (2002) *Schizophrenia: Core Interventions in the Treatment and Management of Schizophrenia in Primary and Secondary Care. Clinical Practice Guideline No. 28.* Online. Available HTTP: www.guidance.nice.org.uk/CG1/guidance/pdf/English (accessed 4 March 2009).

National Institute for Health and Clinical Excellence (NICE) (2003) *Guidance on the Use of Patient-education Models for Diabetes. Technology Appraisal No. 60.* London: NICE.

National Institute for Health and Clinical Excellence (NICE) (2004a) Type 1 Diabetes in Children, Young People and Adults: NICE Guideline. Online. Available at: www.nice.org.uk/nicemedia/pdf/CG015NICEguideline.pdf (accessed 4 April 2009).

National Institute for Health and Clinical Excellence (NICE) (2004b) Type 2 Diabetes Prevention and Management of Foot Problems. Online. Available at: www.nice.org.uk/nicemedia/pdf/CG010NICEguideline.pdf (accessed 4 April 2009).

National Institute for Health and Clinical Excellence (NICE) (2008a) Diabetes – Type 2 (Update): Full Guideline. Online. Available at: www.nice.org.uk/guidance/index.jsp?action=download&o=40803 (accessed 4 April 2009).

National Institute for Health and Clinical Excellence (NICE) (2008b) Continuous Subcutaneous Insulin Function for the Treatment of Diabetes Mellitus (Review of Technology Appraisal Guidance 57). Online. Available at: www.nice.org.uk/nicemedia/pdf/TA151QuickRefGuide.pdf (accessed 2 March 2009).

National Institute for Health and Clinical Excellence (NICE) (2008c) *Diabetes in Pregnancy: Management of Diabetes and its Complications from Pre-conception to the Postnatal Period.* London: NICE.

National Institute for Health and Clinical Excellence (NICE) (2008c) *Diabetes in Pregnancy.* Online. Available at: www.nice.org.uk/Guidance/CG63/NiceGuidance/pdf/English (accessed 4 April 2009).

Panzarino, P.J. (1998) The Costs of Depression: Direct and Indirect, Treatment Versus Nontreatment. *Journal of Clinical Psychiatry*, 59 (suppl. 20), 11–14.

Peet, M. (2004) Diet, Diabetes and Schizophrenia: Review and Hypothesis. *British Journal of Psychiatry*, 184 (suppl. 47), s102–s105.

Phelan, M., Stradins, L. and Morrison, S. (2001) Physical Health of People with Severe Mental Illness. *British Medical Journal*, 322, 443–444.

Pickup, J.C. and Renard, E. (2008) Long-acting Insulin Analogues Versus Insulin Pump Therapy for the Treatment of Type 1 and Type 2 Diabetes. *Diabetes Care*, 31, S140–S145.

Pickup, J.C., Mattock, M.B., Chusney, G.D. *et al.* (1997) NIDDM as a Disease of the Innate Immune System: Association of Acute-Phase Reactants and Interleukin-6 with Metabolic Syndrome X. *Diabetologica*, 40, 1286–1292.

Reaven, G.M. and Reaven, E.P. (1980) Effects of Age on Various Aspects of Glucose and Insulin Metabolism. *Molecular Cell Biochemistry*, 31, 37–47.

Riste, L., Khan, F. and Cruickshank, K. (2001) High Prevalence of Type 2 Diabetes in all Ethnic Groups, Including Europeans, in a British Inner City: Relative Poverty, History, Inactivity or 21st Century Europe? *Diabetes Care*, 24(8), 1377–1383.

Robson, D. and Gray, R. (2009) Physical Health and Severe Mental Illness. In Newell, R. and Gournay, K. (eds) *Mental Health Nursing: An Evidence Based Approach* (2nd edn). London: Elsevier.

Sainsbury Centre for Mental Health (2003) *The Primary Care Guide to Managing Severe Mental Illness*. London: SCMH.

Song, H. (2008) Review: Early Onset Type 2 Diabetes Mellitus: A Condition with Elevated Cardiovascular Risk. *The British Journal of Diabetes and Vascular Disease*, 8(2), 61–65.

UK Prospective Diabetes Study Group (UK PDS) (1998) Intensive Blood Glucose Control with Sulphonylureas or Insulin Compared with Conventional Treatment and Risk of Complications in People with Type 2 Diabetes (UKPDS 33). *Lancet*, 352, 837–853.

Walkinshaw, S. (2004) Type 1 and Type 2 Diabetes and Pregnancy. *Current Obstetrics and Gynaecology*, 14, 375.

Williams, B., Poulter, N., Brown, M. *et al.* (2004) Guidelines for Management of Hypertension: Report of the Fourth Working Party of the British Hypertension Society, 2004 – BHS IV. *Journal of Human Hypertension*, 18, 139–185.

Wood, D., Wray, R. and Poulter, N. (2005) JBS 2: The Joint British Society's Guidelines on Prevention of Cardiovascular Disease. *Heart*, 91 (suppl.), 1–52.

World Health Organisation (1999) *Definition, Diagnosis and Classification of Diabetes Mellitus and its Complications. Report of a WHO Consultation*. Geneva: WHO.

World Health Organisation (2006) *Definition and Diagnosis of Diabetes Mellitus and Intermediate Hyperglycaemia. Report of a WHO/IDF Consultation*. Geneva: WHO.

Wright, J. (2006) *The G.P. and Mental Health in New Ways of Working in Mental Health*. London: Dooher J. Quay Books.

15 Mental health

Steve Trenoweth and Wasiim Allymamod

Introduction

Mental health problems are common in adults (CSIP 2006a). It is estimated that at any one time one in six people may have a mental health problem (DoH 1999). Such problems can be very disabling and potentially have both long- and short-term impacts on the individual and their families. Half of all mental health problems last longer than a year (Jenkins *et al.* 2008). The total economic cost in England alone has been estimated at between £49 and £77 billion through costs of care and losses to the economy (SCMH 2003), while it has been estimated that GPs spend one-third of their time on responding to mental health issues (ODPM 2004). However, mental health problems can often go unrecognised and untreated which may subsequently persist and escalate into seriousness, undermining the quality of an individual's life, increasing suffering, disability (both physical and mental) and premature mortality. Moreover, left untreated, mental ill-health can lead to problems which can be transmitted from one generation to the next (Jenkins *et al.* 2008).

Aetiology of mental health problems

The precise aetiology of mental health problems is unknown and the subject of much debate, but risk factors for particular individuals are likely to be interactive and multi-factorial, comprising social, psychological, biological and environmental issues (Table 15.1 summarises issues which are commonly cited as being implicated in mental distress).

There are several paradigms which seek to account for the development of mental health problems. The biological view sees the development of mental illness as stemming from abnormalities or disease processes within the body. Limosin *et al.* (2003), for example, found that significantly more people diagnosed with schizophrenia had been exposed to the influenza virus during the fifth month of pregnancy, suggesting that prenatal influenza infection is a risk factor for schizophrenia in adult life. Other support for the biological view includes:

- dysfunctional levels of neurotransmitters (chemical messengers responsible for relaying nerve impulses, such as serotonin or dopamine);
- different functional activation of parts of the brain (such as low activation/ glucose metabolism in the prefrontal cortex of people with schizophrenia, especially those with negative symptoms of apathy and a lack of volition);

Table 15.1 Risk factors for mental ill-health

Social
- Bereavement (loss of a close friend, relative or spouse)
- Job loss, redundancy or threat of redundancy
- Relationship difficulties, separation or divorce
- Family stress and parenting styles
- Real or threatened trauma and abuse
- Chronic social adversity (arising from, for example, unemployment, poverty)
- Lack of social support and isolation
- Lack of a sense of belonging
- Stigma, social exclusion and a lack of community acceptance and tolerance

Psychological
- Poor resilience
- Low self-esteem
- Poor coping with stress (such as ambient, background stress as well as specific life event stressors)
- Negative views of self, the world and the future
- Learned behaviour (conditioned responses to stimuli)

Biological risk factors/physical
- Poor nutrition (in general and/or lack of specific nutrients)
- Infection (for example, prenatal influenza)
- Anatomical/physiological issues
- Physical trauma to brain
- Physical health problems/illness
- Genetic/hereditary factors

Environmental
- Poor or unstable living environments and housing
- Unemployment, poor employment prospects and opportunities
- Financial difficulties
- Lack of citizenship and participation in society
- Catastrophic, traumatic, stressful or adverse circumstances
- Urbanisation and overcrowding
- Poor education and training
- Poor access to supportive healthcare and community resources
- Socio-economic deprivation

- apparent links between diet and mental health (see Nutrition and mental health below);
- anatomical and structural differences in the brains of people with mental illness (such as enlarged ventricles in schizophrenia).

The biological approach also points to the fact that there appear to be similar rates of mental illness in identical twins raised apart, suggestive of a high genetic heritability (Kring *et al.* 2007; Butcher *et al.* 2008). However, the biological view does not account for the timing or severity of symptoms (Kring *et al.* 2007). Nor is it clear if such neurobiological changes are the cause or consequence of mental ill-health. Furthermore, the National Institute for Health and Clinical Excellence (NICE) has been unable to recommend the use of structural neuroimaging (such as Magnetic Resonance Imaging (MRI) or Computed Axial Tomography (CT) scanning) as a cost-effective diagnostic test for first-episode psychosis in young adults (NICE 2008), as biological (organic) changes within the brain are not likely to be detectable within this age group.

There are, of course, other paradigms which seek to account for the development of mental distress, including:

- social and sociocultural models which cite social inequalities, deprivation, prejudice, discrimination, industrialisation and a lack of social support as a precursor to ill-health (e.g. Illich 2001);
- cognitive models which suggest that mental distress arises from distortions and biases in one's thinking (Beck 1967) and a pessimistic attributional style (Abramson *et al.* 1989);
- behavioural models which suggest that maladaptive or unhelpful behaviour underpinning mental distress is acquired through learning;
- ecological models (Zubin and Spring 1977) point to environmental factors, such as socio-economic deprivation, overcrowding and social disorganisation as a precursor to the development of mental illness;
- stress models which suggest that mental distress occurs as a result of an inability to respond and adjust to environmental demands (Butcher *et al.* 2008).

It is most likely, however, that the aetiology of mental distress and psychiatric ill-health involves a complex interplay between all or many of these factors at any one time (Gallop and Reynolds 2004). As such, one may conclude that a paradigmatic synergy is required to fully understand the aetiology of mental distress and that neurobiological factors may lead to a predisposition to mental ill-health, but the risk is mediated by stressors and triggers within the environmental context (Zubin and Spring 1977).

It follows, therefore, that the response to mental distress must also be complex and multi-factorial. In 1999, the *National Service Framework for Mental Health* (*NSFMH*) (DoH 1999) introduced what it saw as a 'new vision for mental health'. Its ambition was to set national standards for mental healthcare which would improve quality while achieving realistic and systematic change. Mental healthcare, it envisioned, would be based on 'best' available evidence, guided by values and principles, delivered by appropriately trained, updated and regulated professionals, and standards rigorously monitored. In turn, 'modernised' mental health services would be integrated (from primary care to highly specialised services and across services which provide healthcare and social services), and be safe (affording protection to the public and effective care to those with perceived mental health needs), sound (ensuring access to the full range of services) and supportive (building healthier communities by working with service users, their carers and families). This chapter uses the standards established by the *NSFMH* as its framework for exploring the assessment, care and treatment of people with persistent mental health problems, and in particular will use depression as an example of such modernised care.

Mental health promotion

Standard one of the *National Service Framework for Mental Health* requires that health and social services should:

- promote mental health for all, working with individuals and communities;
- combat discrimination against individuals and groups with mental health problems and promote their social inclusion.

There is evidence that people with existing serious and enduring mental health problems are stigmatised and discriminated against (ODPM 2004) because of their psychiatric diagnosis and symptoms of mental ill-health (DoH 1999; Future Vision Coalition 2008) despite the Disability Discrimination Act (1995) which outlaws discrimination against disabled people. In turn, such people often find that they are socially excluded from communities (Future Vision Coalition 2008). Such exclusion may contribute to the development of mental ill-health and to relapse among those with existing issues (Jenkins *et al.* 2008), and thus represents a significant barrier to their engagement and participation in communities (ODPM 2004). Helping people to claim their rights of citizenship is an important part of contemporary mental health policy (DoH 2001a) and a potentially significant contribution to the maintenance of good mental health and the promotion of recovery.

Promoting recovery

The overall aim of contemporary mental health services is to promote recovery and to help people experiencing mental ill-health get back to living an ordinary life as soon as possible (NICE 2002a). Central to this endeavour is the creation of a hopeful, optimistic, positive approach to the care and treatment of all people who use mental health services (DoH 2001a) who are assisted to live a life of personal value and worth (NIMHE 2005; Jenkins *et al.* 2008). In order to achieve these aims, contemporary policy emphasises:

* the importance of working in partnership within the context of a supportive and empathic professional relationship;
* shared decision-making between mental health service users and healthcare professionals;
* treatments which reflect the service user's preference based on an informed discussion and past experience of treatment;
* responsiveness to previous treatments; a recognition that individuals have personal strengths and assets as well as problems and needs;
* an acknowledgement of expertise which both parties can bring to the health and social care process (DoH 2001b);
* support to deal with the future and cope with challenges that mental health problems may bring (NICE 2002a, 2007a, 2007b; Future Vision Coalition 2008).

Contemporary health services are often seen to be medically dominated and biologically oriented in terms of diagnosis and treatment of mental 'illnesses'. 'Recovery' in this sense is often construed in medical terms – that is, recovery is only 'achieved' if one is symptom free, or to put this another way, when one is 'cured' (Matthews 2008). Many people with mental health problems have, in this sense, not been expected to 'recover'. There have been, however, calls for a more holistic approach which recognises psychological, social, emotional, spiritual as well as biological factors in the aetiology, trajectory, treatment, care and even prognosis of mental distress (NIMHE 2005; Future Vision Coalition 2008). Recently, for example, the Future Vision Coalition (2008) (a coalition of organisations including MIND, Sainsbury Centre for Mental Health, Rethink and the Mental Health Foundation among others) published a paper 'A New Vision for Mental Health' designed to provoke debate about the current mental health policy. It suggests that to realise the approach envisioned by the *National Service Framework for Mental Health* a movement away from an emphasis on diagnosing and treating mental 'disease' and illness to the promotion of positive mental health is required. It suggests that the work of mental health services should be on assisting people with mental health problems to increase their self-determination and self-management by the development of resilience, self-esteem, optimism, a sense of mastery and control, and the ability to develop and maintain satisfying relationships. Such an approach is consistent with the promotion of positive mental *health* (as opposed to responding to mental *illness*) and with supporting the development of subjective well-being (Seligman 2008).

Nutrition and mental health

The role of diet in the care and treatment of people with mental health problems has recently come under scrutiny. There appears to be much evidence of an association between deficiencies between certain nutrients and mental ill-health. For example, a deficiency of vitamin B9 (folic acid) and vitamin B3 (niaicin) has been linked with depression; a deficiency in vitamin B12 may be linked to psychotic disorders; a lack of vitamin B1 (thiamine) is a possible precursor to Korsakoff's Syndrome (symptoms include severe memory loss, confusion, apathy and repetitive behaviour arising from brain damage following long-term excessive alcohol use); and vitamin B9 appears to reduce the risk of dementia (Goodwin *et al.* 1983; Godfrey *et al.* 1990; Gold 1996; Abayomi and Hackett 2004). However, a direct causal link between nutrition, diet and mental illness has yet to be established (Abayomi and Hackett 2004).

In *Feeding Minds*, the Mental Health Foundation draws attention to changes in food consumption over the last 60 years, such as decline in eating vegetables and foods rich in omega-3 fatty acids (such as oily fish, walnuts and flax seeds) and that this has had a possible impact on mental health and may play a contributory role in the development and persistence of depression, schizophrenia and Alzheimer's disease (Mental Health Foundation 2006). The report suggests that a sense of well-being can be promoted by ensuring that a diet provides adequate amounts of complex carbohydrates, essential fats, amino acids, vitamins and minerals and water. More information about the links between food and mental health issues, including 'mood-enhancing' recipes, may be found on Mind's website: www.mind.org.uk/foodandmood/.

Social and economic circumstances

Employment is an important part of our lives not least in terms of the potential for social contacts, meaningful activities and financial rewards. For people with long-term mental health problems, being in paid employment can play a key role in tackling social exclusion and many people with such problems do wish to work (ODPM 2004). However, the 2002 Office for National Statistics (ONS) survey of people with neurotic and psychotic disorders, alcohol use and dependence and drug dependence found that 33 per cent of people in this group were unemployed or economically inactive (ONS 2002). For the subgroup of people with psychotic disorders (for example, those with a diagnosis of schizophrenia) this rate was 72 per cent and of this 60 per cent were in a household with an income of less than £300 per week (compared with 27 per cent of people with no diagnosed mental disorder). Indeed, finding and securing employment can be particularly challenging for people with long-term mental ill-health (Future Vision Coalition 2008) not least because people with such mental health problems are more likely to have left school at age 16 with no qualifications (ONS 2002). A key policy initiative for mental health and social care services, therefore, is the assessment of an individual's occupational status, potential and willingness to work and to assist in the development of employment and training opportunities (NICE 2002a).

The ONS (2002) report also found that people with mental health problems often experienced a severe perceived lack of social support. They are more likely to be single, divorced or separated and are far more likely to be living in rented accommodation with a perceived lack of space (ONS 2002). The five main concerns of people in the ONS (2002) survey were:

- financial problems (20 per cent of the sample);
- lease or contract running out (18 per cent);
- illness (14 per cent);
- domestic problems (8 per cent);
- problems with landlord/agent (8 per cent).

Such social and economic factors are likely to have a detrimental effect on the promotion of positive mental health, placing an onus upon health and social care services to offer practical support in relation to dealing with financial, accommodation and relationship difficulties.

Primary care and access to services

Assessment

Standard two of the *NSFMH* requires that any person who contacts their primary healthcare team with a common mental health problem should:

- have their mental health needs identified and assessed;
- be offered effective treatments, including referral to specialist services for further assessment, treatment and care if they require it.

As such, emphasis in contemporary mental healthcare should be placed on appropriate assessments and referral, along with access to treatment and care which is known to work – that is, based on best available evidence. The National Institute for Health and Clinical Excellence (NICE) has published guidance on mental health treatments based on extensive reviews of research and other materials. Such reviews recognise the central role that primary care services play in the assessment and treatment of people with mental health problems (DoH 1999). However, the emphasis that NICE guidelines have placed on quantitative research inevitably means a bias towards interventions which are amenable to the quantification and measurement of clinical outcomes, such as medication and cognitive behavioural therapy (CBT) (the umbrella term for psychotherapies which are highly structured, problem-oriented and prescriptive) (NICE 2006). It is not possible to examine the various different presentations of mental ill-health or all the various treatment options available, so in this section we will look at the general principles which should be undertaken for the care of an individual with mental health issues, as well as considering the assessment and treatment of depression.

General assessment considerations

NICE recommends (NICE 2002a, 2007a, 2007b) that assessments of health and social care needs should be comprehensive and holistic covering medical/psychiatric symptoms, social functioning, psychological, occupational, economic, physical and cultural/diversity issues. In addition, considerations may need to be given to risk to self/others (including violence, offending) and the presence of co-existing mental health issues, such as those arising from concurrent alcohol and/or drug use. Assessments must also be sensitive to cultural diversity (DoH 1999) which may require developing cultural competence (the knowledge, skills and values required in understanding and working with diverse communities). Furthermore, since the ONS (2002) survey found that 37 per cent of their sample of people with mental disorder had at least one problem with their Activities of Living, issues such as dealing with paperwork and domestic affairs, using transport and money, and household activities need also to be assessed.

However, it is vital that any assessments are person-centred, and attempt to understand the person's subjective world from their own frame of reference. Wherever possible, assessments should be considered a 'purposeful conversation' (Barker 2004) in which the process (that is, the way in which the assessment is conducted focusing on collaboration, partnership working, building trust and developing a therapeutic working alliance) is considered to be as important as the outcome (the clinical information). Likewise, it is important to develop an assessment which balances perceived needs and problems with strengths, assets and abilities that an individual has, such as the ability to cope in the face of a crisis (Watkins 2001).

Physical health

Good mental and physical health is important to our overall sense of positive well-being (Robson et al. 2008). However, people with mental health problems have high rates of physical morbidity and higher mortality rates (DoH 1999) when compared to the general population (Phelan et al. 2001; DoH 2004, 2006). Furthermore, physical health problems tend to occur at a much younger age in people with serious mental ill-health than in the general population, and are pronounced in the 25- to 44-year age range. People with schizophrenia can expect to live, on average, for ten years less than someone without a mental health problem (Mentality/NIMHE 2004) and while suicide or accidental death may account for some of this, death from poor physical health is also a common cause. The risk of cardiac pathology, for example, has been estimated at being three times more likely in patients with schizophrenia compared to the general population (Jindal et al. 2005; Robson et al. 2008). However, physical health problems among those with mental ill-health often go unrecognised (DoH 1999; Cohen and Phelan 2001) or are poorly managed (Inventor et al. 2005; DoH 2006; Robson et al. 2008). Furthermore, people with a diagnosis of schizophrenia tend to have a poorer experience of, and have less access to, medical services (Mentality/

Table 15.2 The annual health check-up

- Calculation of body mass index, and/or body fat measurement and appropriate advice on healthy eating if the patient is obese
- Comprehensive blood tests (e.g. serum electrolytes/complete blood counts (CBC)/Liver function tests (LFT) and so forth)
- Cardiovascular assessment, including blood pressure check
- Assessment of levels of exercise and advice if appropriate
- Cholesterol-level monitoring and advice on preventing cardiovascular disease if appropriate
- Urine analysis for sugar, with fasting blood sugar if positive
- Respiratory assessment, including peak flow readings
- An assessment of smoking status, cessation advice if appropriate
- Annual influenza vaccination and other immunisations as appropriate
- Regular preventive checks such as cervical smear, breast screening, testicular cancer and advice on self-monitoring
- Advice of maintaining good sexual health and family planning with screening for associated infections if appropriate
- Assessment of alcohol use and other drug use with advice and brief intervention if appropriate

---

Source: Robson *et al.* (2008).

NIMHE 2004; DRC 2006) and are less frequently hospitalised for their underlying medical conditions (Mentality/NIMHE 2004).

It is important, therefore, to be alert to co-morbid physical health problems among people with mental health problems. Indeed, there is always a risk of 'diagnostic over-shadowing' with someone with a known mental health problem and care should be taken not to assume that symptoms of physical illness are necessarily related to the person's psychiatric diagnosis. Robson *et al.* (2008) suggest that a proactive strategy is required among primary and secondary healthcare professionals to afford the early detection of physical health problems as a prelude to an effective early medical response. They suggest an annual check-up exploring areas outlined in Table 15.2.

Depression

Depression is the most common mental health issue seen in primary care (CSIP 2006a). Eighty per cent of people with depression are cared for in primary care (NICE 2007a) and the highest rates of depression are to be found in deprived neighbourhoods (ODPM 2004). Depression is more common in women who have an approximately 30 per cent lifetime risk of experiencing a depressive episode (Jenkins *et al.* 2008). While adverse life events are an important risk factor in the development of depression (Jenkins *et al.* 2008), it appears that genetics may also play a role (as evidenced by the fact that depression often runs in families and higher concordance rates are found in identical twins). Possible neurochemical changes in the brain have also been implicated (such as decreased levels of the neu-rotransmitter serotonin) (Martin 2006). Furthermore, people with traumatic brain injury appear to have higher rates of depression (Brown 2004). People with depression also appear to show elevated activity in the amygdala (the structure in the brain associated with assessing the emotional importance of a stimulus) and decreased grey matter volume in the prefrontal cortex (the part of the brain responsible for speech, decision-making and goal-directed behaviour) (Kring *et al.* 2007). As such, it appears that people with depression have an increased awareness of the emotional significance of stimuli but have less ability to plan a response.

People with depression have higher rates of physical health problems and the majority of people with depression often present with physical ailments rather than psychological symptoms which can make detection harder (Harris and Barraclough 1998; Cohen and Hove 2001; NICE 2007a). Moreover, Cohen and Rodriguez (1995) suggest that in people with physical disorders, the complex interplay of several pathways (biological, behavioural, cognitive and social) can result in depression. This model is therefore regarded as *bidirectional* in that depression is seen as both a cause and consequence of physical illness (CSIP 2006a; Margereson 2008), particularly when such illnesses are long term and protracted. For example, in 2006, the Care Services Improvement Partnership (CSIP) drew attention to depression as a co-morbid problem in long-term conditions, such as stroke, coronary heart disease and diabetes, and in the latter case people with diabetes have two to three times the rate of depression than the general population (CSIP 2006a).

The International Classification of Diseases (ICD-10) (WHO 2004) (the medical taxonomy cataloguing medical and psychiatric 'illnesses' for the purposes of diagnosis) distinguishes a wide spectrum of different types of depression of varying severity – from mild single episode to recurrent and psychotic (the latter being characterised by, for example, delusional beliefs, disorganised thinking, bizarre behaviour). Symptoms of depression may include:

- feelings of sadness and despair;
- a loss of hope;
- appetite and sleep disturbances;
- social withdrawal;
- loss of interest or pleasure in activities that are normally pleasurable;
- decreased libido;
- decreased energy;
- an inability to concentrate.

Sometimes people experience feelings of guilt and suicidal thoughts (NICE 2006, 2007a). For a diagnosis to be made the depressed mood must have been present for at least two weeks; be abnormal for the individual; present for most of the day (and almost every day); and largely uninfluenced by environmental circumstances.

People with depression generally respond well to medication and psychological therapies (DoH 1999). NICE (2007a) recommends an incremental stepped-care approach in primary care where initial 'basic' treatments are offered at the start which are escalated in complexity based upon the person's responsiveness to such treatments and subsequent clinical need before referral to specialist secondary psychiatric services.

Step 1: Assessment and recognition of depression in primary care

NICE (2007a) recommends initial recognition and assessment of depression by screening in primary care or general hospital settings of those most at risk (those with a past history of depression, disabling and significant physical illness, or other mental health problems).

Initial screening for depression should include the use of at least two questions concerning mood and interest, such as:

- 'During the past month, have you often been bothered by feeling down, depressed or hopeless?'
- 'During the past month, have you often been bothered by having little interest or pleasure in doing things?'

NICE (2007a) also draws attention to the need to be mindful that the effects or side effects of some types of medication (particularly those which are sedating) and even some physical ailments (such as anaemia) may cause the person to present with symptoms similar to depression.

CSIP (2006a) recommends the use of the Patient Health Questionnaire (PHQ-9) (Kroenke *et al.* 2001) (Table 15.3) in the assessment of depression (available at: www.phqscreeners.com). The PHQ-9 is a validated nine-item inventory designed to capture the severity of depression by assessing an individual's pattern of sleeping, eating and appetite, energy, concentration, negative self-perception, psychomotor slowing or agitation and thoughts of suicide. A total score (the sum of each column) of 0–4 indicates no depression; 5–9 mild depression; 10–14 moderate depression; 15–19 moderately severe depression; and 20–27 indicates severe depression.

Step 2: Managing recognised depression in primary care – mild depression

During this stage, people with depression are offered initial treatment. It is envisaged that this will occur more commonly in primary care. NICE (2007a) recommends during the initial stages of a depressive episode that watchful waiting is undertaken with a two-week follow up, recognising that some symptoms of depression may abate, or to give the chance for other interventions to have an effect. Advice regarding taking exercise (three sessions per week of 45 minutes to one hour duration for ten to 12 weeks is recommended), the promotion of sleep, and anxiety management may also be offered if appropriate. Recently, the Mental Health Foundation has indicated the possible role that diet may play in the development and persistence of depressive episodes, and suggests that dietary advice should be offered particularly in relation to increasing the amount of foods rich in omega-3 fatty acids found in fish and seafood, seeds (especially flax) and nuts (for example, walnuts) and foods which contain vitamin B3, B6, C, folic acid, zinc, magnesium and selenium, for example, wholegrain foods, pulses, fruit, watercress, avocado, liver and chicken (Mental Health Foundation 2006).

In addition, brief psychological interventions, such as CBT, may be offered which can involve individual or group sessions with a therapist. NICE (2007a) recommends six to eight sessions of CBT over ten to 12 weeks. Although some people prefer such therapies, services are currently patchy and demand is high with significant variations in access to services (ODPM 2004). For some people guided self-help over six to nine weeks with follow-up may be appropriate. Here, self-help manuals, audio tapes and videos and/or treatment delivered by a computer package

Table 15.3 Patient Health Questionnaire (PHQ-9)

	Not at all	Several days	More than half the days	Nearly every day
1 Little interest or pleasure in doing things	0	1	2	3
2 Feeling down, depressed or hopeless	0	1	2	3
3 Trouble falling or staying asleep, or sleeping too much	0	1	2	3
4 Feeling tired or having little energy	0	1	2	3
5 Poor appetite or overeating	0	1	2	3
6 Feeling bad about yourself – or that you are a failure or have let yourself or your family down	0	1	2	3
7 Trouble concentrating on things, such as reading the newspaper or watching television	0	1	2	3
8 Moving or speaking so slowly that other people could have noticed, or the opposite – being so fidgety or restless that you have been moving around a lot more than usual	0	1	2	3
9 Thoughts that you would be better off dead or of hurting yourself in some way	0	1	2	3

If you checked off any problems, how difficult have these problems made it for you to do your work, take care of things at home, or get along with other people?

Not difficult at all	
Somewhat difficult	
Very difficult	
Extremely difficult	

Source: Developed by Drs Kurt Kroenke, Robert L. Spitzer, Janet B.W. Williams, and colleagues. Copyright © 2005 Pfizer, Inc. Reproduced with permission.

using CBT principles may be appropriate and in the latter case NICE has recently recommended the 'Beating the Blues' programme as being suitable for people with mild/moderate depression (NICE 2006). Antidepressants are not recommended at step 2 as the risk–benefit ratio is poor unless the person has a known history of moderate or severe depression (NICE 2007a).

Step 3: Managing recognised depression in primary care – moderate to severe depression

If the interventions at step 2 have not been effective and the person appears to be experiencing continued and increasing depressive symptoms, it may be necessary to escalate the amount of support. Moderate or severe depression can be treated in both primary and secondary care and, as with mild depression, the choice of treatment will be influenced by patient preference, past experience of treatment (that is, previous successful interventions) and the fact that the patient may not have benefited from other interventions. The risk of suicide must always be considered and a referral to specialist services may be required if the person is seen to be a high risk. At step 3, and with moderate depression, the NICE guidelines recommend that antidepressant medication of the newer selective serotonin reuptake inhibitor (SSRI) type, such as Fluoxetine and Citalopram, should be offered before psychological interventions (NICE 2007a). SSRIs are the newer type of antidepressants which are not necessarily any more effective than the older, tricyclic antidepressants (such as Amitryptiline) but they tend to have fewer side-effects and are therefore included to be more acceptable to the patient which is likely to promote concordance. In order to promote adherence with prescribed medication, NICE (2009) recommends a patient-centred approach that encourages informed consent based on an open dialogue where patients are encouraged to seek clarification about any medication, and to discuss non-adherence and any doubts or concerns they have about treatment.

The effects of antidepressants may be delayed by up to two weeks during which time the person should be carefully monitored for side-effects (such as increased agitation and anxiety) and suicide risk (especially for those under age 30). For those at particular risk of suicide it may be necessary to restrict the amount of antidepressants given due to toxicity in overdose. Although there is much evidence that the herb St John's Wort, or Hypericum, may be of benefit in mild or moderate depression, NICE (2007a) was unable to recommend its usage due to perceived uncertainty about appropriate doses, the variation in the nature and quality of preparations, and potential interactions with other drugs (including oral contraceptives, anticoagulants and anticonvulsants). At step 3, longer psychological interventions in conjunction with antidepressant medication may be appropriate, and here, 16 to 20 sessions of CBT over six to nine months with a follow-up of two to four sessions over 12 months is recommended (NICE 2007a).

Step 4: Involvement of specialist mental health services including crisis teams

People with depression which appears to be more protracted or resistant to treatment and those with psychotic depression and those at significant risk of harm to self should be referred to specialist mental health services (NICE 2007a). Here, a thorough review of previous treatments for depression will need to be undertaken and consideration should be given to reviewing medication and reintroducing previous treatments with increased monitoring and support. A full comprehensive assessment, including suicide risk, should be undertaken, along with an exploration of possible stressors, personality factors and significant relationship difficulties.

Specialist community mental health teams may be involved, such as crisis resolution and home treatment teams, as a means of supporting those with severe depression. NICE (2007a) recommends that such teams should assist people to continue their normal lives as far as possible without disruption. 'Mindfulness-based CBT' (MCBT) is a therapeutic intervention which assists the individual in becoming aware of, and paying attention to, each present moment experience with an accepting, non-judgemental and non-reactive attitude. This can be delivered in a group format, and may also be considered for people who are currently well as a means of cultivating awareness of the early signs of relapse, stress reduction, acceptance and the development of self-knowledge through dialogue and reflection (Crane 2009).

Step 5: Depression needing inpatient care

In extreme cases, severely depressed people may be admitted to inpatient care especially if there are concerns with self-neglect, and suicide or self-harm risk. Post-discharge care may involve crisis resolution and home treatment teams as a means of intensive follow-up and support. If the person is perceived to need inpatient care, then Standard five of the *NSFMH* requires that each person who is assessed as requiring a period of care away from their home should have:

- timely access to an appropriate hospital bed or alternative bed or place, which is in the least restrictive environment consistent with the need to protect them and the public; and as close to home as possible;
- a copy of a written after-care plan agreed on discharge which sets out the care and rehabilitation to be provided, identifies the care coordinator, and specifies the action to be taken in a crisis.

At this stage, it is possible that electroconvulsive therapy (ECT) may be used to provide short-term and rapid improvement where all other treatment interventions have been unsuccessful, and/or when the condition is considered to be potentially life-threatening (NICE 2003; 2007a). The decision to use ECT should be made jointly by the prescriber and the patient based on an informed discussion, and valid consent should always be obtained where the person has the capacity to do so. An assessment of risk and benefits should also be undertaken (NICE 2003) which weighs up:

- risks associated with the anaesthetic;
- current co-morbidities;
- anticipated adverse events, particularly cognitive impairment such as memory loss;
- the risks of not having treatment.

Transcranial Magnetic Stimulation (TMS) for severe depression is a procedure where an electromagnet is placed over the skull to generate a magnetic field to stimulate parts of the cerebral cortex. According to NICE (2007c), there are no major safety concerns about the procedure but potential adverse events may include local scalp discomfort, headache, nausea, neck stiffness, hearing loss and possible induction of mania. The main concern about TMS, however, is the uncertainty about its effectiveness and what the optimal treatment parameters might be. At present, little is also known about how the procedure may operate within the body (NICE 2007c).

Effective services for people with severe mental illness

Good-quality clinical care is a vital aspect of supporting recovery (Future Vision Coalition 2008). Indeed, creating safe, sound and supportive services which involve people in their care as equal members and citizens of society and a single integrated system of mental health and social care is a central pillar of government policy (DoH 2001a). Over the past ten years, mental health services have been modernised and new GP guidelines are aimed at ensuring that people with mental health problems have their psychological and physical needs met (DoH 2001a). There remains, however, some dissatisfaction with mental health services and the care and treatment offered, particularly acute inpatient services (SCMH 2005).

Many people with mental health problems are treated successfully by their GP and/or other primary care staff without the need for secondary (or specialist) service intervention. In keeping with Standard three of the *NSFMH* (which requires that anyone with common mental health problems should be able to make round-the-clock contact with services) NHS Direct has in recent years provided an additional point of contact and screening. It must be acknowledged that the voluntary sector (e.g. the Samaritans, SANE, Rethink, MIND) also offer extremely valuable information, support and advice. However, people with severe and long-term mental health needs (e.g. chronic depression, schizophrenia, bipolar affective disorders) often have complex needs which require specialist mental health services liaising with other services and agencies (DoH 1999). Some people with serious mental health problems can be difficult to engage, and are at risk of losing contact with services. They are more likely to live in inner city areas, to be homeless, and have high rates of, and vulnerability to, suicide, violence and homicide (DoH 1999) which requires an increased effort from services to provide necessary monitoring and support.

The *National Service Framework for Mental Health* sought to increase the range of community-based assessment and treatments as a response to crises and emergencies and as an alternative to hospital admissions (DoH 1999) such as:

- early intervention in psychosis (those under 35 years with psychosis to receive early and intensive support) (DoH 1999, 2001a, 2001c);
- assertive outreach (intensive case management aimed at managing care in the community for people with serious mental illness who are difficult to engage with an explicit aim of reducing hospital admissions) (DoH 1999, 2001a);
- crisis resolution and home treatment teams (CRHT) (often 24-hour services offering intensive support for acute problems) (DoH 2001a; CSIP 2006b).

Some mental health services also provide specialist care for black and ethnic minorities, mentally disordered offenders, children and adolescents, people with substance use issues, people with mental health problems who are homeless, and women (DoH 2001a).

Central to the provision of effective services for people with mental health problems is the effective care planning and subsequent comprehensive delivery of care based on need within a multi-agency context. The Care Programme Approach (CPA) has been central to government policy since 1991 (DoH 2008). Standard four of the *NSFMH* requires that all mental health service users on CPA should:

- receive care which optimises engagement, anticipates or prevents a crisis, and reduces risk;

- have a copy of their care plan which includes the action to be taken in a crisis by the service user, their carer and their care coordinator, and advises their GP how they should respond if the service user needs additional help and is regularly reviewed by their care coordinator;
- be able to access services 24 hours a day, 365 days a year.

The CPA process aims to ensure that vulnerable people with mental health problems receive the care they need and maintain contact with services. Each person who is subject to CPA arrangements has a named care coordinator who manages their overall care and ensures regular reviews. CPA involves an assessment of health and social care needs and a personalised written care plan drawn up to meet such needs which is agreed with the service user (DoH 2001a, 2008). Such care plans should reflect a whole systems approach, aim to promote independence and should document not only agreed mental healthcare and treatment but also plans to secure employment, occupational activity; accommodation and adequate housing; and entitlement to benefits as appropriate.

Caring about carers

About 50 per cent of people with long-term mental health problems live with family or friends (DoH 1999; Jenkins *et al.* 2008). As such, carers play an essential part in treatment and care (NICE 2002a). In order to fulfil such a role, carers may need support themselves from health and social care services. This could be in the form of practical help and assistance regarding benefit entitlements to information giving about the care and treatment options available to their friend or relative. Certainly, carers will need to know what to do, and who to contact, should a crisis or emergency arise (DoH 1999).

However, while caring can be a rewarding experience, the strains and responsibilities can take their toll, both financially and emotionally (NICE 2008). As a result, carers are twice as likely to have mental health problems themselves if they provide substantial care (DoH 1999, 2001a; ODPM 2004). Standard six of the *National Service Framework for Mental Health* (DoH 1999) requires that all individuals who provide regular and substantial care for a person on CPA should:

- have an assessment of their caring, physical and mental health needs repeated on at least an annual basis;
- have their own written care plan which is given to them and implemented in discussion with them.

Mental health services, therefore, must ensure that carers are provided with information and support to assist them to meet their emotional, mental and physical needs. The CPA care coordinator should inform carers about their rights to request an assessment. Table 15.4 highlights the central features that the carer's plan should address.

A copy of a plan should also be given to the carer's GP, who along with other primary care staff is often in a better position than secondary services to detect early signs of stress, difficulty or deteriorating health.

Table 15.4 The carer's care plan

---

* Information about the mental health needs of the person for whom they have been caring, including information about medication and any side-effects which can be predicted, and services available to support them
* Action to meet defined contingencies
* Information on what to do and who to contact in a crisis
* What will be provided to meet their own mental and physical health needs, and how it will be provided
* Action needed to secure advice on income, housing, educational and employment matters
* Arrangements for short-term breaks
* Arrangements for social support, including access to carers' support groups
* Information about appeals or complaints procedures

Source: DoH (1999).

Preventing suicide

The *National Service Framework for Mental Health* sought to reduce the number of suicides by 2010 by one-fifth to 7.3 per 100,000 (DoH 1999, 2001a, 2002). Standard seven requires that local health and social care communities should prevent suicides by:

* promoting mental health for all, working with individuals and communities (Standard one);
* delivering high-quality primary mental healthcare (Standard two);
* ensuring that anyone with a mental health problem can contact local services via the primary care team, a helpline or an A&E department (Standard three);
* ensuring that individuals with severe and enduring mental illness have a care plan which meets their specific needs, including access to services around the clock (Standard four);
* providing safe hospital accommodation for individuals who need it (Standard five);
* enabling individuals caring for someone with severe mental illness to receive the support they need to continue to care (Standard six).

In 2002 the Department of Health published the *National Suicide Prevention Strategy for England* which sought to reduce the suicide risk in high-risk groups; promote well-being in the wider community; and reduce lethality and availability of suicide methods, such as by reducing the pack size of non-prescription paracetamols (DoH 2002). The latest statistics (ONS 2009) continue to show a downward trend and suicides are currently at their lowest since 1991. In 2007 there were 5377 suicides in adults aged 15 and over – 940 less than in 1991 (6317). The suicide rate in 2007 for men was 16.8 per 100,000 population, and for women 5.0 per 100,000 population (ONS 2009).

Suicide is a complex issue and there is no single approach to suicide prevention (DoH 2002). Central to any risk-reduction strategy is a comprehensive suicide risk assessment which must be undertaken compassionately and sensitively (Watkins 2001; Barker 2004). A careful cataloguing of risk factors needs to be undertaken. It is important to recognise, for example, that most people who commit suicide have

Table 15.5 Suicide risk factors

- Previous history of suicidal attempts
- Family history of suicide
- Negative view of the future – feelings of hopelessness, helplessness, perception of, and plans for the future, if any
- Mental health issues – especially depression, hallucinatory voices commanding self-harm or of persecution, alcohol/drug use
- Social isolation – withdrawal, loss/lack of social support
- Behaviour warning of suicidal intent – for example, procuring means of death, acts in anticipation of death, putting financial affairs in order, general behaviour at interview, plan to commit suicide
- Current stressors – recent bereavement (especially of partner), relationship difficulties or other stressful events, financial problems, terminal illness, accommodation issues

Source: Based on Barker (2004); Cutcliffe and Barker (2004).

mental health problems at the time of their death and are under the influence of alcohol (Jenkins *et al.* 2008). The lifetime suicide rate in people with schizophrenia is 25 per cent (Jenkins *et al.* 2008) and 10 to 15 per cent of people with major depressive disorders eventually kill themselves (NICE 2006). However, social and environmental factors may also play a part. Two-thirds of men under the age of 35 with mental health problems who commit suicide are unemployed (ODPM 2004) and suicide rates increase with age and are higher among those who are single, widowed, divorced or separated (Watkins 2001). Table 15.5 highlights commonly cited risk factors for suicide.

Any risk-reduction strategy must consider the particular factors which appear to underpin the person's feelings of suicidality. In a suicidal crisis, contact should be made via primary care teams or NHS Direct who can advise regarding referral to secondary services where there is a perceived immediate and grave risk of suicide – this could be to crisis resolution and home treatment teams or, in extreme cases, an inpatient admission may need to be arranged. In the case of those who are already known to mental health services, CPA care plans must assess suicide risk and a crisis plan must be developed where there is a perceived risk (DoH 1999). Therapy, treatment and ongoing care may be required to address possible reasons underpinning the suicidal crisis, for example, medication or CBT in response to depressive symptoms or bereavement counselling in the face of grief and loss.

Conclusion

The response to those with long-term mental health problems is likely to require many levels of support from individuals; to neighbourhoods and local communities; to society; to government and statutory intervention. The central message in this chapter is that service users and carers are entitled to support they need *before* they reach crisis point and before their mental distress becomes a long-term condition (ODPM 2004). Where this has not been possible, emphasis must be placed on assisting the *whole person* on the road to recovery and this is likely to involve a multi-factorial and comprehensive response, from clinically effective medical interventions, to improving meaningful employment prospects, to improving diet and physical health, to improving social support and satisfying personal relationships.

Table 15.6 Useful contacts (including helpline support)

NHS Direct	www.nhsdirect.nhs.uk Tel: 0845 4647
The Samaritans	www.samaritans.org Tel: 08457 90 90 90 Email: jo@samaritans.org Post: Chris PO Box 9090 Stirling FK8 2SA
Mind Charity championing the rights of people with mental health problems. Offers support and advice	*MindinfoLine:* Tel: 0845 766 0163 Email: info@mind.org.uk Post: Mind PO Box 277 Manchester M60 3XN Deaf or speech-impaired enquirers can use the same phone number (if you are using BT Textdirect add the prefix 18001) For interpretation, Mind*info*Line has access to 100 languages via language line We are open Monday to Friday, 9 a.m. to 5 p.m. Calls from the UK are charged at local rates
SANE Charity with three primary objectives: increase awareness of mental health issues/research/provide help and information	www.sane.org.uk SANEline – Tel: 0845 767 8000
Rethink A voluntary organisation and charity which campaigns on behalf of, and supports, people with serious and severe mental health problems	www.rethink.org *National Advice Service* Tel: 0207 840 3188 (open 10 a.m. to 3 p.m. Monday, Wednesday and Friday; 10 a.m. to 1 p.m. Tuesday and Thursday) E-mail: advice@rethink.org

Table 15.7 Useful websites

BBC (Mental Health) Useful websites offering information about mental health conditions	www.bbc.co.uk/health/conditions/mental_health/ www.bbc.co.uk/headroom/
Depression Alliance UK charity for people with depression	www.depressionalliance.org/ England Office Depression Alliance 212 Spitfire Studios 63–71 Collier Street London N1 9BE Tel: 0845 1232320 Email: information@depressionalliance.org
Mind Charity in England and Wales providing information and support for people experiencing mental distress	www.mind.org.uk/About+Mind/Contact+us.htm 15–19 Broadway London E15 4BQ Tel: 020 8519 2122 Email: contact@mind.org.uk
Mental Health Foundation UK charity working to improve services for anyone affected by mental health problems	www.mentalhealth.org.uk/welcome/ Mental Health Foundation London Office 9th Floor Sea Containers House 20 Upper Ground SE9 QB
UK Therapists UK directory of psychotherapists and complementary therapists	www.uktherapists.com/

References

Abayomi, J. and Hackett, A. (2004) Assessment of Malnutrition in Mental Health Clients: Nurses' Judgement vs. a Nutrition Risk Tool. *Journal of Advanced Nursing*, 45(4), 430–437.

Abramson, L., Metalsky, G. and Alloy, L. (1989) Hopelessness Depression: A Theory-based Subtype of Depression. *Psychology Review*, 96, 358–372.

Barker, P. (2004) *Assessment in Psychiatric and Mental Health Nursing* (2nd edn). Cheltenham: Nelson Thornes.

Beck, A. (1967) *Depression: Causes and Treatment*. Philadelphia, PA: University of Pennsylvania Press.

Brown, M. (2004) *Coping with Depression after Traumatic Brain Injury*. Online. Available at: www.adap.net/tbi/depression.pdf (accessed: 5 January 2009).

Butcher, J., Mineka, S. and Hooley, J. (2008) *Abnormal Psychology: Core Concepts*. Boston, MA: Pearson.

Care Services Improvement Partnership (CSIP) (2006a) *Long-term Conditions and Depression*. Online. Available at: http://kc.csip.org.uk/viewdocument.php?action=viewdox&pid=0&doc=35063&grp=1 (accessed 12 December 2008).

Care Services Improvement Partnership (CSIP) (2006b) *Crisis Resolution and Home Treatment: Report From A Conference Linking Research, Policy And Practice For Service Development* (5 October 2006). Online. Available at: www.csip.org.uk/silo/files/cris-resolution-home-treatmanet.pdf (accessed 12 December 2008).

Cohen, A. and Hove, M. (2001) *Physical Health of the Severe and Enduring Mentally Ill: A Training Pack for GP Educators.* Online. Available at: www.scmh.org.uk/80256FBD004F6342/vWeb/wpKHAL6G7K9Z (accessed 5 January 2009).

Cohen, A. and Phelan, M. (2001) The Physical Health of Patients With Mental Illness: A Neglected Area. *Mental Health Promotion Update,* 2, 15–16.

Cohen, S. and Rodriguez, M.S. (1995) Pathways Linking Affective Disturbances and Physical Disorders. *Health Psychology,* 14(5), 374–380.

Crane, R. (2009) *Mindfulness-based Cognitive Therapy.* Hove: Routledge.

Cutcliffe, J.R. and Barker, P. (2004) The Nurses' Global Assessment of Suicide Risk (NGASR): Developing a Tool for Clinical Practice. *Journal of Psychiatric and Mental Health Nursing,* 11, 393–400.

Department of Health (DoH) (1999) *National Service Framework for Mental Health: Modern Standards and Service Models.* Online. Available at: www.dh.gov.uk/en/Publicationsandstatistics/Publications/PublicationsPolicyAndGuidance/DH_4009598 (accessed 10 November 2008).

Department of Health (DoH) (2001a) *The Journey to Recovery – the Government's Vision for Mental Health Care.* Online. Available at: www.dh.gov.uk/en/Publicationsandstatistics/Publications/PublicationsPolicyAndGuidance/DH_4002700 (accessed 11 November 2008).

Department of Health (DoH) (2001b) *The Expert Patient – A New Approach To Chronic Disease Management For The 21st Century.* Available at: www.dh.gov.uk/en/Publicationsandstatistics/Publications/PublicationsPolicyandGuidance/DH_4006801 (accessed 11 November 2008).

Department of Health (DoH) (2001c) *The Mental Health Policy Implementation Guide.* London: Department of Health.

Department of Health (DoH) (2002) *National Suicide Prevention Strategy for England.* Available at: www.dh.gov.uk/en/Publicationsandstatistics/Publications/PublicationsPolicyAndGuidance/DH_4009474 (accessed 15 November 2008).

Department of Health (DoH) (2004) *Choosing Health: Making Health Choices Easier.* Online. Available at: www.dh.gov.uk/en/Publicationsandstatistics/Publications/PublicationsPolicyAndGuidance/DH_4094550 (accessed 12 November 2008).

Department of Health (DoH) (2006) *Choosing Health: Supporting The Physical Needs Of People With Severe Mental Illness – Commissioning Framework.* Online. Available at: www.dh.gov.uk/en/Publicationsandstatistics/Publications/PublicationsPolicyAndGuidance/DH_4138212 (accessed 14 November 2008).

Department of Health (DoH) (2008) *Refocusing the Care Programme Approach: Policy and Positive Practice Guidance.* Online. Available at: www.dh.gov.uk/en/Publicationsandstatistics/Publications/PublicationsPolicyAndGuidance/DH_083647 (accessed 14 November 2008).

Disability Rights Commission (DRC) (2006) *Equal Treatment: Closing the Gap.* Available at: www.drc.gov.uk/library/health_investigation.aspx (accessed 15 January 2009).

Future Vision Coalition (2008) *A New Vision for Mental Health: Discussion Paper.* Online. Available at: www.newvisionformentalhealth.org.uk/ (accessed 15 December 2008).

Gallop, R. and Reynolds, W. (2004) Putting It All Together: Dealing with Complexity in the Understanding of the Human Condition. *Journal of Psychiatric and Mental Health Nursing,* 11, 357–364.

Godfrey, P.S., Toone, B.K., Carney, M.W. *et al.* (1990) Enhancement of Recovery from Psychiatric Illness by Methylfolate. *Lancet,* 336, 392–395.

Gold, M.S. (1996) The Risk of Misdiagnosing Physical Illness as Depression. In: Flach, F. (ed.) *The Hatherleigh Guide to Managing Depression, Vol 3.* New York: Hatherleigh Publications.

Goodwin, J.S., Goodwin, J.M. and Garry, P.J. (1983) Association Between Nutritional Status and Cognitive Functioning in a Healthy Elderly Population. *Journal of the American Medical Association,* 249, 2917–2921.

Harris, E.C. and Barraclough, B. (1998) Excess Mortality of Mental Disorder. *British Journal of Psychiatry,* 173, 11–53.

Illich, I. (2001) *Limits to Medicine: Medical Nemesis – The Expropriation of Health.* London: Marion Boyars Publishers Ltd.

Inventor, B., Henricks, J., Rodman, L. *et al.* (2005) The Impact of Medical Issues in Inpatient Geriatric Psychiatry. *Issues in Mental Health Nursing*, 26(1), 23–46.

Jenkins, R., Meltzer, H., Jones, P. *et al.* (2008) *Foresight Mental Capital and Wellbeing Project. Mental Health: Future Challenges.* London: The Government Office for Science.

Jindal, R., Mackenzie, E.M., Baker, G.B. *et al.* (2005) Cardiac Risk and Schizophrenia. *Journal of Psychiatry Neuroscience*, 30(6), 393–395.

Kring, A., Davison, G., Neale, J. *et al.* (2007) *Abnormal Psychology* (10th edn). Hoboken, NJ: John Wiley & Sons.

Kroenke, K., Spitzer, R.L. and Williams, J.B.W. (2001) The PHQ-9: Validity of a Brief Depression Severity Measure. *Journal of General Internal Medicine*, 16(9), 606–613. Online. Available at: www. phqscreeners.com (accessed 1 September 2009).

Limosin, F., Rouillon, F., Pavan, C. *et al.* (2003) Prenatal Exposure to Influenza as a Risk Factor for Adult Schizophrenia. *Acta Psychiatrica Scandinavica*, May, 107(5), 331–335.

Margereson, C. (2008) Physical Illness: Promoting Effective Coping in Clients with Co-morbidity. In: Lynch, J. and Trenoweth, S. (eds) *Contemporary Issues in Mental Health Nursing* (pp. 145–155). Chichester: John Wiley & Sons.

Martin, G. (2006) *Human Neuropsychology* (2nd edn). Harlow: Pearson.

Matthews, J. (2008) The Meaning of Recovery. In: Lynch, J. and Trenoweth, S. (eds) *Contemporary Issues in Mental Health Nursing*. Chichester: John Wiley & Sons.

Mental Health Foundation (2006) *Feeding Minds: The Impact of Food on Mental Health.* Online. Available at: www.mentalhealth.org.uk/campaigns/food-and-mental-health/ (accessed 10 November 2008).

Mentality/NIMHE (2004) *Healthy Body and Mind: Promoting Health Living for People Who Experience Mental Distress.* Online. Available at: www.neyh.csip.org.uk/silo/files/hbhmprimary-care.pdf (accessed 14 December 2008).

National Institute for Health and Clinical Excellence (NICE) (2002a) *Schizophrenia: Core Interventions in the Treatment and Management of Schizophrenia in Primary and Secondary Care.* Online. Available at: www.nice.org.uk/Guidance/CG1/NiceGuidance/pdf/English (accessed 17 January 2009).

National Institute for Health and Clinical Excellence (NICE) (2002b) *Guidance on the Use of Newer (Atypical) Antipsychotic Drugs for the Treatment of Schizophrenia.* Online. Available at: www.nice.org.uk/nicemedia/pdf/ANTIPSYCHOTICfinalguidance.pdf (accessed 17 January 2009).

National Institute for Health and Clinical Excellence (NICE) (2003) *Electroconvulsive Therapy (ECT): Summary.* Online. Available at: www.nice.org.uk/nicemedia/pdf/59ecta4summary.pdf (accessed 17 January 2009).

National Institute for Health and Clinical Excellence (NICE) (2006) *Computerised Cognitive Behaviour Therapy for Depression and Anxiety: Review of Technology Appraisal 51.* Online. Available at: www.nice.org.uk/Guidance/TA97 (accessed 17 January 2009).

National Institute for Health and Clinical Excellence (NICE) (2007a) *Depression (Amended): Management of Depression in Primary and Secondary Care.* Online. Available at: www.nice.org. uk/Guidance/CG23/NiceGuidance/pdf/English (accessed 17 January 2009).

National Institute for Health and Clinical Excellence (NICE) (2007b) *Anxiety (Amended): Management of Anxiety (Panic Disorder (With or Without Agoraphobia), and Generalised Disorder) in Adults in Primary, Secondary and Community Care.* Online. Available at: www.nice.org.uk/ Guidance/CG22/NiceGuidance/pdf/English (accessed 19 January 2009).

National Institute for Health and Clinical Excellence (NICE) (2007c) *Transcranial Magnetic Stimulation for Severe Depression.* Online. Available at: www.nice.org.uk/nicemedia/pdf/ IPG242QRGFINAL.pdf (accessed 20 January 2009).

National Institute for Health and Clinical Excellence (NICE) (2008) *Structural Neuroimaging in First-episode Psychosis.* Online. Available at: www.nice.org.uk/nicemedia/pdf/TA136Guidance.pdf (accessed 20 February 2009).

National Institute for Health and Clinical Excellence (NICE) (2009) *Medicines Adherence.*

Online. Available at: www.nice.org.uk/guidance/index.jsp?action=download&o=43042 (accessed 2 March 2009).

National Institute for Mental Health in England (NIMHE) (2005) *NIMHE Guiding Statement on Recovery.* Online. Available at: www.psychminded.co.uk/news/news2005/feb05/nimherecovstatement.pdf (accessed 9 January 2009).

Office for National Statistics (ONS) (2002) *The Social and Economic Circumstances of Adults with Mental Disorders.* London: TSO.

Office for National Statistics (ONS) (2009) *Suicide Rates in the United Kingdom.* Online. Available at: www.statistics.gov.uk/statbase/Product.asp?vlnk=13618 (accessed 12 February 2009).

Office of the Deputy Prime Minister (ODPM) (2004) *Mental Health and Social Exclusion: Social Exclusion Unit Report.* Wetherby: OPDM Publications.

Phelan, M., Stradins, L. and Morrison, S. (2001) Physical Health of People With Severe Mental Illness. *British Medical Journal*, 322, 443–444.

Robson, H., Trenoweth, S. and Margereson, C. (2008) Co-morbidity in Physical and Mental Ill Health. In: Lynch, J. and Trenoweth, S. (eds) *Contemporary Issues in Mental Health Nursing.* Chichester: John Wiley & Sons.

Sainsbury Centre for Mental Health (SCMH) (2003) *Economic and Social Costs of Mental Illness in England.* London: SCMH.

Sainsbury Centre for Mental Health (SCMH) (2005) *Acute Care 2004: A National Survey of Adult Psychiatric Wards in England.* London: SCMH.

Seligman, M. (2008) Positive Health. *Applied Psychology: An International Review*, 57, 3–18.

Watkins, P. (2001) *Mental Health Nursing: The Art of Compassionate Care.* Edinburgh: Butterworth-Heinemann.

World Health Organisation (WHO) (2004) *International Statistical Classification of Diseases and Related Health Problems Tenth Revision (ICD-10) Volume 2*, Geneva: World Health Organisation.

Zubin, J. and Spring, B. (1977) Vulnerability – A New View of Schizophrenia. *Journal of Abnormal Psychology*, 86(2), 103–126.

16 Cancer

Clair Sadler and Jacquie Woodcock

Introduction

One in three people in the UK will receive a cancer diagnosis at some stage in their lives and one in four individuals will die as a result of cancer. It is a devastating diagnosis that affects not only the lives of those with cancer but also their family and friends. There is often an experience of uncertainty regarding the trajectory of the disease and clinical outcomes (Schroevers *et al.* 2008). For those living with cancer the journey can be particularly trying and as each phase is navigated there will be multiple needs that must be considered and met if care is to be truly holistic. Support is required to help the person meet both psychological and emotional needs but there will also be the need for clear information, advice and guidance. Carers too, both professional and non-professional alike, may attempt to make sense of what is happening to the person with cancer during times that often lack meaning and coherence, and they will often need appropriate knowledge so that they are able to support individuals throughout their cancer experience (Hinnen *et al.* 2008).

Attitudes towards cancer

There have been many advances in cancer treatment and an overall increase in survival rates over recent years. However, cancer remains for many synonymous with death and suffering in the minds of the British population (Cancer Research UK 2007) and it is clearly, and understandably, a major concern in modern society (Murray and McMillan 1993).

The attitudes of the general public towards cancer can lead to delays in detection and access to treatment (Kearney *et al.* 2003). There are a number of reasons for such attitudes. Media coverage and the reporting of cancer will often include headlines which use combative words, such as battle, fight, victim, survival, war against cancer and so forth. In Susan Sontag's *Illness as Metaphor* first published in 1978 the use of such military metaphors is challenged but 30 years later they remain prevalent (Sontag 2002). Such language can reinforce negative attitudes towards the disease and many people with cancer state how unhelpful they feel such language to be. Lance Armstrong, Tour de France winner and cancer survivor, for example, famously wrote in his autobiography that he changed his oncologist when the first doctor he saw stated that he would be hit so hard with chemotherapy that it would virtually kill him (Armstrong 2001). This chapter will provide factual information and insight for those caring for individuals with cancer and aims to develop more realistic and optimistic views of the illness.

Aetiology

Cancer is not a single disease, as there are estimated to be over 200 different types of cancer, and it is a disease that can develop in any cells within the body. It is caused by changes occurring in normal cells which result in uncontrolled growth. Cancer cells lose those attributes that usually result in orderly growth and function. Normal cells are able to respond to external signals regulating growth but cancer cells do not respond to such signals and continue to grow in an unregulated manner. Although normal cells recognise when their life cycle is at an end and die (a process called apoptosis) cancer cells do not recognise these signals and are able to evade cell death. Cells are also normally able to recognise the limits of their growth in relation to other structures. For example, a liver cell will stop replicating when the structure has sufficient cells, while the cancer cell will continue growing, thereby invading surrounding healthy tissues. All cells require a sufficient blood supply in order to thrive and cancer cells have the ability to develop their own blood supply by producing signals that stimulate the production of a new blood supply (called angiogenesis). Cancer cells are also able to travel to other parts of the body via the blood system and the lymphatic system (that is, to metastasise) where they can then infiltrate other organs (Souhami and Tobias 2005).

Epidemiology

Although the past two decades have seen an increase in the incidence of cancer there has also been a noticeable decrease in death rates. Over 289,000 people are diagnosed with cancer in the UK each year with more than 150,000 deaths. Therefore most families in the UK will have experiences of people who have or have had cancer (Cancer Research UK 2007). Cancers can be classified as 'common' or 'rare' and the four most common causes of cancer death in descending order are lung, colorectal, breast and prostate.

Treatment success in cancer is often related to early detection and intervention. Lung cancers, however, are often detected late with first presentation often in the advanced stages of the disease. Early signs and symptoms such as cough, hoarseness and breathlessness can be linked to many respiratory complaints and often be attributed to the expected effects of smoking. Diagnosis in lung cancer is therefore often problematic and treatment challenging. Another reason for the gradual increase in cancer incidence is that cancer is a disease predominately of older people and the UK has an ageing population. It has been estimated that 65 per cent of all cancers are diagnosed in individuals over the age of 60 and that the average age of diagnosis in this country is currently 64 years of age. Cancer can, however, affect people at any age and while cancer in children is rare there are still approximately 1500 new cases diagnosed in the UK each year. Whereas many cancers in older people can be attributed to lifestyle factors, for example, smoking, diet and alcohol, the majority of childhood cancers are related to developmental changes before birth, often involving chromosomal abnormalities.

With one in three people developing cancer at some time in their lives it remains high on the political agenda and there are many government initiatives to improve cancer care, including the *Cancer Reform Strategy* (DoH 2007) and *The NHS Cancer Plan* (DoH 2000). The aim of such initiatives is to set a clear direction for the development and implementation of cancer services in the UK. The *Cancer Reform Strategy* is divided into distinct areas and includes impact on patients, the role of healthcare professionals and patterns of care delivery.

Cancer prevention

It must be noted that over the past decade there has been increasing evidence of a strong genetic predisposition to cancer (Vogelstein and Kinzler 2004). However, there are a number of lifestyle factors which are known to be directly related to the development of cancer. For example, there have been year-on-year increases in the incidence of cancer of the uterus and endometrium with overweight women estimated to have three times the risk. As obesity becomes an increasing issue in the UK it is anticipated that the incidence of such cancers will continue to rise. It is important to remember that over half of all cancers are preventable by lifestyle changes (American Cancer Society 2006) and health promotion plays an important role. However, in a recent survey of 4000 people less than 20 per cent were aware that over half of all cancers are preventable by lifestyle changes (Cancer Research UK 2007).

Smoking

Smoking accounts for almost 30 per cent of all cancer deaths and 90 per cent of deaths from lung cancer in the UK each year. While smoking has an acknowledged link with lung cancer clearly demonstrated in the 1950s (Doll and Hill 1956) it is also responsible for cancers of the oesophagus, pharynx and larynx, oral cavity, cervix, stomach, liver and pancreas. Smoking cessation, even well into middle age, has wide-ranging health benefits and can significantly reduce the risk of lung cancer (Peto *et al.* 2000).

Though smoking rates in the UK have reduced considerably over the past few decades one in four people continue to smoke. A particular challenge for any disease prevention campaign is that smoking is most prevalent in lower social economic groups with one-third of men in manual work compared with 18 per cent of their professional counterparts. Health-promotion campaigns therefore need to acknowledge the demographic of this group and choose health messages appropriate to them. Nor is the impact of tobacco limited to cigarette smoking. The UK is becoming increasingly multicultural and is continually adopting practices from other countries. Chewing tobacco, for example, a common pursuit in Southern Asia, is becoming increasingly prevalent in this country and there have been marked increases in the diagnosis of oral cancers. Increases in this relatively rare cancer have been particularly marked in young Asian men.

Diet

After smoking, diet and weight are the second most significant lifestyle factors that increase the risk of developing cancer (World Cancer Research Fund 2007). Cancers of the bowel, uterus, kidney, gall bladder and breast cancer in post-menopausal women are all directly linked to obesity. With increasing obesity prevalence in our somewhat sedentary and convenience food society, a rise in these cancers can be anticipated. The recommended diet to minimise cancer risk is one which is high in fibre, fruit and vegetables and low in red and processed meats and salt (see Chapter 10). The *Cancer Reform Strategy* (DoH 2007) has highlighted the need for a change in dietary habits among children as a way of protecting against cancers in later life, including the teaching of food and nutrition in schools.

Alcohol consumption

Alcohol is directly attributable to the development of cancers of the mouth, larynx, pharynx, oesophagus, breast, liver and bowel. Six per cent of cancer deaths each year are caused by excessive alcohol. When combined with smoking, consuming excessive levels of alcohol can double the risk of developing cancer.

Sun exposure

Skin cancer is one of the most common cancers in the UK, and is usually caused by ultraviolet damage. Skin cancer can be divided into two main classifications – non-melanoma and the less common and more aggressive malignant melanoma. Sunburn or intense sun exposure in childhood increases the risk of developing melanoma in later life. Adequate sun protection in children, particularly the under-fives, is therefore imperative. Melanoma tends to occur in people in their fifties and older. However, the incidence is increasing in younger people and appears to be connected with lifestyle factors such as intense sun exposure with subsequent sunburn particularly among those with fair, pale and often freckled skin which is more prone to burning. It is important to note that one-third of all melanomas develop following changes to an existing mole. Therefore individuals need to be familiar with any moles on the body and to take prompt action when there is notice-able change, particularly where a mole grows in size, changes shape and colour, becomes painful, itches or bleeds.

Viruses

Ten to 20 per cent of cancers are attributable to viruses (Crawford 2005) and are responsible for some cancers of the liver, skin, anus, penis and nasopharyngeal area as well as some haematological cancers. Recently a human papilloma virus (HPV) vaccination programme was launched, as 99 per cent of all invasive cervical cancers are caused by HPV which is a virus spread by sexual contact. The vaccination pro-gramme aims to protect against two strains of the virus that are responsible for 70 per cent of all cervical cancers (Davis 2008). The vaccination is offered to 12- and 13-year-old girls with a two-year catch-up programme currently running.

Screening and early diagnosis

Late diagnosis is known to be a poor prognostic factor in most cancers. The UK has well-respected screening programmes for breast, bowel and cervical cancer. The *Cancer Reform Strategy* (DoH 2007) builds on the success of these programmes and intends to extend the age range at which people are invited to take part. There is also currently much discussion in relation to the introduction of a national screening programme for other major cancers such as lung, prostate and ovarian cancer. National screening programmes are, however, costly, and are not appropriate in detecting all cancers.

Reluctance to engage in national screening programmes or to seek help where there are early symptoms may account for poorer survival rates among people with mental health problems. Social deprivation is a major factor in the development of cancer. This is due in part to lifestyle cancers such as smoking-related conditions, but it is also acknowledged that lower socio-economic groups are less likely to attend screening and seek medical advice. Among people with mental health problems Kisley *et al.* (2008) found that while incidence of cancer was similar (and in some cases lower) compared with the general population, the mortality rate was higher. The possible explanation proposed was that that this group had delays in initial presentation and diagnosis and therefore presented at a more advanced stage of the illness. Possible difficulties with communication and access to healthcare were also thought to be contributing factors. Wereneke *et al.* (2006) found that women with severe mental health problems, specifically those with psychosis or who have had repeated admission for psychiatric illnesses, were significantly less likely to engage in breast-screening programmes. This therefore presents major challenges for those caring for this client group but, if detected early, breast cancer is an eminently treatable condition.

While screening programmes can be effective, they are not sufficient in isolation. There also needs to be public awareness of the signs and symptoms of cancer. Individuals or those caring for them need to be familiar with their own bodies and aware of changes. Any of the following changes could be a sign of cancer and therefore worthy of seeking medical advice:

- abnormal bleeding or discharge;
- lumps (e.g. in breast, testicles, groin, neck, arm pit);
- bowel and urinary changes;
- weight loss and lethargy;
- changes in appearance of moles;
- persistent hoarseness or cough;
- difficulties in swallowing and digestion.

Health professionals need to be alert to warning signs and particularly vigilant when caring for vulnerable people, such as those with learning disabilities, for example, who have higher rates of certain cancers (e.g. childhood leukemia, gastrointestinal and gonadal cancers). The Royal Society for Mentally Handicapped Children and Adults document *Death by Indifference* (Mencap 2007) highlighted the story of Emma, a young woman with severe learning disabilities. Healthcare professionals at Emma's district general hospital did not respond to the symptoms that she presented with and the delay in treatment for the cancer subsequently diagnosed was attributed to her lack of compliance and difficult behaviour. This report has led to greater understanding of the needs of this vulnerable group. It has also resulted in the *Treat Me Right* campaign which has led to annual routine health checks for all adults with learning disabilities (Mencap 2004). Carers need to be aware of possible warning signs. It is interesting to note, however, that there is a lower rate of cancer in people with Downs syndrome compared with the general population, particularly breast cancer, and more research is currently being undertaken in this area (Hasle *et al.* 2000).

Assessment and decision-making

The treatment an individual will require following assessment and diagnosis will depend on the site, the type of cells the cancer has originated from and whether the cancer is localised or has spread to other body systems or organs (metastasised). These factors considered together help clinicians identify the stage of the cancer and assist in choosing the appropriate treatment. In order to establish the stage of the cancer prior to treatment various investigations will take place and may involve the sampling of tissue and the use of imaging techniques. By examining cancer cells under the microscope (histology) it is possible to identify how closely they resemble the cell from which they have originated. For example, if a breast cancer cell can be easily identified as a breast cell this is thought to be 'well differentiated'. However, if the breast cancer cell bears little resemblance to its cell of origin then it is considered to be 'poorly differentiated'.

Histological distinction is very relevant in terms of treatment pathway and overall prognosis. The other main staging criteria include spread of the cancer to other parts of the body and there are agreed international staging systems available for specific cancers. The most common and internationally recognised way of identifying cancer stage is the 'TNM' system, where 'T' refers to tumour size, 'N' relates to possible nearby lymph node involvement and 'M' to the presence or absence of metastatic spread. Part of any staging process may involve a range of imaging techniques including plain X-rays, ultra-sounds, Computerised Tomography (CT scan) and Magnetic Resonance Imaging (MRI) and bone scans. The most current technology is Positron Emission Tomography (PET) scanning which offers an even more sensitive image than MRI but is only available in a few specialist centres.

Other points that need to be considered prior to any decision regarding treatment will be the individual's physical state, the effectiveness of available treatment options and of course the individual's wishes. Keating *et al.* (2002) found that while 64 per cent of patients with early stage breast cancer wished to be included regarding decisions relating to their treatment, only 33 per cent felt that the process involving clinicians was truly collaborative. As treatments for cancer continue to develop, the decision-making process becomes more complex and can be difficult to comprehend. This may be particularly so for vulnerable adults within the community, such as older people, those with learning difficulties or mental health problems (Aziz and Rowland 2002; Tuffrey-Wijne *et al.* 2006). Those faced with low-level literacy can also struggle to understand the complexities of information about treatment options (Kim *et al.* 2001). Perhaps as a consequence, vulnerable groups may not receive the same quality of care as the general population. Mateen *et al.* (2008) have shown that individuals with a known diagnosis of schizophrenia receive poorer treatment when presenting with co-morbid symptoms of lung cancer. Inagaki *et al.* (2006) also argue that for people with mental health problems the support of a psychiatrist is needed when they are faced with making decisions regarding cancer treatment.

Treatment

Where cancer is diagnosed at an early stage then only one treatment mode may be needed, such as a woman diagnosed in the early stage of cervical cancer requiring total abdominal hysterectomy but no additional treatment. However, many individuals will require treatment involving different modes of anti-cancer therapy (multi-modal therapy). This may be because they have presented with a cancer at an advanced stage. The main treatments used are surgery, radiotherapy and chemotherapy. Other treatments may involve giving hormones (endocrine therapy) or biological therapies to assist the body's immune system in killing the cancer cells (see below). These treatments may be delivered singularly or more commonly in combination. For example, women with a diagnosis of breast cancer may have surgery to remove the tumour within the breast followed by chemotherapy to treat any known or anticipated spread to other organs. Such multi-modal treatment is often in response to the ability of the disease to metastasise.

Surgery

Surgery is the single most common treatment for adults with a cancer diagnosis and may be used at a number of stages during the trajectory of the illness. Surgery is usually used as a primary treatment to remove the cancer and some surrounding healthy tissue. However, over the past decade there has been a move away from major radical surgery which often left individuals with physical changes altering their body image and impacting dramatically and negatively on their quality of life. The introduction of laparoscopic surgery and lasers, and more recently robotic surgery, along with the improvements in X-ray and scanning techniques, has allowed for less radical surgical techniques which help to preserve function and body image while removing the cancer.

Surgery may also be used as a prophylactic treatment in individuals who carry a genetic mutation that places them at a high risk of developing cancer. This is most commonly seen in families with a genetic predisposition to breast cancer where the removal of the whole breast or breasts (mastectomy) may be considered. However, this needs careful consideration, as surgery results in significant changes in body image and associated psychological implications. Women contemplating this type of surgery require access to genetic counselling in order for them to be able to make informed decisions (Lobb and Meiser 2004) and will be offered breast reconstruction either at the time of the original surgery or at a later date.

Surgery may also be used for palliation (that is, to relieve suffering rather than to halt the cancer) where it may be used to relieve obstruction (for example, of the bowel) or to relieve pain where fractures have occurred due to bone metastases. Surgery may also be used to remove isolated metastatic deposits, such as within the lung, and more recently an impact has been made on survival in those diagnosed with colorectal cancer where there is liver metastases. Many individuals with a diagnosis of cancer will require other supportive surgical interventions, for example, long-term intravenous access in the form of central venous lines (Hickman lines) which require surgical insertion. Nutritional support may also require the insertion of special feeding tubes.

Chemotherapy

Chemotherapy uses cytotoxic drugs which disrupt cellular replication. It is a systemic treatment in that once administered the drugs are able to travel throughout the blood system to many target sites. It may be used as a treatment option at all stages of the cancer experience whenever the cancer is known to or is likely to have spread from its primary site. It may be used as the primary treatment of choice; for example, in the management of haematological cancers which require a systemic treatment at the point of diagnosis. Following surgical removal of a primary tumour, chemotherapy may be used to remove any remaining cells or micro metastases that may be present (known as adjuvant chemotherapy). It may also be given at the same time as another treatment option which is commonly radiotherapy and this combined treatment is known as chemo radiation. There may be occasions when chemotherapy is given prior to another treatment option such as surgery or radiotherapy in order to reduce the bulk of the tumour and therefore reduce the surgery required.

Chemotherapy is often considered to be the most feared of cancer treatments carrying associated unpleasant side-effects such as fatigue, nausea, vomiting and alopecia, all of which can impact adversely on quality of life. Commonly, cells most affected by the drugs are those that are rapidly dividing as the more cells are replicating at any one time then the more cells will be damaged by the drug. This also includes mucosal cells of the gastrointestinal system leading to mucositis (pain, inflammation and ulceration along the digestive tract). It is therefore important that regular mouth care is carried out, as once breakdown of the mucosal membrane occurs there is a potential for infection to be introduced. Nausea and vomiting occur when the receptors are stimulated in the brain by the cytotoxic drugs which act on the vomiting centre. It is an unpleasant side-effect and requires prompt intervention with the administration of appropriately prescribed anti-emetic drugs. However, it can also be aided by the use of cognitive behavioural interventions such as guided imagery or complementary therapies such as acupressure.

Some chemotherapeutic drugs will lead to hair loss, although this is by no means true of all drugs. Therefore it is important that individuals receive accurate information from healthcare professionals. Scalp cooling is a method of using cold caps to prevent the action of the drug administered on the hair follicles. However, not everyone is suitable to receive this treatment and even for those who are it is not always totally successful and cannot be tolerated by everyone.

The side-effects of chemotherapy may not only impact on the individual's quality of life but can also be potentially dangerous, particularly in relation to the effect that these drugs have on the blood system. Cytotoxic drugs will affect all blood cells but the impact on the white blood cells that fight infection may mean that there is increased risk from minor infections such as the common cold. It is therefore very important that early signs of infection are recognised early and medical advice sought at the first opportunity.

Radiotherapy

Radiotherapy destroys cancer cells by using radiation to interfere with the replication of cancer cells and leads to either immediate or eventual cell death. Radiotherapy can be given by external beams often using a linear accelerator (which uses electricity to produce ionising radiation) or alternatively, a solid source of radiation (e.g. caesium) can be inserted into a part of the body such as the vagina or buccal mucosa of the mouth. In cancer of the thyroid gland treatment may involve the ingestion of radioactive iodine 131. Like surgery, radiotherapy is a localised treatment and some site-specific cancers may be treated by radiotherapy alone (e.g.

small superficial skin cancers). Commonly, radiotherapy will be used as part of a multi-modal approach to cancer treatment as mentioned earlier.

Side-effects of radiotherapy are generally localised and occur as a result of the inflammatory response. Particular care needs to be taken of the skin in the area receiving treatment, as damage may occur and can lead to treatment having to be postponed allowing recovery to take place. Advice needs to be given on appropriate skin care and regular observation made of the skin for reddening, itchiness or breakdown, and where this occurs the doctor or nurse should be informed (Faithfull and Wells 2003).

Hormonal therapy

Some cancers are known to rely on hormones that are naturally produced within the body, such as breast and prostate cancer. This means that hormonal manipulation can prevent further growth of the cancer and hormonal therapies used as an antagonist to the naturally produced hormone. These treatments, while less toxic than cytotoxic drugs, are not without side-effects and may include induction of early menopausal symptoms in women and the development of female secondary sex characteristics in men, all of which need to be managed sensitively.

Managing pain

Pain is one of the most feared symptoms following a cancer diagnosis and there is evidence to suggest that this distressing symptom remains poorly managed in half of all people experiencing pain as a result of cancer (Menzies *et al.* 2000). Pain is a complex, multi-dimensional phenomenon encompassing physical, emotional, social and spiritual aspects (World Health Organisation 1990). In order to achieve good pain control comprehensive holistic assessment and ongoing evaluation of interventions, whether pharmacological or non-pharmacological, is very important. Those involved in pain management need to be knowledgeable about basic pain theories and analgesic regimens available. Prescribed drugs to relieve pain need to be administered regularly and the World Health Organisation (WHO) analgesic ladder offers a simple framework to guide healthcare professionals in the management of pain (WHO 2004). Following initial assessment drugs such as oral non-opioids or non-steroidal anti-inflammatories may be effective at first. However, where pain control is not achieved then moving up the analgesic ladder will involve the selection of mild and then stronger opioids to ensure individuals are not in distress.

Complementary therapies

Many people with cancer find the loss of control one of the most difficult challenges of a cancer diagnosis. There is a real need to gain some control over their own destiny and this may lead to searches for various complementary therapies, some regulated with potential benefit, others non-regulated and offering no benefit whatsoever. Some authors (Downer *et al.* 1994; Paltiel 2001) suggest that those who access complementary therapies may do so as a result of experiencing higher levels of anxiety and distress. However, Corner and Harewood (2004) suggest that those with cancer who use these therapies may be more likely to believe that they have internal control over their illness. Davidson *et al.* (2005) highlight other characteristics of individuals turning to complementary therapies where decisions may be influenced by socio-economic status and gender with well-educated younger women being those who most frequently access these therapies.

The number of people with cancer using complimentary therapies is estimated to be 30 per cent (Cancer Research UK 2007). Currently, however, there is a lack of evidence for the use of complementary therapies in cancer care and this can result in confusion over their efficacy and safety. In 2004 the National Cancer Research Institute established the Complementary Therapies Clinical Studies Development Group to encourage further development of research underpinning the use of complementary therapies in cancer care, and reviews are being carried out on the use of hypnotherapy, yoga, acupuncture and reflexology (see Chapter 11). Where individuals express an interest in using a complementary therapy alongside their traditional cancer treatment, they should be advised to seek guidance from the multi-disciplinary specialist team.

Psycho-social support

A diagnosis of cancer can be a psychologically traumatic experience for many and can have profound effects on function, self-image, subjective well-being and mental health (Humphris and Ozakinci 2008). However, as cancer survival rates continue to increase there is a concomitant large and growing population who are living with the fear and threat of recurrence (Humphris and Ozakinci 2008; Schroevers *et al.* 2008), and up to 50 per cent of people recovering from head/neck cancer may experience depressive symptoms and psychological distress (Humphris and Ozakinci 2008). The challenge for the professional helper is to assist people to maintain hope (Herth 2000; Hinds 2004) while maintaining an alertness to the possibility of a recurrence of their illness and to take effective steps in monitoring without exacerbating psychological fears. To this end, there are specialist interventions available such as Humphris and Ozakinci (2008) AFTER (Adjustment to the Fear, Threat and Expectation of Recurrence) programme which involves six structured sessions of one hour using cognitive behavioural principles delivered by a specialist nurse. The programme targets recurrence fears, and facilitates discussion regarding illness beliefs, inappropriate checking behaviours, stress management via progressive muscle relaxation (PMR) and beliefs about cancer.

There are, of course, differences among individuals who are faced with a diagnosis of cancer and beliefs about illness and treatment can impact on coping strategies (Llewellyn *et al.* 2007). For many people perceptions of cancer can be affected by media coverage of cancer, both in news reports and popular fictional television. For example, a woman may find a lump in her breast which she believes could be symptomatic of cancer. If her previous experience is of women who have had similar problems due to cancer but with a poor outcome, she is less likely to seek early support or have a positive view compared to a woman who has had more positive experiences. Personality and social roles may also play an important part in accounting for such differences in reactions to a diagnosis of cancer. Frieswijk and Hagedoorn (2009) found that a diagnosis of breast cancer was potentially more devastating for those women who are more focused on the needs of others or who define themselves in terms of their social roles. Such women may seek to maintain interpersonal relationships by suppressing their own feelings about their diagnosis while being more concerned about the impact of their diagnosis on others than they are for themselves. In so doing, Frieswijk and Hagedoorn (2009) argue, such women may potentially ignore and neglect their own personal and self-care needs and not take sufficient time to rest.

There will be a need for adjustment for the partner of the person with a diagnosis of cancer. Manne *et al.* (2009) found that partners experience significantly higher levels of depression on diagnosis of a wife's early stage breast cancer. Maintaining a satisfactory personal relationship with significant others is a crucial issue in coping with cancer. Hinnen *et al.* (2008) argue that while a cancer diagnosis is not necessarily a risk factor for relationship problems, tension within a relationship coupled with an inability to express thoughts and feelings may be harmful in times of threat. This seems particularly true for assertive women who are more likely to be dissatisfied with partners who provide support in a defensive and avoidant manner (such as dismissing negative feelings). As such, partner support which is open and responsive can promote relationship satisfaction under such circumstances and this finding has implications for the professional helper in preventing relationship distress and enhancing relationship satisfaction.

Personal goals give us a sense of meaning in our life and our psychological well-being can be affected when we are confronted with obstacles in the way of our attainment of goals, both in terms of experiencing depressive symptoms and a loss of purpose in life. Chronic illness such as cancer often places limitations in the way of achieving personal goals, such as impairments in social functioning, the experience of being healthy and being able to carry out daily tasks, having a sense of self-confidence and competence and feeling connected to others (Jim and Andersen 2007; Schroevers *et al.* 2008). Schroevers *et al.* (2008) found that the psychological well-being of people with cancer can be improved by strategies which assisted them to disengage from unrealistic or unattainable goals, and to re-engage with meaningful personal goals:

> [A]s long as cancer patients find it difficult to let go of unattainable goals and to put effort into alternative goals, they are caught up in a process of continuously thinking about cancer, explicitly emphasising the negative aspects, and overlooking pleasant experiences.
>
> (Schroevers *et al.* 2008, 58)

An important role for professional helpers, Schroevers *et al.* (2008) argued, was to assist the person to identify alternative realistic personal goals as well as cognitive emotion-regulation strategies (not engaging in catastrophising, rumination and positive refocusing). As such, therapies which assist the person to focus on positive experiences and present-moment thoughts and feelings can be beneficial in improving psychological well-being.

Living with and beyond cancer

There can be many potential crisis points along the cancer trajectory – at diagnosis, on commencement of treatment and relapse. A major crisis point for many, however, is when cancer treatment is completed. A cancer survivor is defined by the cancer charity Macmillan Cancer Support as someone who is 'living with and beyond cancer' when the treatment may be completed and there is no sign of active disease, but there may be ongoing psychological issues. According to Macmillan Cancer Support (2008) this accounts for two million people in this country rising by 3 per cent each year. There is, for example, increasing acknowledgement of the concept of 'survivor's guilt'. This can be best defined as the feeling a person experiences once their treatment is successfully completed when remembering those people who have not had such successful outcomes. This can also be experienced by those who have a close relative or friend who has died. David Rieff (2008) in his book *Swimming in the Sea of Death: A Son's Memoir* eloquently discusses the gnawing sense of guilt felt following the death of his mother and summed up in his comment 'I can still not believe that there was nothing I could do to help her'.

The need for targeted information together with good communication and counselling skills is imperative at all stages (see Chapter 8). Coulter (2003) highlights the need for patients' concordance with treatments and that deficits in information are the major cause of complaints and litigation. Coulter also identifies that not all cancer patients want to know everything and that while access to information is essential, 'health professionals must remain sensitive to patients' varying needs'. Assessment is therefore vital. Information is available from a range of sources – through advice centres, leaflets, help lines, charities and increasingly significantly the Internet. There, however, remain a large group of the general public who are 'information poor'. These are people who do not, cannot or will not access relevant healthcare-related information. This may be for a range of reasons such as a learning disability, age, or practical constraints to access.

This is an issue that needs to be addressed at both national and local levels. As previously discussed, the government-initiated *Cancer Reform Strategy* highlights the political backing for the focus of cancer care to be not only on the diagnosis and treatment of cancer but also through a greater emphasis on prevention through targeted information and support. The specific needs of the groups to be accessed need to be assessed. The charity Macmillan Cancer Support, for example, is endeavouring to address the issue of practical access through mobile centres. This scheme uses buses that travel across the country and which park in shopping areas so that information and support can be easily accessed by many more people. The way that information is delivered also needs to be considered. The Royal College of Psychiatrists and St George's, University of London have developed a useful series of books aimed at individuals with communication difficulties and those who care for them (Royal College of Psychiatrists 2008). The 'Books Beyond Words' series deals with issues such as breast and testicular self-examination. Using pictures, they can form the basis of discussion with adults who have learning or communication difficulties.

Conclusion

The care of each individual coping with a cancer diagnosis requires a multi-disciplinary approach in order that the best outcomes both in relation to medical treatment and quality-of-life issues can be achieved. Carers need to be knowledgeable about the major issues that individuals may struggle with across the cancer trajectory from diagnosis through to end of life. An understanding of the impact of a cancer diagnosis and the various treatments necessary will contribute to meeting individual needs more effectively.

Table 16.1 Useful contacts (including helpline support)

Macmillan Cancer Support A charity which provides practical, medical, emotional and financial support and push for better cancer care	www.macmillan.org.uk/ Macmillan Cancer Support 89 Albert Embankment London SE1 7UQ Tel: 020 7840 7840 Email: webmanager@macmillan.org.uk
The Cancer Counselling Trust National charity providing free specialist counselling for those affected by cancer and their family and friends	www.cancercounselling.org.uk/ The Cancer Counselling Trust Edward House, 2 Wakley Street London EC1V 7LT Tel: 020 7843 2292 Email: support@cctrust.org.uk
Marie Curie Cancer Care Charity which employs nurses, doctors and other health professionals who provide care to terminally ill patients in the community and in hospices. Services are always free of charge to patients and their families	www.mariecurie.org.uk/ Marie Curie Cancer Care 89 Albert Embankment London SE1 7TP

References

American Cancer Society (2006) *Cancer Prevention and Early Detection – Facts and Figures.* Atlanta: American Cancer Society.

Armstrong, L. (2001) *It's Not About the Bike: My Journey Back to Life.* London: Yellow Jersey Press.

Aziz, N.M. and Rowland, J.H. (2002) Cancer Survivorship Research Amongst Ethnic Minority and Medically Underserved Groups. *Oncology Nursing Forum,* 29(5), 789–801.

Cancer Research UK (2007) *Cancer is Our Number One Fear But Most Don't Understand How Many Cases Can be Prevented.* Cancer Research UK. Online. Available at: http://info.cancerresearchuk.org/news/archive/pressreleases/2007/april/316684 (accessed 23 March 2009).

Corner, J. and Harewood, J. (2004) Exploring the Use of Complementary and Alternative Medicine by People with Cancer. *Nursing Research,* 9(2), 101–109.

Coulter, A. (2003) Patient Information and Shared Decision-making in Cancer Care. *British Journal of Cancer,* 89 (suppl. 1), S15–S16.

Crawford, D.H. (2005) An Introduction to Viruses and Cancer. *Microbiology Today,* 32(3), 110–112.

Davidson, R., Geoghegan, L., McLaughlin, L. *et al.* (2005) Psychological Characteristics of Cancer Patients who use Complementary Therapies. *Psycho-Oncology,* 14(3), 187–195.

Davis, C. (2008) Stopping Cervical Cancer in its Tracks. *Cancer Nursing Practice,* 7(5), 19–21.

Department of Health (DoH) (2000) *The NHS Cancer Plan: A Plan for Investment, a Plan for Reform.* London. Online. Available at: www.dh.gov.uk/en/Publicationsandstatistics/Publications/PublicationsPolicyAndGuidance/DH_4009609 (accessed 25 March 2009).

Department of Health (DoH) (2007) *Cancer Reform Strategy.* London. Online. Available at: www.dh.gov.uk/en/Publicationsandstatistics/Publications/PublicationsPolicyAndGuidance/DH_081006 (accessed 26 March 2009).

Doll, R. and Hill, A.B. (1956) Lung Cancer and other Causes of Death in Relation to Smoking. *British Medical Journal,* 2, 1071–1081.

Downer, S.M., Cody, M.M. and McCluskey, P. (1994) Pursuit and Practice of Complementary Therapies. *British Medical Journal,* 309, 86–89.

Faithfull, S. and Wells, M. (2003) *Supportive Care in Radiotherapy*. Edinburgh: Churchill Living-stone.

Frieswijk, N. and Hagedoorn, M. (2009) Being Needy versus Being Needed: The Role of Self-Regulatory Focus in the Experience of Breast Cancer. *British Journal of Health Psychology*, 14, 69–81.

Hasle, H., Clemmensen, I.H. and Mikkelsen, M. (2000) Risks of Leukaemia and Solid Tumours in Individuals with Downs Syndrome. *Lancet*, 355, 165–169.

Herth, K. (2000) Enhancing Hope in People with a First Recurrence of Cancer. *Journal of Advanced Nursing*, 32(6), 1431–1441.

Hinds, P.S. (2004) The Hopes and Wishes of Adolescents with Cancer and the Nursing that Helps. *Oncology Nursing Forum*, 31(5), 927–933.

Hinnen, C., Hagedoorn, M., Ranchor, A. *et al.* (2008) Relationship Satisfaction in Women: A Longitudinal Cross-control Study about the Role of Breast Cancer, Personal Assertiveness and Partners' Relationship-Focused Coping. *British Journal of Health Psychology*, 13, 737–754.

Humphris, G. and Ozakinci, G. (2008) The AFTER Intervention: A Structured Psychological Approach to Reduce Fears of Recurrence in Patients with Head and Neck Cancer. *British Journal of Health Psychology*, 13, 223–230.

Inagaki, T., Yasukawa, R., Okazaki, S. *et al.* (2006) Factors Disturbing Treatment for Cancer in Patients with Schizophrenia. *Psychiatry and Clinical Neurosciences*, 60(3), 327–331.

Jim, H. and Andersen, B. (2007) Meaning in Life Mediates the Relationship Between Social and Physical Functioning and Distress in Cancer Survivors. *British Journal of Health Psychology*, 12, 363–381.

Kearney, N., Paul, J., Smith, K. *et al.* (2003) Oncology Health Care Professionals' Attitudes to Cancer: A Professional Concern. *Annals of Oncology*, 14(1), 57–61.

Keating, N., Guadagnoli, E., Landrum, M.B. *et al.* (2002) Treatment Decision Making in Early-Stage Breast Cancer: Should Surgeons Match Patients' Desired Level of Involvement? *Journal of Clinical Oncology*, 20(6), 1473–1479.

Kim, S.P., Knight, S.J., Tomori, C. *et al.* (2001) Health Literacy and Shared Decision Making for Prostate Care Patients with Low Socioeconomic Status. *Cancer Investigation*, 19(7), 684–691.

Kisley, S., Sadek, J., Mackenzie, A. *et al.* (2008) Excess Cancer Mortality in Psychiatric Patients. *Canadian Journal of Psychiatry*, 53(11), 753–761.

Llewellyn, C., McGurk, M. and Weinman, J. (2007) The Relationship Between the Patient Generated Index (PGI) and Measures of HR-QoL Following Diagnosis with Head and Neck Cancer: Are Illness and Treatment Perceptions Determinants of Judgment-Based Outcomes? *British Journal of Health Psychology*, 12, 421–437.

Lobb, E. and Meiser, B. (2004) Genetic Counselling and Prophylactic Surgery in Women from Families with Hereditary Breast or Ovarian Cancer. *Lancet*, 363(9424), 1841–1842.

Macmillan Cancer Support (2008) Our Ambition. London. Online. Available at: www.macmillan.org.uk/About_Us/Our_ambition/Our_ambition.aspx (accessed 27 March 2009).

Manne, S., Ostroff, J., Fox, K. *et al.* (2009) Cognitive and Social Processes Predicting Partner Psychological Adaptation to Early Stage Breast Cancer. *British Journal of Health Psychology*, 14, 49–68.

Mateen, F.J., Jataoi, A., Lineberry, T.W. *et al.* (2008) Do Patients with Schizophrenia Receive State-of-the-art Lung Cancer Therapy? A Brief Report. *Psycho-Oncology*, 17(7), 721–725.

Mencap (2004) *Treat Me Right*. London: Mencap.

Mencap (2007) *Death by Indifference*. London: Mencap.

Menzies, K., Murray, J. and Wilcock, A. (2000) Audit of Cancer Pain Management in a Cancer Centre. *International Journal of Palliative Nursing*, 6, 443–447.

Murray, M. and McMillan, C.L. (1993) Gender Differences in Perceptions of Cancer. *Journal of Cancer Education*, 8(1), 53–62.

Paltiel, O., Avitzour, T.P. and Peretz, N. (2001) Determinants of the Use of Complementary Therapies by Patients with Cancer. *Journal of Clinical Oncology*, 19(9), 2493–2448.

Peto, R., Darby, S., Deo, H. *et al.* (2000) Smoking, Smoking Cessation, and Lung Cancer in the UK Since 1950: Combination of National Statistics with Two Case-Control Studies. *British Medical Journal*, 321(7257), 323–329.

Rieff, D. (2008) *Swimming in the Sea of Death: A Son's Memoir*. New York: Simon & Schuster.

Royal College of Psychiatrists (2008) Books Beyond Word Series. London. Online. Available at: www.rcpsych.ac.uk/publications/booksbeyondwords.aspx (accessed March 2009).

Schroevers, M., Kraaij, V. and Garnefski, N. (2008) How Do Cancer Patients Manage Unattainable Goals and Regulate Their Emotions? *British Journal of Health Psychology*, 13, 551–562.

Sontag, S. (2002) *Illness as Metaphor and Aids and its Metaphors*. London: Penguin Classics.

Souhami, R. and Tobias, J. (2005) *Cancer and its Management* (5th edn). Oxford: Blackwell Publishing.

Tuffrey-Wijne, I., Bernal, J., Jones, A. *et al.* (2006) People with Intellectual Disabilities and their Need for Cancer Information. *European Journal of Oncology Nursing*, 10(2), 106–116.

Vogelstein, B. and Kinzler, K.W. (2004) Cancer Genes and the Pathways they Control. *Nature Medicine*, 10(8), 789–799.

Wereneke, U., Horn, O., Maryon-Davis, A. *et al.* (2006) Uptake of Screening for Breast Cancer Patients with Mental Health Problems. *Journal of Epidemiology and Community Health*, 60(7), 600–605.

World Cancer Research Fund (2007) *Food, Nutrition, Physical Activity and the Prevention of Cancer: A Global Perspective*. Washington, DC: American Institute for Cancer.

World Health Organisation (1990) *Cancer Pain Relief and Palliative Care*. Geneva: WHO.

World Health Organisation (2004) Palliative Care: Symptom Management and End of Life Care. Geneva. WHO. Online. Available at: www.who.int/hiv/pub/imai/genericpalliative-care082004.pdf (accessed March 2009).

17 Coronary artery disease

Katie Burke and Jillian Riley

Introduction

The term cardiovascular disease (CVD) is used to include coronary artery disease (CAD), hypertension and stroke, but this chapter will focus on CAD, a disease that accounts for almost half of all cardiovascular deaths (Allender *et al.* 2008). The pathological processes of CAD can lead to the cardiovascular disorders known as angina, myocardial infarction (MI) (heart attack) and heart failure. In 2000 the *National Service Framework for Coronary Heart Disease* (*CHD NSF*) was published detailing 12 standards for improving prevention, diagnosis, treatment and rehabilitation (DoH 2000) (see Table 17.1). An eighth chapter was added in 2005 outlining quality requirements for the prevention of arrhythmias (abnormal heart rhythms) and sudden cardiac death (DoH 2005). In 2008 the seventh progress report on the *CHD NSF* highlighted the tremendous progress made including 22,000 fewer premature deaths per year (DoH 2008). Since the publication of the NSF the term coronary artery disease (CAD) has been adopted and is therefore used throughout this chapter.

Given the high prevalence of CAD, carers across a variety of settings are likely to encounter individuals who have already been diagnosed or who have several risk factors increasing their susceptibility. Although hospitalisation is warranted for acute episodes, most people receiving treatment for CAD are cared for in the community. For those at high risk of CAD early recognition and referral is important so that diagnosis can be made and treatment initiated without delay. Carers also need to be aware of specific treatment regimens so that they can contribute to effective symptom control and recognise when there is deterioration. Lifestyle modification can reduce risk significantly before and following the onset of disease and knowledge of modifiable risk factors is crucial.

Table 17.1 NSF for coronary heart disease

	Areas covered	Standard
1	Reducing heart disease in the population	1 and 2
2	Preventing CHD in high-risk populations	3 and 4
3	Heart attack and other acute coronary syndromes	5, 6 and 7
4	Stable angina	8
5	Revascularisation	9 and 10
6	Heart failure	11
7	Cardiac rehabilitation	12

Epidemiology

Cardiovascular disease (CVD) is a major health problem globally and a major contributor to premature mortality and morbidity (World Health Organisation (WHO) 2004). In the United Kingdom (UK) it is the single commonest form of premature death, accounting for just under 57,000 deaths before the age of 75 years and overall there are 208,000 deaths annually, although death rates for CAD have fallen by approximately 40 per cent in those under age 75 (Allender *et al.* 2008; DoH 2008). For many years CAD was thought of as a predominantly 'male' problem despite the fact that one in six women die from the disease. At time of presentation women tend to be older with fewer specific symptoms, which can make diagnosis and management more difficult (Clarke *et al.* 1994; Lockyer 2005; Mikhail 2005).

Despite a decrease in premature deaths from CAD there are marked regional differences in the prevalence of CAD within the UK, with death rates consistently higher in Scotland and Northern England (Allender *et al.* 2008). Socio-economically, CAD exemplifies inequality and despite much progress the premature death rate for men in the most deprived groups is around twice that found in the least deprived group (Allender *et al.* 2008). Similar findings are seen in South Asian people born in India, Bangladesh, Pakistan or Sri Lanka who are approximately 50 per cent more likely to die prematurely from CAD than the general population (Fox 2004).

Differences are also seen in those with mental health problems. Risk of sudden unexpected death from cardiac problems is reported as being three times greater in those with schizophrenia compared to the general population (Jindal *et al.* 2005) with survival of more than five years less likely once a diagnosis of CAD is made (Disability Rights Commission 2006). It has been suggested that the long-term use of antipsychotic medication leading to weight gain and hyperlipidaemia may contribute to greater risk of developing a number of physical disorders including CAD and type 2 diabetes (Allison *et al.* 2003; Dixon *et al.* 2004). A range of factors may contribute to these differences found in those with mental health problems including unhealthy lifestyles such as smoking, lack of exercise, poor diet as well as poverty, social deprivation and exclusion, poor housing and unemployment (Mentality/ NIMHE 2004). Evidence also reveals that a diagnosis of schizophrenia or bipolar disorder often means that physical health problems are overlooked or ignored (Friedli and Dardis 2002) with stigma of a psychiatric diagnosis also making it less likely that this group receive optimum healthcare (Phelan *et al.* 2001).

Pathophysiology of coronary artery disease

The coronary circulation to the heart consists of three major arteries, the right and left coronary arteries and the circumflex artery, which ensures that there is a constant blood supply to the myocardium (heart muscle). These major arteries then branch to form progressively smaller vessels called arterioles and capillaries which extend through the myocardium for the delivery of oxygen. Carbon dioxide and waste products are removed by the coronary veins.

Atherosclerosis affecting the arteries is now recognised as a chronic inflammatory disorder (Spagnoli *et al.* 2007) with many complex processes involved, including the development of fatty lesions (plaques) within the inner layers of the coronary artery. These processes result in injury to the innermost layer of the artery called the endothelium attracting more inflammatory cells (e.g. macrophages) and, as the plaque and muscle cells enlarge, the artery narrows, which can lead to obstruction. Our knowledge of what causes this endothelial damage is incomplete but factors contributing to athero-sclerosis involve not only high blood pressure, high cholesterol levels and smoking but environmental factors along with complex immune responses (Hansson 2005).

As the atherosclerotic plaque develops, the surface can crumble and crack with possible rupture and, as blood platelets enter, a thrombus (blood clot) can form. This thrombus will decrease blood flow through the coronary artery and where the blood vessel diameter is reduced significantly (>80 per cent) may lead to critical impairment of blood flow resulting in myocardium ischaemia. This can be precipi-tated where there is increased energy expenditure and therefore oxygen demand, and occurs during exercise or where the body is similarly stressed.

Cardiovascular disorders

Angina pectoris

One of the most common manifestations of CAD is angina pectoris or cardiac chest pain and in more than 90 per cent of cases this is due to a reduction in coronary blood flow caused by atherosclerosis. 'Stable' angina is usually predictable, occurs when the heart works faster, thus requiring more oxygen, and can usually be relieved with simple medication or by removing the 'trigger'. Stable angina should resolve within 15 minutes. The term 'unstable' angina is used when the chest pain is unexpected (occurring at rest or during sleep) and is often more severe, prolonged and more serious. Unstable angina typically occurs when the fatty plaque in the cor-onary arteries ruptures with thrombus formation and although blood flow is reduced there is no total obstruction.

In a minority of cases angina pectoris is attributed to coronary artery spasm or when the oxygen supply to the myocardium is reduced due to anaemia, cardiomy-opathy (enlarged heart) or stenosis (hardening) of a heart valve. In these cases there is no evidence of serious amounts of plaque in the coronary arteries.

Recognition of angina and care principles

With angina increasing steeply with age, the prevalence is likely to increase as more people live longer. Angina can often be disabling and affects the quality of life in all its dimensions, often leading to early retirement (Steg and Himbert 2005). Usually individuals complain of chest pain which is 'heavy', 'tight' or 'crushing' in nature. Typically, this pain often radiates to the arms (especially the left), neck, lower jaw and abdomen. The chest pain can range from a mild ache or discomfort to a severe pain that is induced by exertion, cold weather and emotional triggers; any activities that increase the myocardial oxygen demand. Shortness of breath may accompany angina and there may also be less specific symptoms such as fatigue or faintness, nausea, burping, restlessness or a sense of impending doom (Fox *et al.* 2006).

Although diagnosis can be made on history alone, where individuals are experi-encing these symptoms for the first time, further investigation is required. Physical and clinical assessment with specific cardiac investigations will confirm the diagnosis and assess the severity of underlying disease. When angina is severe and physically limiting then, following investigation, there may be a need for heart surgery or balloon angioplasty.

The immediate management of angina is glycerine trinitrate (GTN) which dilates the blood vessels and improves blood flow to the myocardium. This is usually given as a spray with one or two puffs under the tongue (sublingual). Chest pain is also relieved by stopping the activity that brought on the attack; for example, an angina attack may come on with exercise and so stopping the activity, sitting down and resting is likely to stop the chest pain. Close relatives and other associates should be aware of the possible presentation of angina and the use of sublingual medication. Initially there may be faintness and headache when taking GTN although this often disappears with time. However, side-effects may be more problematic in older people where different drugs are taken and medical therapy can be a challenge, leading quite often to a need for revascularisation (Pfisterer 2004).

As angina is an indicator of coronary heart disease, secondary prevention measures should be started. These include lifestyle advice on exercise, optimising body weight, smoking cessation and eating a low-fat diet. In addition, medication to reduce blood cholesterol levels should be started (usually this is a statin) and there is evidence that a beta blocker (drug to reduce heart rate and myocardial work) should also be commenced.

Acute coronary syndrome

The term acute coronary syndrome (ACS) is used to group together the ischaemic pathological processes of CAD (Webster et al. 2007) and includes unstable angina and myocardial infarction. These are life-threatening disorders and can result in sudden death, and so emergency medical care is essential. A major cause is the rupture of an atherosclerotic plaque with a resulting thrombus contributing to ischaemia or infarction (muscle death). Interestingly, there is mounting evidence to suggest that depression, anxiety and hostility/anger may each be an independent risk factor for acute coronary syndrome occurrence (Davidson 2008).

Myocardial infarction

Myocardial infarction (MI), or heart attack, is a common cause of death. There are an estimated 227,000 people suffering myocardial infarctions each year and about 20 per cent of those will die following this event (Allender et al. 2007). Myocardial infarction occurs when there is a severe obstruction of blood flow in a major coronary artery with death (necrosis) of myocardial cells within 15 to 30 minutes. Total occlusion of the coronary artery for more than four to six hours can result in irreversible damage but early re-establishment of blood flow (reperfusion) may salvage regions of the myocardium (Camm and Bunce 2005).

Early recognition of MI and care principles

Classically, patients present with severe chest pain that has lasted for more than 20 minutes that is not resolved with rest or with removal of the 'trigger' (cold weather, emotional distress). As with angina pectoris the pain may radiate to the arm, lower jaw, neck or abdomen and where the pain is severe there may be a fear of impending death with individuals appearing pale, sweaty and grey (Camm and Bunce 2005). However, in some cases, especially in older people, women or in those with diabetes, presentation may be atypical with breathlessness, fatigue, nausea, confusion, dizziness and fainting. In some there may be no pain and the term 'silent' MI is used. Unfortunately there may be few or no warning signs, and onset may be sudden with cardiac arrest and death. Needless to say, all non-specialist carers should have basic life support skills for when these events occur.

Chest pain not relieved by rest or GTN should be treated as an emergency and the individual should be encouraged to sit or lie down. An emergency ambulance should be called and the control room should be told that the person has chest pain so that skilled paramedics can attend. While waiting for the emergency service to arrive, individuals if sufficiently awake should be encouraged to take an aspirin (300 mg) either chewed or dissolved in water to increase absorption, as this helps to dissolve the blood clot in the coronary artery. Further acute management is required, however, including a drug to dissolve the blood clot (thrombolytic) or a balloon angioplasty to open the blocked artery.

Heart failure

In the UK there are 38,000 new cases of heart failure in men each year and 30,000 in women. In total there are around 707,000 in the UK with definite heart failure: 393,000 men aged 45 years and over, and 314,000 women (Allender *et al.* 2008). It has been described as one of the most important causes of morbidity and mortality in society today, with a prevalence ranging from 0.4 to 2 per cent in the general European population (Cowie *et al.* 1997). In younger patients, heart failure is often a consequence of myocardial infarction with damage to the left ventricle (heart chamber), while in older patients a number of additional factors are responsible including hypertension, valvular heart disease and atrial fibrillation (Gillespie 2006). Heart failure is a common, progressive and disabling condition, and is associated with a poor prognosis (Cowie *et al.* 2000).

Heart failure is a complex syndrome resulting from any structural or functional disorder that impairs the heart's ability to pump blood at a rate that adequately supports the body's requirements (Camm and Bunce 2005). The condition may be caused by a slowly developing inability of the myocardium to contract (cardiomyopathy), factors that place excessive demands on the heart (fluid overload, myocardial infarction, long-standing hypertension) resulting in impaired ventricular filling or by the heart muscle becoming increasingly stiff, as occurs with age (Schoen 2004). In order to maintain an adequate volume of blood pumped from the heart each minute (cardiac output) to the tissues (peripheral perfusion), there are a number of complex compensatory mechanisms activated by the nervous and endocrine systems. However, as heart failure progresses these compensatory changes are no longer helpful and can ultimately worsen cardiac function (Klabunde 2007).

Recognition of heart failure and care principles

Carers need to be alert not only for signs of heart failure in those presenting with problems for the first time, but for signs of possible deterioration in those already diagnosed. Acute decompensated heart failure where response to treatment is poor

Table 17.2 Signs and symptoms in heart failure

Left-sided heart failure Caused by CAD, hypertension, cardiomyopathy, valve disease	Right-sided heart failure Caused by pulmonary hypertension, valve disease, pulmonary embolism
• Exertional breathlessness • Fatigue • Breathlessness on lying down • Episodes of sudden breathlessness during the night • Pulmonary oedema (fluid in the lungs) • Cough • Third heart sound (normally two) • Tachycardia (fast heart rate)	• Exertional breathlessness • Fatigue • Nausea • Oedema (swelling) in feet, ankles, legs, sacrum or abdomen • Cold peripheries • Anorexia • Jaundice • Raised jugular venous pressure

is a common and growing medical problem associated with major morbidity and mortality and is the leading reason for hospital admissions among patients over age 65 (Allen and O'Connor 2007). The two major heart chambers that can be affected in heart failure are the right and left ventricles and either one or both can be involved. The right ventricle pumps deoxygenated blood from the right side of the heart into the pulmonary arteries and to the lungs so that it can be oxygenated. The right ventricle can be affected by high pressure in the pulmonary artery (pulmonary hypertension), valve disease as well as by blood clots which can sometimes block the pulmonary artery and its branches (pulmonary emboli). The left ventricle pumps oxygenated blood into the aorta and around the body and can be affected by high blood pressure, diseases which affect the muscle size of the myocardium (cardiomyopathy), damage to heart valves as well as following cardiovascular disease. Table 17.2 outlines the signs and symptoms of both right- and left-sided heart failure.

Assessment issues in CAD

CAD may have been present for many years before there are symptoms. It may also only be diagnosed during routine medical screening or following a clinical examination as part of preparation for surgery or during examination for another illness. Following diagnosis, deterioration may occur, with signs that the disease is progressing. Chapter 5 offers a detailed overview of how a systematic assessment should proceed and only specific issues relating to CAD will be outlined here. The clinical diagnosis of CAD is made on the basis of presenting symptoms, a comprehensive assessment including history, a physical examination and various diagnostic tests. Gathering of subjective data including a detailed history is important and this should be documented carefully, allowing comparisons to be made later.

After obtaining biographical details a personal history should then focus on the individual's perception of their overall health status and the meaning attributed to the current presenting problem. The following should be documented:

- The current problem (documented in their own words).
- Family history; history of premature unexplained death or of coronary artery disease.
- Symptom exploration (e.g. chest pain) (used to obtain information regarding

Table 17.3 Common presenting symptoms of CAD

- Chest pain/discomfort
- Breathlessness
- Fainting/dizziness
- Fatigue
- Palpitations
- Swollen ankles (peripheral oedema)

Onset, Provocation/Palliation, Quality/Quantity, Radiation, Site, Timing and Understanding – OPQRSTU); see Table 17.3.

- Past medical history (prior history of CAD and other physical and mental health problems/surgery).
- Risk factors (e.g. smoking, diet, weight, physical activity, alcohol).
- Treatment – current medication including vaccination history and use of medical equipment.
- Allergies.
- Social history (education, occupation, marital status, living circumstances).
- Psychological status (see Chapter 5).

There are many different factors which can contribute to poor coping in someone with CAD. There may be varying degrees of disability and it is important to perform a functional assessment to determine how current health problems are impacting across the activities of living (ALs).

Physical assessment

Gathering objective data involves the recording of vital observations such as blood pressure, temperature, pulse and respirations as well as a physical examination where each body system is reviewed systematically. Assessment skills of inspection, palpation, percussion and auscultation are utilised by experienced health practitioners. However, the focus here will be on the cardiovascular system and inspection and palpation, as these two techniques are relatively easy to perform yet can yield a great deal of information about the current health status. Only the cardiovascular system will be outlined here and the reader will find other body systems outlined in Chapter 5.

General observations

Individuals presenting with CAD may be extremely distressed not only due to pain but because of the fear and anxiety often generated with cardiac-related disorders. Where there is a cardiac problem the body attempts to compensate by diverting blood from the skin (peripheries) to the essential organs and as a result there is often pallor/greyness with sweating and cold, clammy skin. Poor oxygenation in the lungs and a falling cardiac output will also result in poor oxygenation of tissues, and a bluish discolouration (cyanosis) may be seen under the tongue, ear lobes and fingertips. Poor oxygenation will result in profound breathlessness with increased respirations, and individuals may appear to be gasping for breath.

Observation of the lower legs, feet and ankles may reveal swelling due to fluid retention (oedema) and occurs with worsening heart failure. If severe, such fluid retention may be seen in the lower back region (sacral area) and if abdominal girth is increasing then fluid may be accumulating in the abdominal cavity (ascites). Observation of general appearance may also offer clues regarding individual lifestyle and possible risk, with overweight and nicotine-stained fingers being two examples. The presence of scars may also suggest earlier surgery with a vertical scar over the breastbone possibly the result of a sternotomy (sternal splitting) performed for open heart surgery.

As heart failure worsens and fluid retention increases then pressure in the veins returning blood to the heart increases due to obstruction, and this back pressure can result in distended neck veins, visible when the individual is lying in bed at a 45-degree angle. Increased pressure in the left ventricle can result in similar back flow through the blood vessels to the lungs and can result in fluid accumulating in the air sacs (alveoli) referred to as pulmonary oedema. A productive cough often accompanies pulmonary oedema with 'frothy' sputum and specks of blood common. Audible 'bubbling' sounds may be heard as the individual breathes and pulmonary oedema can be heard with a stethoscope placed on the lower posterior chest wall where crackles can be heard.

Problems with oxygenation in the lungs often develop into severe heart failure and this may be detected by using a simple finger probe called a pulse oximeter which can measure the proportion of haemoglobin in the blood saturated with oxygen. Normal saturation values should be 95 per cent and more, although it is important to know the baseline value. Diminishing urine output may also reflect worsening heart failure where, because of a falling cardiac output, blood pressure in the kidneys is too low to result in filtration. When accompanied by falling blood pressure, increased pulse rate, fluid retention and other signs outlined earlier, this suggests that cardiovascular status is seriously compromised.

Diagnostic tests

Physical examination performed by an experienced health professional is often enough for confident diagnosis of cardiac problems. Additional objective data through diagnostic tests will provide more information on the underlying disease process and ensure that the most appropriate treatment intervention is selected.

Electrocardiogram (ECG)

An ECG is a recording of the electrical activity of the heart from the body surface and is non-invasive and often performed as an outpatient. A baseline ECG is always performed but if a cardiac diagnosis is suspected or confirmed, serial ECGs are repeated as often as every 30 minutes to monitor progression (Webster *et al.* 2007).

Blood tests

A number of blood tests may be requested and baseline values allow useful future comparison. A range of biochemical data can be obtained. Damaged cardiac muscle releases various biomedical markers and these can be detected and measured in the blood. Where there has been death (necrosis) of myocardial muscle, for example, biomedical markers routinely measured are: troponin T, troponin I and creatinine kinase (CK). Urea is a waste product of the body and elevated blood urea levels may

Table 17.4 Diagnostic tests in coronary artery disease

Exercise tolerance tests	ECG monitored while treadmill walking to detect exertion-induced changes
Ambulatory (Holter) monitoring	Miniature ECG worn on chest for 24 to 48 hours allows continuous monitoring. Analysed for abnormalities
Chest X-ray (CXR)	Enlarged heart (cardiomegaly) a common feature of some cardiac conditions. Aorta also evaluated and pulmonary oedema can be detected
Echocardiography	Non-invasive use of sound waves to assess cardiac structure, function and blood flow. Often used to assess left ventricular function. May involve passing probe down oesophagus (gullet) with local anaesthesia
Magnetic resonance imaging (MRI)	Non-invasive use of magnetic field (harmless although noisy) to identify cardiac damage. Need to lie flat for 30 minutes in an enclosed space
Coronary angiogram	Performed in catheter laboratory where catheter inserted (local anaesthetic used) through the groin or arm and advanced to the coronary arteries. Dye injected to detect any narrowing (stenosis) and pictures taken

reflect renal dysfunction. Electrolytes are electrically charged salt particles (e.g. sodium and potassium) in body fluids and a number of conditions can result in blood levels falling outside the normal range. Effective cardiac function is especially dependent on normal potassium levels with low or high levels possibly contributing to abnormal heart rhythms. Diuretic therapy is a major component in treatment regimens for heart failure and helps to decrease fluid retention by increasing urine output, but may result in electrolyte imbalance.

Coagulation studies involve determining how well or not the blood is clotting. Increased stickiness (viscosity) of the blood can precipitate clot formation in the calf muscle (deep vein thrombosis or DVT), lungs (pulmonary embolus or PE), heart (MI) or brain (cerebral thrombus resulting in stroke). Anticoagulation therapy (e.g. warfarin) is often indicated for some with CAD but excessive doses can result in increased bleeding. Lipid profiling contributes to risk evaluation where the various fats carried in the blood including cholesterol and triglycerides are measured. In heart failure not well controlled the cardiac cells release increasing amounts of a small protein called brain natriuretic peptide (BNP) and this can be used as a prognostic indicator.

Haematological blood tests can also be useful. A full blood count provides information on the haemoglobin content and the number of red and white blood cells (called erythrocytes and leucocytes respectively). Low haemoglobin content may suggest that anaemia is contributing to fatigue and an increase in white cells may indicate underlying infection. Erythrocyte sedimentation rate is a blood test which can be performed to detect if there is a focus of inflammation in the body.

Additional diagnostic tests may be required and these are outlined in Table 17.4.

Treatment interventions

The decline in CAD prevalence can be largely attributed to improved secondary prevention measures (measures undertaken once an individual is diagnosed with a disease) and increased access to rapid diagnosis and management. Examples include the widespread introduction of predominantly nurse-led chest pain clinics, better implementation of national and international guidelines for care and the development of primary percutaneous coronary intervention (PPCI) centres to rapidly treat patients following a myocardial infarction (DoH 2008).

Thrombolytic therapy

Thrombolytic therapy is given intravenously to patients diagnosed with a myocardial infarction. It is predominantly administered in the A&E department of an acute hospital although some paramedics may administer pre-hospital thrombolysis. The patient's vital signs need to be carefully monitored following administration of the drug therapy. It acts as a 'clot buster' and so dissolves the blockage in the coronary artery and re-establishes blood flow (Hatchett and Thompson 2007).

Primary percutaneous coronary intervention (PPCI)

PPCI is undertaken in a specialist hospital and is rapidly becoming the treatment of choice following a myocardial infarction. Similar to a coronary angiogram, a catheter is passed into the coronary artery and a small balloon at the tip is inflated to reduce the blockage (Hatchett and Thompson 2007).

Cardiac surgery

Cardiac surgery is sometimes required. This is undertaken in a specialist centre. One of the patient's arteries (usually from the arm) or a vein (from the leg) is grafted to the blocked coronary artery to act as a bypass (Margereson and Riley 2003).

Drug therapy

- Lipid lowering therapy such as simvastatin, atrovastatin or pravastatin.
- Antiplatelet therapy such as aspirin 75 mg daily or clopidogrel.
- Beta blocker such as carvedilol or bisoprolol.
- ACE inhibitors such as ramipril.
- Diuretics such as furosemide or bumetanide.

Risk factors in cardiovascular disease

There are many risk factors for CAD identified by epidemiologists over the years and the puzzle has become increasingly complex. What is agreed is that the cause of CAD is multifactorial and it is likely that a combination of factors is responsible for disease progression. Some risk factors are non-modifiable and include increasing age, ethnicity, sex, family history and premature menopause. A number of risk factors are modifiable so that a knowledge of these is necessary if any contribution is to be made in reducing risk.

Smoking

Smoking is a major cause of CAD and is clearly linked to poor health outcomes in those with coronary heart disease. Individuals who continue to smoke following MI have a 50 per cent higher risk of recurrent coronary events compared to non-smokers (Rea *et al.* 2002; Twardella *et al.* 2004). Evidence suggests that the risk from smoking declines to almost normal after ten years of abstinence. Smoking rates are consistently higher in people with serious mental health problems (McCloughen 2003) and health promotion may be problematic, with individuals often feeling that smoking offers them relaxation, pleasure and social contact, and a significant number of mental health workers believing that smoking is helpful in terms of creating therapeutic relationships (Robson and Gray 2005).

Diet

Diet has long been associated with CAD risk particularly where there is high saturated fat, salt and sugar and low antioxidants (fruit and vegetables) (WHO 2002). A diet of saturated fats can increase blood lipid levels (hyperlipidaemia), and sedentary activity, familial hyperlipidaemia and metabolic conditions such as diabetes can also influence cholesterol levels. Risk may be further increased in those with mental health problems where antipsychotic treatment, particularly with atypical antipsychotics, may contribute to atherosclerosis as a result of high levels of blood triglycerides and weight gain (Sarandol *et al.* 2007). High levels of lipids contribute significantly to the development of atherosclerosis and measurement of a fasting lipid profile (total cholesterol, low- and high-density lipoproteins) should be undertaken in all patients with suspected CVD. High-density lipoproteins offer some protection in that they encourage the removal of fat away from blood vessels. Although cholesterol-lowering drugs have been found to offer benefit for some, there is evidence to show that in those with mental health problems prescription of these drugs is less frequent (Redelmeier *et al.* 1998). Table 17.5 outlines dietary modification which can increase cholesterol levels.

It is recommended that children eat five portions of fruit and vegetables a day and adults should eat at least five portions a day. High-calorie meals rich in processed, easily digestible, quickly absorbable foods and drinks can lead to exaggerated elevations in blood glucose and triglycerides following meals, and it is argued that specific dietary strategies can dramatically and immediately improve glucose and lipid levels, inflammation and endothelial function, with improved cardiovascular health (O'Keefe and Bell 2007; O'Keefe *et al.* 2008).

Obesity and sedentary lifestyle

Sedentary lifestyle leads to weight gain and obesity and is an independent CAD risk factor that is also linked to high blood pressure and raised cholesterol. People who have higher levels of physical activity have a lower risk of CAD. Other benefits include the reduction in the risk of developing diabetes, hypertension and obesity.

Table 17.5 Dietary modifications to improve cholesterol levels

- Reduce intake of saturated fats (butter, cream, fatty meat, cakes, ghee)
- Cut down on total fat intake
- Cut down on trans-fats (fats often found in processed foods such as cakes and biscuits)
- Eat oily fish (sardines, mackerel, fresh tuna)

Table 17.6 Measuring weight gain

Body mass index (BMI)	Significance
BMI less than 18.5	Underweight – may need to gain weight
BMI 18.5–25 (23 in South Asian population)	Normal – attempt to stay at this level
BMI 25–30	Overweight – should attempt to lose weight or stop gaining any more weight
BMI >30	Obese – losing weight may improve health

Measuring waist circumference
Place a tape measure midway between the lower ribs and the top of the hip bone and measure. Increased risk to health if measurement:
>94 cm (men) >80 cm (women)

The current recommendation for adults is 30 minutes of moderate exercise (walking, cycling, running) at least five days of the week (DoH 2004). Exercise can improve inflammation directly by lowering glucose levels following meals and indirectly by reducing excess abdominal fat (Healy *et al.* 2007).

Ability to evaluate weight gain is important, and body mass index (BMI) as well as waist measurements can be useful in identifying those who are overweight. In healthy athletic individuals with greater muscle mass, BMI may give a misleading higher value. The adverse effect of weight is more pronounced when fat is concentrated around the waist (see Table 17.6).

Hypertension

Raised blood pressure beyond acceptable levels is called hypertension and is almost always without symptoms. Individuals with raised blood pressure are just under twice as likely to suffer a heart attack as those with normal blood pressure (Allender *et al.* 2007). The main modifiable causes of hypertension are dietary intake (especially salt), physical activity and alcohol. The maintenance of blood pressure within the normal range remains challenging as a result of an ageing population, improved survival following MI, the prevalence of diabetes and increases in obesity and inactivity levels, but in general risk is reduced by achieving a systolic blood pressure of below 140 mmHg (Pepine *et al.* 2006).

Alcohol

Excess alcohol can be detrimental to the heart, directly causing damage to the heart muscle. Levels of alcohol use may vary greatly across different groups but in those with serious mental health problems as many as 36 per cent are reported as having some form of substance abuse over the course of a year (Primhe *et al.* 2005). However, light to moderate alcohol consumption can improve the prognosis in CAD even in those with associated heart failure as long as intake remains moderate (Cooper *et al.* 2000). Men are encouraged to drink no more than three to four units of alcohol a day and women two to three units a day. A unit is defined as a 25 ml single measure of spirit, a third of a pint of beer or half a standard (175 ml) glass of wine.

Diabetes

Diabetes is closely associated with vascular disease and strongly magnifies the effect of other CAD risk factors particularly where blood glucose control is poor. It substantially increases the risk of CAD (Allender *et al.* 2008). In type 2 diabetes risk is increased by the presence of the metabolic syndrome where there is obesity, impaired fasting glucose, hypertension, low high-density lipoprotein (HDL) cholesterol and elevated triglycerides (Meigs *et al.* 2007) (see Chapter 14).

Psychosocial factors in CAD

Epidemiological studies over the years have identified a number of risk factors contributing to heart disease, some of which have been outlined earlier. However, there is increasing interest in how individual risk is influenced by biological, behavioural and psychosocial processes across the life course or across generations (Kuh and Ben-Shlomo 2004). Despite an earlier focus on smoking, high blood pressure and high cholesterol there is increasing evidence to show that emotions play a role in the progression of atherosclerosis and development of coronary heart disease (Blazer and Hybels 2004). Negative emotions generally are associated with an increased risk of coronary heart disease and depressive symptoms present a degree of relative risk comparable to traditional risk factors (Rugulies 2002). Indeed, it is argued that not only emotional factors including major depression and anxiety disorders as well as hostility and anger are involved, but also chronic stressors such as low social support, low socio-economic status, work stress, marital stress and caregiver strain (Rozanski *et al.* 2005).

Not only do psychosocial factors contribute to the development of CAD but they can also affect progression of the disease following diagnosis. The prevalence of depression in medically ill people ranges from 20 per cent to 50 per cent with milder depression even more common (Jiang 2008). Depression and heart disease often coexist where risk for complications and death is increased (Pozuelo *et al.* 2009). There is often an emphasis on lifestyle modification such as overeating and physical inactivity but, as Rozanski *et al.* (2005) argue, given the strong and robust relation between psychosocial risk factors and CAD a more proactive role is needed in this area.

Facilitating recovery with CHD

Cardiac rehabilitation is recognised as being an effective multidisciplinary treatment for those with cardiac disease (Ades 2001) and is addressed in Standard 12 of the KSF CHD. GP practice surgeries are required to keep registers of individuals with long-term conditions and this includes CHD and heart failure. Identifying those who might benefit from cardiac rehabilitation is important and should be offered to all those following myocardial infarction or cardiac intervention. Those with stable angina and heart failure can also benefit from rehabilitation. Following initial assessment it may be found that there are complex needs, and where necessary there should be referral to social workers, occupational therapists, physiotherapists, cardiologists and mental health workers.

A number of studies have shown that participation in a rehabilitation programme for those with heart disease can reduce hospitalisation rates, increase exercise and improve quality of life. Cardiac rehabilitation is considered in four stages including inpatient care, early post discharge, exercise training and long-term follow up (Scottish Intercollegiate Guidelines Network (SIGN) 2002). It is during phase 2 in the early discharge period where there may be psychological distress and insecurity. Although phase 3, involving structured exercise routines, has traditionally been delivered in a hospital setting, more community interventions are being developed. Once progress has been made, phase 4 involves long-term maintenance of lifestyle changes which need to be continued for maximum benefit.

Risk factors need to be reviewed and appropriate action taken to reduce risk further by lifestyle modification. Individuals will need information on specific cardiac conditions and the treatment necessary, including reasons for prescribed medication. Those with heart failure, for example, should understand the implications of diuretic therapy and be given advice regarding fluid balance and monitoring effectives of therapy (daily weights), salt reduction, smoking cessation as well as influenza and pneumococcal vaccination. If there is a tendency towards abnormal cardiac rhythms then caffeine reduction may also be beneficial. Where symptom relief is still considered poor then referral to a specialist practitioner should be made for review of therapy.

Information giving alone will not necessarily result in healthy behaviours, and rehabilitation programmes which have a psychological and educational component as well as an exercise regimen offer better results (Dusseldorp *et al.* 1999). Time needs to be taken in both clearing up any misconceptions individuals may have and in allaying anxieties. There may be uncertainty in a number of areas including activity levels, return to employment, diet, alcohol consumption, sexual function, travel and insurance issues. Psycho-educational interventions and counselling techniques including motivational interviewing (Miller and Rollnick 2002; Brodie and Inoue 2005) and cognitive behavioural therapy (CBT) have been found to be particularly useful in facilitating lifestyle modification (see Chapter 7).

Uptake of cardiac rehabilitation and other health promotion initiatives can be low in some groups including older people, ethnic minority groups, women, and those with physical disability or mental health problems. Seymour (2003) found that mental health service users have concerns about their physical health and would value helpful and effective health promotion information and advice, but this is largely lacking within existing primary and secondary care services. The stigma of a psychiatric diagnosis may also make it less likely that this group receive optimum healthcare (Phelan *et al.* 2001) and there is considerable evidence that receiving a diagnosis of schizophrenia or bipolar disorder often means that physical health is overlooked or ignored, or takes second place to their mental healthcare (Friedli and Dardis 2002).

A major shift in healthcare focus and government policy over recent years has promoted the idea of collaboration and partnership in the facilitation of self-management. The Expert Patients Programme (EPP) (DoH 2001, 2006) is based on the work of Kate Lorig at Stanford University in the USA and provides training for people with a chronic condition where training is led by people who have personal experience of living with a long-term illness. Such initiatives are used to reduce severity of symptoms and can improve confidence, resourcefulness and self-efficacy.

Standard 11 of the *CHD NSF* (DoH 2000) sets out milestones for improving care and services of those with heart failure, and further guidelines by the Royal College of Physicians (2003) are available on the NICE website. Key aims are helping people to live longer and achieve a better quality of life and, where heart failure is unresponsive, to ensure that appropriate palliative care support is delivered (DoH 2003). Those with heart failure can feel isolated once discharged from hospital and depression is high compared to the general population (Friedman and Griffin 2001).

Table 17.7 Useful contacts (including helpline support)

British Heart Foundation Charity which supports pioneering research, vital prevention activities and also ensures quality care and support for those living with heart disease	www.bhf.org.uk Head Office British Heart Foundation Greater London House 180 Hampstead Road London NW1 7AW Tel: Main 02075540000 Heart helpline: 03003303311 (Mon.–Fri. 9 a.m. to 6 p.m.)
The British Cardiac Patients Association Charity run by volunteers for cardiac patients and their carers. Offers support, reassurance and practical advice	www.bcpa.co.uk BCPA Head Office 15 Abbey Road Bingham Nottingham NG13 8EE Tel: 01949 837070 Email: Enquiries@BCPA.co.uk
HEART UK Charity offering information, advice and support in preventing premature deaths caused by high cholesterol and cardiovascular disease	www.heartuk.org.uk/ HEART UK 7 North Road Maidenhead Berkshire SL6 1PE Helpline: 0845 450 5988 Helpline hours: Tuesday and Thursday from 10 a.m. to 4 p.m. Email: ask@heartuk.org.uk
ASH (Action on Smoking and Health) Campaigning public health charity that works to eliminate the harm caused by tobacco	www.ash.org.uk Action on Smoking and Health First Floor 144–145 Shoreditch High Street London E1 6JE Tel: 0207 739 5902 Email: enquiries@ash.org.uk
Grown Up Congenital Heart Patients Association Helps adults who were born with a heart condition cope with their condition and champions their rights within all aspects of life	www.guch.org.uk/ GUCH Patients Association Saracen's House 25 St Margaret's Green Ipswich IP4 2BN Helpline: 0800 854759 Email: admin@guch.org.uk

Conclusion

This chapter has briefly reviewed the common diseases associated with CAD – angina, myocardial infarction and heart failure – and has outlined the common treatment options. Patients with CAD are not only cared for in the acute hospital setting so it is important that the common diseases and their manifestations are widely understood. Equally much may be done to reduce the risk of developing CAD and the likelihood of it worsening. However, the presence of acute chest pain should always be taken seriously and the individual referred to a specialist centre.

References

Ades, P.A. (2001) Cardiac Rehabilitation and Secondary Prevention of Coronary Heart Disease. *New England Journal of Medicine*, 345, 892–902.

Allen, L.A. and O'Connor, C.M. (2007) Management of Acute Decompensated Heart Failure. *Canadian Medical Association Journal*, 176, 797–805.

Allender, S., Peto., V., Scarborough, P. *et al.* (2007) *Coronary Heart Disease Statistics 2007 Edition*. London: British Heart Foundation.

Allender, S., Peto, V., Scarborough, P. *et al.* (2008) *Coronary Heart Disease Statistics 2008 Edition*. London: British Heart Foundation.

Allison, D.B., Mackell, J.A. and McDonnell, D.D. (2003) The Impact of Weight Gain on Quality of Life Among Persons with Schizophrenia. *Psychiatric Services*, 54(4), 565–567.

Blazer, D.G. and Hybels, C.F. (2004) What Symptoms of Depression Predict Mortality in Community Dwelling Elders? *Journal of the American Geriatrics Society*, 52, 2052–2056.

Brodie, D.A. and Inoue, A. (2005) Motivational Interviewing to Promote Physical Activity for People with Chronic Heart Failure. *Journal of Advanced Nursing*, 50, 518–527.

Camm, A.J. and Bunce, N.H. (2005) Cardiovascular Disease. In Kumar, P. and Clark, M. (eds) *Clinical Medicine* (6th edn). London: Elsevier Saunders.

Clarke, K.W., Gray, D., Keating, N.A. *et al.* (1994) Do Women with Acute Myocardial Infarction Receive the Same Treatment as Men? *British Medical Journal*, 309, 563–566.

Cooper, H.A., Exner, D.V. and Domanski, M.J. (2000) Light-to-moderate Alcohol Consumption and Prognosis in Patients with Left Ventricular Systolic Dysfunction. *Journal of the American College of Cardiology*, 35, 1753–1759.

Cowie, M.R., Mosterd, A., Wood, D.A. *et al.* (1997) The Epidemiology of Heart Failure. *European Heart Journal*, 18(2), 208–225.

Cowie, M.R., Wood, D.A., Coats, A.J.S. *et al.* (2000) Survival of Patients with a New Diagnosis of Heart Failure: A Population Based Study. *Heart*, 83, 505–510.

Davidson, K.W. (2008) Emotional Predictors and Behavioral Triggers of Acute Coronary Syndrome. *Cleveland Clinic Journal of Medicine*, 75 (suppl. 2), S15–S19.

Department of Health (DoH) (2000) *Coronary Heart Disease: National Service Framework for Coronary Heart Disease: Modern Standards and Service Models*. London: DoH.

Department of Health (DoH) (2001) *The Expert Patient. A New Approach to Chronic Disease Management for the 21st Century*. London: DoH.

Department of Health (DoH) (2003) Developing Services for Heart Failure. London. Online. Available at: www.dh.gov.uk/en/Publicationsandstatistics/Publications/PublicationsPolicyAndGuidance/DH_4069457 (accessed 17 March 2009).

Department of Health (DoH) (2004) *At Least Five a Week: Evidence on the Impact of Physical Activity and its Relationship to Health*. London: DoH.

Department of Health (DoH) (2005) *National Service Framework for Coronary Heart Disease. Chapter Eight. Arrhythmias and Sudden Cardiac Death*. London. Online. Available at: www.dh.gov.uk/en/Healthcare/NationalServiceFrameworks/Coronaryheartdisease/DH_4117048 (accessed 18 March 2009).

Department of Health (DoH) (2006) *Supporting People with Long Term Conditions to Self Care: A Guide to Developing Local Strategies and Good Practice*. London: DoH.

Department of Health (DoH) (2008) *The Coronary Heart Disease National Service Framework. Building for the Future. Progress Report 2007*. London: DoH.

Disability Rights Commission (DRC) (2006) Equal Treatment: Closing the Gap. Online. Available at: www.equalityhumanrights.com/en/publicationsandresources/Documents/Disability/Health_FI_part1.pdf (accessed March 2009).

Dixon, L.B., Kreyenbuhl, J.A., Dickerson, F.B. *et al.* (2004) A Comparison of Type 2 Diabetes Outcomes among Persons with and without Severe Mental Illnesses. *Psychiatric Services*, 55, 892–900.

Dusseldorp, E., van Elderen, T., Maes, S. *et al.* (1999) A Meta-analysis of Psychoeducational Programs for Coronary Heart Disease Patients. *Health Psychology*, 18, 506–519.

Fox, C. (2004) *Heart Disease and South Asians. Delivering the National Service Framework for Coronary Heart Disease*. London: DoH. Online. Available at: www.dh.gov.uk/en/Publicationsandstatistics/Publications/PublicationsPolicyAndGuidance/DH_4098586 (accessed 18 March 2009).

Fox, K., Garcia, M., Ardissino, D. *et al.* (2006) Guidelines on the Management of Stable Angina Pectoris; Executive Summary: The Task Force on the Management of Stable Angina Pectoris of the European Society of Cardiology. *European Heart Journal*, 27, 1341–1381.

Friedli, L. and Dardis, C. (2002) Smoke Gets on their Eyes. *Mental Health Today*, January, 18–21.

Friedman, M.M. and Griffin, J.A. (2001) Relationship of Physical Symptoms and Physical Functioning to Depression in Patients with Heart Failure. *Heart and Lung*, 30, 98–104.

Gillespie, N.D. (2006) The Diagnosis and Management of Chronic Heart Failure in the Older Patient. *British Medical Bulletin*, 75–76, 49–62.

Hansson, G.K. (2005) Inflammation, Atherosclerosis, and Coronary Artery Disease. *New England Journal of Medicine*, 352, 1685–1695.

Hatchett, R. and Thompson, D. (eds) (2007) *Cardiac Nursing. A Comprehensive Guide* (2nd edn). Philadelphia, PA: Churchill Livingstone.

Healy, G., Dunstan, D., Salmon, J. *et al.* (2007) Objectively Measured Light Intensity Physical Activity is Independently Associated with 2-h Plasma Glucose. *Diabetes Care*, 30, 1384–1389.

Jiang, W. (2008) Impacts of Depression and Emotional Distress on Cardiac Disease. *Cleveland Clinic Journal of Medicine*, 75, S20–S25.

Jindal, R., MacKenzie, E.M., Baker, G.B. *et al.* (2005) Cardiac Risk and Schizophrenia. *Journal of Psychiatry Neuroscience*, 30(6), 393–395.

Klabunde, R.E. (2007) Cardiovascular Physiology Concepts. Online. Available at: www.cvphysiology.com/Heart%20Failure/HF002.htm (accessed 18 March 2009).

Kuh, D. and Ben-Shlomo, Y. (2004) *A Life Course Approach to Chronic Disease Epidemiology*. New York: Oxford University Press.

Lockyer, L. (2005) Women's Interpretation of their Coronary Heart Disease. *European Journal of Cardiovascular Nursing*, 4(1), 29–36.

McCloughen, A. (2003) The Association between Schizophrenia and Cigarette Smoking: A Review of the Literature and Implications for Mental Health Nursing Practice. *International Journal of Mental Health Nursing*, 12, 119–129.

Margereson, C. and Riley, J. (2003) *Cardiothoracic Surgical Nursing: Current Trends in Adult Care*. Oxford: Blackwell Publishing.

Meigs, J.B., Rutter, M.K., Sullivan, L.M. *et al.* (2007) Impact of Insulin Resistance on Risk of Type 2 Diabetes and Cardiovascular Disease in People with Metabolic Syndrome. *Diabetes Care*, 30, 1219–1225.

Mentality/NIMHE (2004) Healthy Body and Mind: Promoting Healthy Living for People who Experience Mental Distress. Online. Available at: www.neyh.csip.org.uk/silo/files/hbhm-primarycare.pdf (accessed 18 March 2009).

Mikhail, G. (2005) Coronary Heart Disease in Women. *British Medical Journal*, 331, 467–468.

Miller, W.R. and Rollnick, S. (2002) *Motivational Interviewing. Preparing People for Change*. London: The Guilford Press.

O'Keefe, J. and Bell, D. (2007) The Post-prandial Hyperglycemia/Hyperlipemia Hypothesis: A Hidden Cardiovascular Risk Factor? *American Journal of Cardiology*, 100, 899–904.

O'Keefe, J.H., Gheewala, N.M. and O'Keefe, J.O. (2008) Dietary Strategies for Improving Post-prandial Glucose, Lipids, Inflammation, and Cardiovascular Health. *Journal of the American College of Cardiology*, 51, 249–255.

Pepine, C.J., Kowey, P.R., Kupfer, S. *et al.* (2006) Predictors of Adverse Outcome Among Patients with Hypertension and Coronary Heart Disease. *Journal of the American College of Cardiology*, 47, 547–551.

Pfisterer, M. (2004) Trial of Invasive Versus Medical Therapy in Elderly Patients Investigators. Long-Term Outcome in Elderly Patients with Chronic Angina Managed Invasively Versus by Optimized Medical Therapy: Four-year Follow-up of the Randomized Trial of Invasive Versus Medical Therapy in Elderly Patients (TIME). *Circulation*, 110, 1213–1218.

Phelan, M., Stradins, L. and Morrison, S. (2001) Physical Health of People with Severe Mental Illness. *British Medical Journal*, 322, 443–444.

Pozuelo, L., Jianping, Z., Franco, K. *et al.* (2009) Depression and Heart Disease: What Do We Know, and Where are We Headed? *Cleveland Clinic Journal of Medicine*, 76, 59–70.

Rea, T.D., Heckbert, S.R., Kaplan, R.C. *et al.* (2002) Smoking Status and Risk for Recurrent Coronary Events after Myocardial Infarction. *Annals Internal Medicine*, 137, 500.

Redelmeier, D.A., Tan, S.H. and Booth, G.L. (1998) The Treatment of Unrelated Disorders in Patients with Chronic Medical Diseases. *New England Journal of Medicine*, 338, 1516–1520.

Rethink. (2005) *Running on Empty: Building Momentum to Improve Wellbeing in Severe Mental Illness*. London: Rethink.

Robson, D. and Gray, R. (2005) Can we Help People with Schizophrenia Stop Smoking? *Mental Health Practice*, 9(4), 14–18.

Royal College of Physicians (2003) *Chronic Heart Failure. National Clinical Guidelines for Diagnosis and Management in Primary and Secondary Care*. The National Collaborating Centre for Chronic Conditions. Online. Available at: www.nice.org.uk/nicemedia/pdf/Full_HF_Guideline.pdf (accessed March 2009).

Rozanski, A., Blumenthal, J.A., Davidson, K.W. *et al.* (2005) The Epidemiology, Pathophysiology and Management of Psychosocial Risk Factors in Cardiac Practice: The Emerging Field of Behavioural Cardiology. *Journal of the American College of Cardiology*, 45, 637–651.

Rugulies, R. (2002) Depression as a Predictor for Coronary Heart Disease: A Review and Meta-analysis. *American Journal of Preventive Medicine*, 23, 51–61.

Sarandol, A., Kirli, S., Akkaya, C. *et al.* (2007) Coronary Artery Disease Risk Factors in Patients with Schizophrenia: Effects of Short Term Antipsychotic Treatment. *Journal of Psychopharmacology*, 21, 857–863.

Schoen, F.J. (2004) *The Heart*. In Kumar, V., Abbas, A. and Fausto, N. (eds) *Robbins and Cotran Pathologic Basis of Disease* (7th edn). Philadelphia, PA: Elsevier Saunders.

Scottish Intercollegiate Guidelines Network (SIGN) (2002) 57. *Cardiac Rehabilitation. A National Guideline*. Edinburgh: SIGN. Online. Available at: www.sign.ac.uk/pdf/sign57.pdf (accessed 18 March 2009).

Seymour, L. (2003) Not All in the Mind: The Physical Health of Mental Health Service Users. Mentality. Online. Available at: www.scmh.org.uk/pdfs/not+all+in+the+mind.pdf (accessed 18 March 2009).

Spagnoli, L.G., Bonanno, E., Sangiorgi, G. *et al.* (2007) Role of Inflammation in Atherosclerosis. *Journal of Nuclear Medicine*, 48, 1800–1815.

Steg, P. and Himbert, D. (2005) Unmet Medical Needs and Therapeutic Opportunities in Stable Angina. *European Heart Journal Supplement*, 7, H7–H15.

Stewart, S., Jenkins, A., Buchan, S. *et al.* (2002) The Current Cost of Heart Failure to the National Health Service in the UK. *European Journal of Heart Failure*, 4, 361–371.

Twardella, D., Kupper-Nuybelen, J., Rothenbacher, D. *et al.* (2004) Short-term Benefit of Smoking Cessation in Patients with Coronary Heart Disease: Estimates Based on Self-reported Smoking Data and Serum Cotinine Measurements. *European Heart Journal*, 25, 2101–2108.

Webster, R., Hatchett, R. and Waring, E. (2007) Coronary Heart Disease: Stable Angina and Acute Coronary Syndromes. In Hatchett, R. and Thompson, D. (eds) *Cardiac Nursing. A Comprehensive Guide* (2nd edn). Philadelphia, PA: Churchill Livingstone.

World Health Organisation (WHO) (2004) *The Atlas of Heart Disease and Stroke*. Online. Available at: www.who.int/cardiovascular_diseases/resources/atlas/en/print.html (accessed 10 July 2008).

World Health Organisation (WHO) (2002) *The World Health Report 2002 – Reducing Risks, Promoting Healthy Life*. Online. Available at: www.who.int/whr/2002/en/ (accessed 12 July 2008).

18 Asthma and chronic obstructive pulmonary disease

Samantha Prigmore and Carl Margereson

Introduction

Respiratory disease is the third most commonly reported long-term condition in the United Kingdom (UK) with more people dying from a respiratory condition (117,456 in 2004) than from ischaemic heart disease (106,081) (British Thoracic Society (BTS) 2006). Two common respiratory diseases are asthma and chronic obstructive pulmonary disease (COPD). Asthma affects 5.2 million people in the UK and was responsible for 80,593 hospital admissions in 2006 to 2007, costing the NHS an estimated £61 billion. Drug therapy in asthma is very effective and it is believed that 75 per cent of all hospital admissions could have been avoided through good asthma management and routine care (Asthma UK 2008).

Nearly 900,000 people in the UK have been diagnosed with COPD (National Institute for Health and Clinical Excellence (NICE) 2004), although it is argued that the real figure is likely to be 3.7 million (Shahab *et al.* 2006) with 2.8 million unaware that they have this disease and referred to as the 'missing millions' (British Lung Foundation (BLF) 2007). With respiratory disease the second most common illness responsible for emergency medical admissions, over one million bed days are occupied by individuals with COPD (Commission for Healthcare Audit and Inspection 2006) and the direct cost of providing care in the NHS is almost £500 million a year.

But it is the personal cost of respiratory disease that is enormous and which needs to be considered. Troublesome breathlessness can be profoundly disabling, leading to loss of independence and poor quality of life. People with severe COPD often report that they feel invisible and seldom have the energy or the confidence to challenge those in authority (BLF 2007). With worsening symptoms, all aspects of life can be affected, and with increasing loss of independence and increased isolation it is hardly surprising that psychological distress is experienced by many with COPD (Dowson *et al.* 2004; Wagena *et al.* 2005).

In those with asthma, undertreatment can result in disturbed sleep, time off work, reduced exercise tolerance, and inability to enjoy previously enjoyed leisure activities. Management of symptoms may be particularly challenging in those living alone/socially isolated, and where there is physical disability, learning difficulties or mental health problems. In severe asthma, where there are one or more behavioural or psychosocial factors, the risk of death is high (British Thoracic Society/Scottish Intercollegiate Guidelines Network (BTS/SIGN) 2008).

Professional and non-professional carers alike must be aware of those individuals diagnosed with a respiratory disorder and, as well as having an understanding of the disease process, should be familiar with management principles and the agreed care plan. Although this chapter focuses on those already diagnosed with asthma or COPD, carers need to be vigilant for progressive symptoms which may indicate the early onset of respiratory disease. A significant number of individuals have undiagnosed COPD and early detection is crucial so that a diagnosis can be made and appropriate care given.

Pathophysiology of obstructive lung disease

Asthma and COPD are referred to as obstructive lung diseases. The respiratory tract facilitates the movement of air in and out of the lungs and is made up of airways (passages) called bronchi and smaller bronchioles, terminating in small air sacs (alveoli) where oxygen and carbon dioxide between lungs and blood are exchanged. The process of breathing drives air through the airways, and in health, little effort is required as there is no obstruction to flow. A number of factors can contribute to airway obstruction, and in diseases such as asthma and COPD it is inflammation of the delicate inner lining of the airways. Irritation of this inner lining (respiratory epithelium) results in a great number of inflammatory cells (e.g. neutrophils and eosinophils) contributing to increased narrowing as a result of tissue swelling and muscle spasm. This narrowing of the airways makes the work of breathing much harder and there is increased awareness of the effort involved with each breath. We will consider asthma and COPD separately.

Asthma

Asthma is regarded as a chronic inflammatory disorder of the airways, and recognition of the inflammatory basis of this disorder is crucial if management is to be understood. Airway inflammation causes recurrent episodes of wheezing, breathlessness, chest tightness and coughing, particularly at night or in the early morning. These episodes are usually associated with widespread but variable airflow obstruction that is often reversible either spontaneously or with treatment (BTS/SIGN 2008). The inflammation also causes increased sensitivity of the airways (bronchial hyper-reactivity) which is triggered by a variety of stimuli. What initiates and promotes this ongoing inflammation has generated many different theories. A history of allergy (atopy) is typical, however, and specific allergens may be known (e.g. house dust mites, cat dander, food items, pollen) with allergen avoidance being an important part of self-management.

Chronic obstructive pulmonary disease (COPD)

The term COPD includes chronic bronchitis, emphysema and chronic asthma, but a recent survey highlights confusion over the name and inconsistency around diagnosis and explanation by healthcare workers (BLF 2006). The airway obstruction in COPD also has an inflammatory component, but in contrast to asthma, obstruction is not reversible and the airflow limitation tends to be progressive (Barnes 2000). With emphysema there is destruction and breakdown of the air sac walls by digestive enzymes released by neutrophils, and this eventually results in impaired gas exchange. Initially there may be few symptoms with mild COPD, but as the disease worsens there is cough, increased sputum production, breathlessness and disability. Eventually there will be difficulty in oxygenation and the removal of carbon dioxide from the blood and lungs, and the development of respiratory failure.

The major cause of COPD is smoking. It has been found that those at risk of future hospital admission from COPD live mostly in social housing and have, or have had, industrial or semi-skilled jobs, uncertain employment, low levels of disposable income and considerable health problems, and by using postcodes, 'hotspot' areas of high-risk groups in the UK have been identified (BLF 2007). These reflect areas where health inequalities exist, and in the main are urban areas of former industrial landscapes where factories, steelworks, dockyards and mines once existed.

Assessment issues

Chapter 5 offers frameworks for comprehensive assessments and here we will focus on issues specifically relating to asthma and COPD. Most individuals will probably have a periodic assessment of their respiratory status by either a doctor or nurse specialist and this should take place at least annually, depending on the severity of their symptoms and disease. With severe COPD, review by an experienced health professional may be needed every six months. However, once diagnosed, ongoing monitoring of the effectiveness of any prescribed treatment regimen, as well as recognition of any deterioration should be encouraged. The extent to which individuals are involved in self-management activities will vary depending on ability, but in overcoming disability, individual strengths need to be identified so that, however small, individuals have a role to play, thus promoting self-efficacy. Assessment always provides an ideal opportunity to assess individual ability to use a prescribed inhaler.

Ensuring that the correct diagnosis is made is important, as individuals may have been incorrectly 'labelled' as having asthma rather than COPD, and Table 18.1 outlines the main differences in the presenting symptoms with each disorder. These should be considered when assessing and reviewing individuals.

Subjective data

This part of the assessment involves taking a history and gathering information about the individual's respiratory problem and presenting symptoms. In some

Table 18.1 Differences in presentation: asthma and COPD

Presentation/symptom	Asthma	COPD
Dominant inflammatory cells in airways	Eosinophils, lymphocytes, mast cells	Neutrophils, macrophages
Childhood symptoms	Common	Occasional
Allergies	Common	Occasional
Family history	Common	Occasional
Smoking history	Less common	Usual
Breathlessness on effort	Intermittent	Progressive
Nocturnal waking	Common	Occasional
Cough	Common	Always
Sputum	Sometimes	Always
Wheeze	Intermittent	Often present

instances information may need to be obtained from primary carers/relatives. Initially the data collected should be comprehensive so that all necessary details are readily available and simply updated as necessary. Too often the only focus is on whether or not medication is being taken as prescribed. Activities of living should be explored, as symptoms can often impact, for example, on sleeping patterns, work and leisure, personal hygiene and the ability to cope generally with household activities.

In this initial part of the assessment the following areas should be explored and documented:

- Personal and social history with details of primary carer/s.
- Major health problem/s in the individual's own words.
- Review of symptoms (see OPQRSTU assessment in Chapter 5) and in particular noting breathlessness, cough, sputum, pain and any recent changes.
- Triggers precipitating wheeze and breathlessness.
- Medication prescribed and level of understanding. 'Over-the-counter preparations' and any recreational drugs should be documented.
- Dates of vaccines (e.g. influenza and pneumococcal).
- Equipment used (e.g. inhalers, nebulisers, oxygen therapy) together with contact details of suppliers and specialist support.
- Allergies (asthmatics may have other allergy-driven conditions, such as eczema or hay fever, which if treated appropriately may improve their asthma control).
- Tobacco and alcohol use.
- Medical history (e.g. medical conditions, mental health problems, surgical procedures, hospitalisations and frequency).
- Occupational history (some respiratory diseases may be linked to occupational exposure (e.g. coal-mining, noxious fumes (soldering) and irritants (chemicals)).

With increasing age the presence of several diseases may be a reality for some and is referred to as co-morbidity. Many factors contribute to the development of diseases such as COPD and may also be implicated in the development of heart disease and diabetes. Being aware of other conditions is important, as these may impact on how the respiratory problem is experienced and managed. Additional symptoms may arise not only due to other conditions but from the side-effects of prescribed medication. Readers should refer to other relevant chapters in this section for guidance on how other health conditions should be assessed and managed.

Psychosocial assessment either during an episodic assessment or as part of ongoing care should be undertaken but although the psychological impact of COPD can be profound, depression is often not detected. Assessment of those with depression is addressed in Chapter 15.

Objective data

This is where objective measurements are obtained to complement the subjective data so that there is a more complete picture and includes physical examination. Temperature, pulse, respiratory rate and blood pressure readings are often routinely taken as part of any assessment. Height and weight should be recorded and the body mass index (BMI) recorded (normal adult range 18.5 to 25). Excessive weight gain may contribute to breathing difficulties, and studies show that significant weight loss (low BMI) along with the degree of airway obstruction, breathlessness and exercise performance can predict morbidity and mortality risk in COPD (Celli et al. 2004).

The measurement of breathlessness in respiratory disease is quite difficult, as so many factors contribute to this distressing symptom. However, there are several measurement tools available including the Medical Research Council (MRC) Breathlessness Scale (Fletcher 1960) (see Chapter 6) used in COPD and scores allow future comparisons so that judgements can be made regarding progress and rate of decline.

Observation of sputum is an important aspect to discuss with clients, as changes in colour, amount and consistency may indicate possible deterioration and infection. The British Lung Foundation has published a useful self-management booklet for those with COPD which contains a colour chart to aid early detection. Although many respiratory infections are caused by viruses where antibiotics are not indicated, green sputum may signify a higher bacterial load (Stockley et al. 2000) and antibiotics are usually prescribed.

Oxygenation of the blood can be measured simply and painlessly by using pulse oximetry and in COPD oxygen saturations of 88 to 92 per cent are acceptable. In controlled asthma, oxygen saturations should be greater than 95 per cent with levels below 92 per cent possibly indicating acute severe asthma, or worse still, life-threatening asthma. Health professionals who are caring for those with COPD and asthma on a regular basis should be able to utilise pulse oximetry in the assessment of clients and be competent in interpreting values. If appropriate, lung function measurements may be taken to estimate the degree of airway obstruction, and this involves the use of spirometers and peak expiratory flow rate (PEFR) meters, which although used in initial diagnosis are important in ongoing review and assessment.

Measuring airway obstruction

Peak expiratory flow rate (using a peak flow meter) expressed in litres per minute (L/min) measures the rate of airflow through the airways and is a useful measurement in the management of asthma but of less benefit in COPD. An increase in peak flow rate reveals that lung function has improved with a decrease indicating possible deterioration. Spirometry measures the amount of air expelled from the lungs in the first second of a forced expiration known as forced expiratory volume 1 (FEV_1). The forced expiratory volume in one second (FEV_1) and the maximum volume of air expired from the lungs during a forced and complete expiration from a position of full inspiration (forced vital capacity or FVC) are recorded. This requires the individual to breathe in as deeply as possible, and then, using a one-way mouthpiece attached to a spirometer, blowing out forcibly and as hard and as fast as possible until no more air can be expelled, which for some can take as long as 15 seconds (BTS COPD Consortium 2005). Spirometry is the gold standard of classifying the severity of airflow obstruction, and the recording of the FEV_1 level of someone with COPD is performed annually by GPs and practice nurses.

With healthy lungs, most of the air during a forced expiratory effort can be removed during the first second (i.e. over 80 per cent of the total volume of the lungs). This indicates that air can be removed from the lungs during expiration with very little obstruction to airflow. However, in obstructive lung diseases, like asthma and COPD, FEV_1 typically falls below the 80 per cent level and in COPD FEV_1 is used to classify disease severity (see Table 18.2). As FEV_1 continues to fall, symptoms become more noticeable and troublesome, but there are steps that may be taken to slow the rate of decline, for example, by stopping smoking.

Peak expiratory flow rate (PEFR)

PEFR can be a useful measure where control of asthma is not achieved. Peak flow meters manufactured since 2004 conform to a new European standard referred to as the new 'EU' scale providing greater accuracy than earlier models. To obtain a peak flow reading a maximum deep breath is taken, the lips then close around the mouthpiece attached to the peak flow meter and the air blown out as hard and as fast as possible. The pointer must be at zero (that is, 0 litres per minute or 0 L/min) before each manoeuvre.

One-off peak flow readings can be helpful, although clients may also be asked to keep a diary of their morning and evening peak flow values for a two-week period. From these recorded values the degree of change or variability between morning and evening readings can be calculated. Slight variability is normal but where this is greater than 20 per cent and occurring on two or more days each week then symptom control is likely to be suboptimal (Case Study 18.1). Accompanying symptoms may include disturbed sleep, increasing cough/wheeze, chest tightness and reduced exercise tolerance, and the management plan should be reviewed by the GP or an experienced practice nurse.

Peak flow values along with presenting symptoms may also be used to identity the severity of asthma in clients where control is poor and where the current PEFR is calculated (Box 18.1) as a percentage of the client's normal value when well or predicted value (that is, the value obtained from a chart of what we may predict as being normal). 'Normal' and 'predicted' values provide a reference point with predicted values based on gender, age and height. If someone has never used a peak flow meter before then they will not know their normal value. Predicted values along with other useful information on peak flow monitoring may be accessed from the Clement Clarke international website (www.peakflow.com/top_nav/home/index.html) as well as the BTS/SIGN (2008) asthma guidelines (www.brit.thoracic.org.uk).

Table 18.2 Severity of airflow obstruction in COPD

Mild obstruction = FEV_1 between 50 and 80%
Moderate obstruction = FEV_1 between 30 and 49%
Severe obstruction = FEV_1 less than 30%

Source: NICE (2004).

Note
Values given are percentages of normal or predicted.

Box 18.1 Calculating peak expiratory flow rate values in asthma

PEFR variability (usually less than 20 per cent variability where asthma is well controlled):

$$\frac{\text{Highest reading} - \text{lowest reading}}{\text{Highest reading}} \times 100$$

PEFR as a % of client's normal value:

$$\frac{\text{Current reading}}{\text{Normal or predicted}} \times 100$$

Values in asthma
Greater than 80% = good control
50 to 80% = mild to moderate asthma
33 to 49% = acute severe asthma
Less than 33% = life-threatening asthma

Case study 18.1   Poorly controlled asthma

John is 28 years old and has had asthma since childhood. During his asthma review by the practice nurse John was asked to keep a diary of his morning and evening peak flow values over a two-week period. When well, John's best peak flow reading is 600 L/ min but reviewing his diary the nurse notes that the lowest reading is 400 L/min and highest is 550 L/min. She calculates a variability of 27 per cent which is occurring several times each week:

$$\frac{550 - 400}{550} \times 100 = 27\%$$

During his review the nurse requests another peak flow reading so that she can observe his technique. He repeats this three times and the best value obtained is 450 L/min. Calculated as a percentage of his normal value (600 L/min), this is 75 per cent, indicating mild to moderate severity.

$$\frac{450}{600} \times 100 = 75\%$$

His peak flow readings demonstrate that current treatment is not adequate. The nurse increases the dose of inhaled corticosteroid and checks John's inhaler technique. On his next visit his peak values have improved along with his symptoms.

Physical examination of the respiratory system

Although physical examination involves inspection, palpation, percussion and auscultation, non-specialists do not usually complete full physical examinations. However, even where carers have limited training, inspection skills can be really useful in detecting relevant changes. Non-specialist nurses will also find that developing basic skills in auscultation will enable them to obtain a more comprehensive picture.

Inspection

Although inspection may be part of an episodic assessment in a clinic setting, ongoing inspection of clients in other residential and healthcare settings will enable significant change to be detected. During the routine care of clients (e.g. when assisting with hygiene needs) ongoing observation should be purposeful so that subtle respiratory changes, possibly denoting early deterioration, can be picked up.

Inspection of someone with a respiratory problem begins during history-taking and a great deal of information may be obtained by direct observation. In well-controlled asthma there should be no abnormal visible signs. In COPD this will depend on the severity, and baseline data should be documented and updated regularly so that comparison can be made. An increase in the resting respiratory rate (adult rate is usually 12 to 20) accompanied by signs of distress will indicate that the work of breathing has increased, possibly due to worsening of the respiratory condition. A resting rate of 24 or more in someone with asthma would be very serious but in someone with moderate to severe COPD may be acceptable. An obvious wheeze during inspiration and expiration may also be heard. Observation of individuals when walking or carrying out simple tasks/activities of living may indicate that exercise tolerance has reduced, but in COPD the significance of this will only be known if baseline data (when stable) are documented. This is where the MRC Breathlessness Scale (Fletcher 1960) is useful with scores documented for later comparison. Observation of chest expansion may also reveal inequality with one side expanding less than the other. Reduced expansion on one side can be due to a collapsed lung or to consolidation of lung tissue.

Observation of the skin may detect signs of weight loss, swollen ankles (indicating possible fluid retention), dehydration, bruising or skin thinning secondary to long-term corticosteroid use. Bluish discolouration (cyanosis) of the tissues may also be evident where there is difficulty with oxygenation. Central cyanosis (due to heart and/or lung disease) can affect the lips, oral mucosa, tongue and conjunctivae, and peripheral cyanosis (poor circulation) results in a bluish tinge to the fingers, nose and earlobes. COPD can result in chronically low levels of oxygen in the blood (chronic hypoxaemia) which the body can adjust to over time. Oxygenation is normal in well-controlled asthma but cyanosis during an acute episode is a serious sign. However, cyanosis can be a late sign and difficult to detect, and other signs of respiratory distress must be monitored. As many as 26 per cent of individuals with stable COPD have heart failure (Rutten *et al.* 2005) and increasing breathlessness, fatigue, reduced exercise tolerance and swollen ankles and legs of recent onset should be investigated

Because breathing can be controlled voluntarily, the respiratory rate is often counted after taking the radial pulse (with fingers still on the pulse). An increase in resting respiratory rate (>24) with also an increase in the pulse (>110) should be of concern, as this may indicate serious respiratory problems. These are the body's attempts to try to maintain effective oxygenation but unfortunately results in much greater effort, and the need for even more energy and oxygen. At rest and during health the main muscle used for breathing is the diaphragm with very little energy needed for breathing. Where breathing is difficult, other muscles (accessory muscles) are also used and include those in the neck (sternocleidomastoids) as well as the shoulder girdle (e.g. trapezius and pectorals). The use of accessory muscles suggests difficulties in breathing, as does nasal flaring (Kennedy 2007) and action should be taken to avoid fatigue which can result in respiratory failure, where oxygen pressures in the blood fall below acceptable levels and where carbon dioxide can also accumulate because the individual is too tired to adequately ventilate

Palpation and percussion

Only a brief overview of these two techniques performed during a physical examination can be given here. Palpation involves the use of the examiner's sense of touch. The skin may feel very warm where there is infection, or cool where the ambient temperature is too low, or perhaps when the circulation is poor. Care should be taken when gently palpating the anterior and posterior chest when searching for possible tender areas (e.g. due to fractured ribs). Experienced practitioners may obtain further information by performing percussion which can detect areas of the lung that may have underlying pathology. Percussion involves tapping the surface of the anterior and posterior chest which produces a sound described as either resonant (underlying hollow, air-containing structures) or dull (where, for example, there is consolidation, as in pneumonia).

Auscultation

Auscultation of the chest involves listening with the help of a stethoscope to the sounds produced by air moving through the airways. The diaphragm rather than the bell of the stethoscope is used, and although the skill of auscultation may seem complex initially, with practice some mastery can be achieved to enhance pulmonary assessment by providing additional data. Appreciation of normal breath sounds is paramount as a first step in acquiring skills in auscultation so that possible abnormalities can be detected, such as wheezes and crackles.

Treatment

Smoking cessation

Maternal smoking during pregnancy can affect infant lung function with increased infant wheezing (Dezateau *et al.* 1999) and direct or passive exposure to cigarette smoke adversely affects quality of life, lung function and long-term control with inhaled steroids in asthma (Chalmers *et al.* 2002). Risk for COPD is increased with a pack year figure of around 20 (Pack years = Number of cigarettes smoked per day × years/20) (see Chapter 5), and the single most important management strategy is smoking cessation if the rate of lung function deterioration is to be reduced.

A number of factors may contribute to the development of respiratory problems in those who smoke. As we saw in Chapter 1, the development of long-term disorders including COPD may be associated with risk accumulation over an individual's life stages, where not only genetic predisposition but socio-economic disadvantage and psychosocial stress increase vulnerability. People with serious mental health problems tend to be in poorer physical health than those without mental illness and studies show that respiratory illness is the most prevalent physical health problem (Amaddeo *et al.* 1995; Kamara *et al.* 1998; Jones *et al.* 2004). Yet in this group and in many institutional settings, higher smoking rates contribute to the increased risk of respiratory problems. The culture within the mental healthcare system generally often promotes smoking, although research has shown that many mental health service users are concerned about their physical health and would like help and advice on looking after themselves more effectively (Seymour 2003). Appropriate health promotion strategies are needed for specific groups where perhaps smoking is a coping mechanism they use in stressful situations.

With smoking the biggest cause of COPD and also an important cause of poor control in asthma, smoking cessation is an important goal. For non-smokers with respiratory problems smoky environments should be avoided and UK legislation in 2007, banning smoking in public places, has been a positive public health measure. Smokers should be encouraged to stop but many will have a physical, psychological and emotional dependence and will need support.

Quitting can be difficult with side-effects troublesome, making behavioural support a vital component in successful smoking cessation and it is here that tailored advice with follow-up by motivated healthcare professionals can be very effective (Lewis 2007). Success improves with pharmacological interventions and effects of nicotine withdrawal reduced with nicotine replacement therapy (NRT) available as gum, patches and lozenges. Other non-nicotine-based treatments are available but further guidance should be sought from pharmacists and experienced health professionals.

NHS Choices is a useful website which can help individuals locate local support services for specific postcodes (www.smokefree.nhs.uk/) and QUIT is an independent charity offering support by experienced counsellors (www.quit.org.uk/). Although complementary approaches (e.g. hypnosis and acupuncture) offer benefit for some, studies demonstrate limited effectiveness over conventional treatment (Abbott *et al.* 1998; White *et al.* 2006).

Drug therapy in asthma

Drug treatment in asthma is very effective and should result in no daytime symptoms, no early awakening, no limitations on activity and normal lung function (BTS/SIGN 2008). Because COPD in contrast is an irreversible condition, management goals are different and include prevention of disease progression, relief of symptoms, improved exercise tolerance and health status (NICE 2004). Maintenance drug therapy usually involves administration using the inhaled and occasionally the oral route. In acute situations, as well as increased doses of inhaled medication, intravenous therapy is often required.

Two groups of drugs used in asthma are commonly referred to as relievers and preventers. Examples of 'reliever' drugs are salbutamol (beta2 agonist) and ipratropium (anti-cholinergic), short-acting bronchodilators used to open the airways and reduce wheeze. In mild asthma the occasional use of a reliever such as a salbutamol (more effective than ipratropium) may be enough to control symptoms. However, where control is not achieved, drugs are prescribed to reduce the airway inflammation such as inhaled corticosteroids (ICS) (e.g. beclomethasone) and these are 'preventers'. The prescribed daily inhaled steroid is best taken in two doses, morning and evening, and, when first prescribed, encouragement and perseverance is needed as it can often take several days for any benefit to be seen.

Where asthma control is still not achieved, review by a specialist nurse or doctor is important so that additional treatment may be prescribed. A stepwise approach to drug therapy in asthma management is adopted and the step selected which is most appropriate to initial severity (BTS/SIGN 2008). Although this may involve increasing the dose of inhaled corticosteroids, the use of another preventer such as a long-acting beta2 agonist (LABA) is often far more effective. For some, combination therapy delivered with an inhaler containing both a LABA and a corticosteroid gives better results than doses of ICS alone (GINA 2008). Examples of inhalers providing combination therapy are Symbicort (budesonide and formoterol) and Seretide (fluticasone and salmeterol).

Where control is still not achieved, further doses of corticosteroids may be needed as well as additional drugs to suppress airway inflammation (e.g. anti-leukotrienes and immuno-modulators). For maintenance therapy the inhaled route is preferred, as lower drug doses may be used so that drug particles can reach the lung tissue directly. Oral bronchodilators and steroids are sometimes necessary, however, but with larger doses there is a greater risk of side-effects. Where asthma is poorly controlled then, in addition to medication, diaphragmatic and nasal breathing techniques taught by a physiotherapist may combat dysfunctional breathing such as hyperventilation and shallow breathing (Thomas *et al.* 2009).

Drug treatment in COPD

Inhaled bronchodilators such as ipratropium or salbutamol are also useful in COPD for relief of symptoms. If needed, greater symptom relief can be achieved by using a once-daily dose of inhaled ipratropium (e.g. Tiotropium) (Niewoehner *et al.* 2005). Where there is worsening lung function (FEV_1 < 50 per cent predicted: see Table 18.2) and symptoms, then inhaled combination therapy with a LABA is often more effective than either drug alone (Szafranski *et al.* 2003). Inhaled corticosteroid use in COPD is controversial, as inflammation is not suppressed by steroids as effectively as in asthma; however, studies have demonstrated that when given in a combination preparation, there is a reduction in exacerbation rates and an improved quality of life for individuals, who have two or more exacerbations a year, with moderate to severe COPD (Jones *et al.* 2003).

Productive cough can be troublesome in COPD and a drug may be prescribed (mucolytic) to aid sputum clearance which may benefit some. During the winter months there can be increased risk for those with respiratory diseases such as asthma and COPD. Infections with either the influenza virus or streptococcus pneumonia may increase morbidity and mortality, and carers need to ensure that the appropriate vaccinations are given.

Further information regarding management may be accessed from the BTS/SIGN (2008) asthma guidelines and the NICE (2004) guidelines on COPD. The Department of Health has worked closely with clinicians, patients and carers to develop a National Clinical Strategy for COPD (to be published later in 2009), which reflects the need to prevent the disease where possible and to identify its development early so that appropriate treatment may be given.

Oxygen therapy

In acute severe asthma it is often difficult to achieve effective oxygenation, and where oxygen saturations are less than 94 per cent high-concentration oxygen therapy is needed. Oxygen therapy also plays a role in the treatment of acute episodes of COPD where oxygenation is difficult to maintain, but caution is needed and only low concentrations administered. In severe COPD where blood gases are abnormal and chronic respiratory failure is diagnosed by a pulmonary specialist, long-term oxygen therapy for at least 15 hours each day can improve morbidity and mortality (Nocturnal Oxygen Therapy Trial Group 1980; Medical Research Council Working Party 1981) (see Chapter 6 for further information on breathlessness and oxygen therapy).

Achieving better control

Where symptom control is not achieved, every effort should be made to identify possible factors responsible. There may be lack of understanding regarding the differences between 'reliever' and 'preventer' medication, and information should be given on the underlying disease process and why specific drugs are needed. Steroids often cause concern, and reassurance regarding the small dose usually needed for inhaled compared to oral therapy explained. Side-effects of inhaled steroids include hoarseness and oral thrush (candidiasis), but can be minimised by gargling with water following each dose. Of course, where steroid dose needs to be increased, risk is also increased. There are many possible side-effects including osteoporosis, diabetes, raised blood pressure and weight gain. The resulting distress can be significant and listening to individual concerns is important, as is ongoing review of medication and monitoring for side-effects.

Side-effects with bronchodilators such as salbutamol and terbutaline (beta2 agonists) include muscle tremor, dizziness, nervousness, palpitations and sleeplessness. In some cases of obstructive pulmonary disease a drug called aminophylline is prescribed and blood levels of the drug are monitored to ensure appropriate treatment levels and to minimise side-effects such as nausea, vomiting, sleeplessness, headaches and convulsions.

Ineffective inhaler technique is a common reason for poor symptom control and this should be checked at regular intervals. There are many different devices used including metered dose inhalers, breath-activated devices, dry powder devices and compressors that nebulise a liquid form of the drug into a fine mist, which can then be inhaled. Musculoskeletal disorders, weakness, poor manual dexterity and visual problems can affect inhaler use, in the elderly who may be unable to gain optimum benefit from their inhaler (Jarvis *et al.* 2007).

Carers should familiarise themselves with specific devices prescribed, and Asthma UK has a useful website with interactive resources on basic respiratory physiology and inhaler technique (www.asthma.org.uk/). A volume spacer used with an inhaler device not only helps where there is coordination difficulty but facilitates better drug delivery to the lungs. Specialist advice should be sought where there are ongoing problems so that the most appropriate device can be selected to optimise symptom control.

Self-management in asthma and COPD

Self-management and the use of written action plans in asthma are very effective in improving knowledge, self-efficacy and confidence (Lahdensuo *et al.* 1996; Osman *et al.* 2002). Where hospitalisation has been necessary, prior to discharge self-management education that focuses on individual needs should be offered and supported by a written action plan (BTS/SIGN 2008). Understanding of medication, allergen/trigger avoidance and recognition and management of worsening symptoms are important areas. Asthma UK has developed a useful asthma action pack called 'Be in Control' which is easily accessible (www.asthma.org.uk/control). The pack consists of a personal asthma action plan, peak flow diary, medicine card and guidance on making the most of each asthma review. This material should be discussed with the doctor or practice nurse.

Studies regarding use of self-management plans for COPD exacerbations, while less conclusive, have shown increases in the use of oral corticosteroids and oral antibiotics (Effing *et al.* 2007), reduction in the use of short-acting bronchodilators (Gallefoss and Bakke 1999) and an increase in appropriate treatment interventions for exacerbations (Wood-Baker *et al.* 2006). Many studies define self-management in a rather limited way and the use of a management plan alone is likely to be of limited benefit. As other chapters show, self-management strategies need to address issues on a number of levels including not only symptoms but behavioural, cognitive and social/environmental factors. Self-management approaches should incorporate five core skills which need to be developed if confidence is to be increased (DoH 2001):

1   Problem-solving.
2   Decision-making.
3   Resource utilisation.
4   Developing effective partnerships with health providers.
5   Taking action.

The British Lung Foundation has produced a comprehensive self-management booklet for those with COPD which may be ordered, and contact details may be found at the end of this chapter. The General Practice Airways Group (GPIAG) has developed a useful opinion sheet including an example of a COPD action plan, accessible from its website www.gpiag.com.

Pulmonary rehabilitation

Pulmonary rehabilitation is an evidence-based, multidisciplinary and comprehensive intervention for patients with chronic respiratory diseases who are symptomatic and often have decreased daily life activities (Nici *et al.* 2006). Benefits include reduced breathlessness and healthcare utilisation as well as improved exercise tolerance and quality of life, and all those who consider themselves disabled by COPD should be offered rehabilitation (NICE 2004). It is not appropriate, however, in those who are unable to walk, have unstable angina or for those who have had a recent myocardial infarction. Programmes should run over a minimum of six weeks and a maximum of 12 weeks and include physical exercise, disease education and psychological and social interventions. Programmes typically include aerobic training involving both upper and lower extremities exercises and some of these should be incorporated into day-to-day activities. Home-based rehabilitation for those with COPD compares well with hospital based programmes (Maltais *et al.* 2008).

There may be dietary difficulties experienced by those with COPD that need to be addressed and low body mass index (BMI) is a serious problem (Congleton 1999). There are several factors contributing to weight loss, reduced exercise tolerance and muscle weakness including greater energy expenditure due to breathlessness, particularly during acute episodes, and reduced energy intake from food (Slinde *et al.* 2002; Vermeeren *et al.* 2006). COPD is no longer considered as a disorder where only lung tissue is affected but as a systemic problem where a number of complex biological processes are involved.

Where there are weight problems, dietetic advice should be sought and nutritional supplements offered where there is significant loss. Conversely, excessive weight gain can increase ventilatory demands and breathlessness. Regular, high-calorific meals should be encouraged as large portions, especially with excessive carbohydrate, can result in 'bloating' and increased breathlessness. Oxygen masks and non-invasive ventilation can interfere with dietary intake and simple measures such as using nasal cannulae and scheduling 'time off' from ventilators may facilitate eating and drinking without the individual feeling unduly distressed.

Coping with breathlessness can be a challenge for individuals with COPD and strategies should be taught to reduce this distressing symptom. Increased breathlessness, prolonged expiratory time and increased respiratory rate results in breaths being taken before air from the previous breath has been exhaled (ZuWallack 2007). This leads to hyperinflated lungs and is a major cause of breathlessness on effort. Once again, a multidisciplinary approach is important and guidance from a chest physiotherapist should be sought so that exercises may be continued and encouraged. Improving the strength and endurance of respiratory muscles, purse lip breathing (a breathing manoeuvre similar to blowing out a candle), diaphragmatic breathing and exercises to strengthen the diaphragm can lower ventilatory requirement and reduce breathlessness (Casaburi 1995; Ambrosino and Strambi 2004).

Reviewing daily routines and if necessary modifying these to pace activities more effectively can reduce exertional breathlessness significantly. Breathlessness can increase levels of anxiety and this cycle can be difficult, with over-breathing and hyperventilation precipitating further problems.

Psychosocial factors

Psychosocial factors can be a significant cause of poor coping in those with asthma and COPD. There is a clear relationship between psychosocial factors and allergic disorders such as asthma, with negative mood associated with decreases in lung function and airway inflammation (Chida *et al.* 2008; Kullowatz *et al.* 2008). A large national survey showed a clear relationship between asthma and mental health symptoms with poor mental health increasing risk for asthma (Chun *et al.* 2008). A high rate of psychiatric disorders has been found among inner-city asthma patients with mental health problems associated with greater perceived impairment from asthma (Feldman *et al.* 2005), and psychosocial factors are linked with near fatal attacks and attendance at A&E departments.

Higher rates of anxiety and depression are found in COPD and although estimates vary widely are higher than those reported in some other advanced chronic diseases, and can have a significant impact on individuals, their families, society and the course of the disease, resulting in greater physical disability and ill-health (Van Manen *et al.* 2006; Maurer *et al.* 2008; Quint *et al.* 2008). There is also evidence to suggest that psychological distress may be greater in women with COPD (Laurin *et al.* 2007). Yet despite the high risk of developing depression in COPD, only a small number interact with a mental health professional and it is suggested that more referrals and better care coordination with mental health specialty care could lead to a significant reduction in mortality risk (Jordan *et al.* 2008). Depression can be associated with under-treatment of COPD (Dahlen and Janson 2002), highlighting the importance of early detection and intervention.

Non-concordance with treatment for chronic diseases such as COPD and asthma is common, contributing to increased morbidity and mortality, more frequent hospitalisation and reduced quality of life. Examples of non-concordance include overuse, underuse and alteration of schedule and doses of medication, continued

Table 18.3 Useful contacts (including helpline support)

ASH (Action on Smoking and Health) Campaigning public health charity that works to eliminate the harm caused by tobacco	www.ash.org.uk Action on Smoking and Health First Floor 144–145 Shoreditch High Street London E1 6JE Tel: 0207 739 5902 Email: enquiries@ash.org.uk
British Lung Foundation UK charity supporting people affected by lung disease. Provides comprehensive and clear information on paper, on the web and on the telephone. Support also provided by nationwide network of Breathe Easy support groups. Works for positive change in lung health by campaigning, raising awareness and funding world-class research	www.lunguk.org British Lung Foundation 73–75 Goswell Road London EC1V 7ER Helpline: 08458 50 50 20 Email: enquiries@blf-uk.org
British Thoracic Society Charity whose objective is to improve standards of care of people who have respiratory disease. Carries out research and provides national guidelines. Web pages contain information of interest to those with respiratory disease.	www.brit-thoracic.org.uk BTS 17 Doughty Street London WC1N 2PL Tel: 0207 831 8778
Asthma UK Charity which provides independent, confidential advice and support to people living with asthma, their families, friends and carers, and also professionals	www.asthma.org.uk Asthma UK Summit House 70 Wilson Street London EC2A 2DB Tel: 0800 121 62 44, Monday–Friday 9 a.m. to 5 p.m. Email: info@asthma.org.uk

smoking and lack of exercise with care providers playing a critical role in helping patients understand the nature of the disease, potential benefits of treatment, addressing concerns regarding potential adverse effects and events, and encouraging patients to develop self-management skills (Bourbeau and Bartlett 2008). Concordance with medication in optimising both physical and mental health can be particularly challenging, especially in people with mental health problems such as schizophrenia. Increasing motivation by using problem-solving strategies as part of proactive telenursing intervention (nursing support via telephone) has been shown to improve adherence to both psychiatric and non-psychiatric medications (Beebe *et al.* 2008).

Conclusion

Respiratory disease causes significant mortality and morbidity, and conditions such as COPD and asthma can result in poor quality of life. Long-term support is often needed and this places a considerable health burden not only on family and carers but on the National Health Service. Where there is poor control the psychosocial impact can be huge, resulting in a great deal of distress. Asthma and COPD are often misdiagnosed, under-diagnosed and under-treated, and carers need to be alert for respiratory symptoms, so that either diagnosis can be made and effective treatment prescribed or management plans reviewed where there is poor control and deterioration.

References

Abbot, N.C., Stead, L.F., White, A.R. *et al.* (1998) Hypnotherapy for Smoking Cessation. *Cochrane Database of Systematic Reviews*, Issue 2. Art. No.: CD001008. DOI: 10.1002/14651858. CD001008.

Amaddeo, F., Bisoffi, G., Bonizzato, P. *et al.* (1995) Mortality Among Patients with Psychiatric Illness: A Ten Year Case Register Study in an Area with a Community Based System of Care. *British Journal of Psychiatry*, 166, 783–788.

Ambrosino, N. and Strambi, S. (2004) New Strategies to Improve Exercise Tolerance in Chronic Obstructive Pulmonary Disease. *European Respiratory Journal*, 24, 313–322.

Asthma UK (2008) Wish You Were Here? – UK Report www.asthma.org.uk/how_we_help/world_asthma_day/index html (accessed 16 October 2008).

Barnes, P. (2000) Chronic Obstructive Pulmonary Disease. *New England Journal of Medicine*, 343, 269–280.

Beebe, L.H., Smith, K., Crye, C. *et al.* (2008) Telenursing Intervention Increases Psychiatric Medication Adherence in Schizophrenia Outpatients. *Journal of the American Psychiatric Nurses Association*, 14(3), 217–224.

Bourbeau, J. and Bartlett, S.J. (2008) Patient Adherence in COPD. *Thorax*, 63(9), 831–838.

British Lung Foundation (2006) *Lost in Translation. Bridging the Communication Gap in COPD. A Report by the British Lung Foundation.* London: BLF.

British Lung Foundation (2007) *Invisible Lives. Chronic Obstructive Pulmonary Disease (COPD) – Finding the Missing Millions.* London: BLF.

British Thoracic Society COPD Consortium (2005) *Spirometry in Practice. A Practical Guide to Using Spirometry in Primary Care.* London: BTS COPD Consortium.

British Thoracic Society (2006) *Burden of Lung Disease Report.* Online. Available at: www.brit-thoracic.org.uk/Portals/0/Library/BTS%20Publications/burdeon_of_lung_disease2007.pdf (accessed 6 April 2009).

British Thoracic Society/Scottish Intercollegiate Guidelines Network (BTS/SIGN) (2008) British Guidelines on the Management of Asthma. A National Clinical Guideline. *Thorax*, 63 (suppl. 4), iv1–iv121.

Casaburi, R. (1995) Mechanism of the Reduced Ventilatory Requirement as a Result of Exercise Training. *European Respiratory Review*, 5 (25), 42–46.

Celli, B.R., Cote, C.G., Marin, J.M. *et al.* (2004) The Body Mass Index, Airflow Obstruction, Dyspnoea and Exercise Capacity Index in Chronic Obstructive Pulmonary Disease. *New England Medical Journal*, 350(10), 1005–1012.

Chalmers, G.W., MacLeod, K.J., Little, S.A. *et al.* (2002) Influence of Cigarette Smoking on Inhaled Corticosteroid Treatment in Mild Asthma. *Thorax*, 57(3), 226–230.

Chida, Y., Hamer, M. and Steptoe, A. (2008) A Bidirectional Relationship Between Psychosocial Factors and Atopic Disorders: A Systematic Review and Meta-analysis. *Psychosomatic Medicine*, 70(1), 102–116.

Chun, T.H., Weitzen, S.H. and Fritz, G.K. (2008) The Asthma/Mental Health Nexus in a Population-based Sample of the United States. *Chest*, 134(6), 1176–1182.

Commission for Healthcare Audit and Inspection (2006) *Clearing the Air: A National Study of Chronic Obstructive Pulmonary Disease*. London: Healthcare Commission.

Congleton, J. (1999) Pulmonary Cachexia Syndrome: Aspects of Energy Balance. *Proceedings of the Nutrition Society*, 58(2), 321–328.

Dahlen, I. and Janson, C. (2002) Anxiety and Depression are Related to Outcomes of Emergency Treatment in Patients with Obstructive Lung Disease. *Chest*, 122(5), 1633–1637.

Department of Health (DoH) (2001) *The Expert Patient. A New Approach to Chronic Disease Management for the 21st Century*. London: The Stationery Office.

Department of Health (DoH) (2008) *High Quality Care for All – NHS Next Stage Review Final Report*. London: The Stationery Office.

Dezateau, C., Stocks, J., Dundas, I. *et al.* (1999) Impaired Airway Function and Wheezing in Infancy: The Influence of Maternal Smoking and a Genetic Predisposition to Asthma. *American Journal of Respiratory and Critical Care Medicine*, 159(2), 403–410.

Dowson, C.A., Kuijer, R.G. and Mulder, R.T. (2004) Anxiety and Self Management Behaviour in Chronic Obstructive Pulmonary Disease: What Has Been Learned? *Chronic Respiratory Disease*, 1, 213–220.

Effing, T.W., Monninkhof, E.M. and van der Valk, P.D.L. (2007) Self-management Education for Patients with Chronic Obstructive Pulmonary Disease. *Cochrane Database of Systematic Reviews*, Issue 4. Art. No.: CD002990. DOI: 10.1002/14651858.CD002990.pub2.

Feldman, J.M., Siddique, M.I., Morales, E. *et al.* (2005) Psychiatric Disorders and Asthma Outcomes Among High-risk Inner-city Patients. *Psychosomatic Medicine*, 67(6), 989–996.

Fletcher, C.M. (Chairman) (1960) Standardised Questionnaire on Respiratory Symptom: A Statement Prepared and Approved by the MRC Committee on the Aetiology of Chronic Bronchitis (MRC Breathlessness Score). *British Medical Journal*, 2, 1665s.

Gallefoss, F. and Bakke, P.S. (1999) How Does Patient Education and Self Management Amongst Asthmatics and Patients with Chronic Obstructive Pulmonary Disease Affect Medication? *American Journal of Respiratory and Critical Care Medicine*, 160, 2000–2005.

Global Initiative for Asthma (GINA) (2008) Global Strategy for Asthma Management and Prevention. URL: www.ginasthma.com/GuidelinesResources,asp??li=2&l2=1&intId=1561 (accessed 2 February 2009).

Jarvis, S., Ind, P.W. and Shiner, R.J. (2007) Inhaled Therapy in Elderly COPD Patients: Time for Re-evaluation? *Age and Ageing*, 36, 213–218.

Jones, D.R., Macias, C., Barreira, P.J. *et al.* (2004) Prevalence, Severity, and Co-occurrence of Chronic Physical Health Problems of Persons with Serious Mental Illness. *Psychiatric Services*, 55(11), 1250–1257.

Jones, P.W., Willits, C.R., Burge, P.S. *et al.* (2003) Disease Severity and the Effect of Fluticosone Propionate on Chronic Obstructive Pulmonary Disease Exacerbations. *European Respiratory Journal*, 21(1) 68–73.

Jordan, N., Lee, T.A., Valenstein, M. *et al.* (2008) Effect of Depression Care on Outcomes in COPD Patients with Depression. *Chest*, 10.1378/chest.08–083910.1378/chest.08–0839.

Kamara, S.G., Peterson, P.D. and Dennis, J.L. (1998) Prevalence of Physical Illness Among Psychiatric Inpatients who Die of Natural Causes. *Psychiatric Services*, 49, 788–793.

Kennedy, S. (2007) Detecting Changes in the Respiratory Status in Ward Patients. *Nursing Standard*, 21(49), 42–46.

Kullowatz, A., Rosenfield, D., Dahme, B. *et al.* (2008) Stress Effects on Lung Function in Asthma are Mediated by Changes in Airway Inflammation. *Psychosomatic Medicine*, 70(4), 468–475.

Lahdensuo, A., Hannhtela, T., Herrala, J. *et al.* (1996) Randomised Comparison of Guided Self Management and Traditional Treatment of Asthma over One Year. *British Medical Journal*, 312(7033), 748–752.

Laurin, C., Lavoie, K.L, Bacon, S.L. *et al.* (2007) Sex Differences in the Prevalence of Psychiatric Disorders and Psychological Distress in Patients with COPD. *Chest* 132(1), 148–155.

Lewis, K. (2007) Smoking Cessation – Making Quitting a Real Option. *Respiratory Medicine: COPD update*, 3, 128–134.

Maltais, F., Bourbeau, J., Shapira, S. *et al.* (2008) Effects of Home-based Pulmonary Rehabilitation in Patients with Chronic Obstructive Pulmonary Disease: A Randomized Trial. *Annals of International Medicine*, 149(12), 869–878.

Maurer, J., Rebbapragada, V., Borson, S. *et al.* (2008) Anxiety and Depression in COPD: Current Understanding, Unanswered Questions, and Research Needs. *Chest*, 134(4), (suppl.), 435–456.

Medical Research Council Working Party (1981) Long Term Domiciliary Oxygen Therapy in Chronic Hypoxic Cor Pulmonale Complicating Chronic Bronchitis and Emphysema. *Lancet*, I, 681–686.

National Institute for Clinical Excellence (NICE) (2004) Chronic Obstructive Pulmonary Disease: National Clinical Guideline for the Management of Chronic Obstructive Pulmonary Disease in Primary and Secondary Care. *Thorax* (suppl. 1), 1–232.

Nici, L., Donner, C., Wouters, E. *et al.* (2006) American Thoracic Society/European Respiratory Society Statement on Pulmonary Rehabilitation. *American Journal of Respiratory Critical Care Medicine*, 173(12), 1390–1413.

Niewoehner, D.E., Rice, K., Cote, C. *et al.* (2005) Prevention of Exacerbation of Chronic Obstructive Pulmonary Disease with Tiotropium; A Once Daily Inhaled Anticholinergic Bronchodilator. A Randomised Trial. *Annals of Internal Medicine*, 143(5), 317–326.

Nocturnal Oxygen Therapy Trial Group (1980) Continuous or Nocturnal Oxygen Therapy in Hypoxic Chronic Obstructive Pulmonary Disease: A Clinical Trial. *Annals of International Medicine*, 93, 391–398.

Osman, L.M., Calder, C., Godden, D.J. *et al.* (2002) A Randomised Controlled Trial of Self Management Planning for Adult Patients Admitted to Hospital with Acute Asthma. *Thorax*, 57(10), 869–874.

Quint, J.K., Baghai-Ravary, R., Donaldson, G.C. *et al.* (2008) Relationship Between Depression and Exacerbations of COPD. *European Respiratory Journal*, 32, 53–60.

Rutten, F.H., Cramer, M.J. and Grobbee, D.E. (2005) Unrecognised Heart Failure in Elderly Patients with Stable Chronic Obstructive Pulmonary Disease. *European Heart Journal*, 26 (18), 1887–1894.

Seymour, L. (2003) *Not All in the Mind. The Physical Health of Mental Health Service Users.* London: Mentality.

Shahab, L., Jarvis, M.J., Britton, J. *et al.* (2006) Prevalence, Diagnosis and Relation to Tobacco Dependence of Chronic Obstructive Pulmonary Disease in a Nationally Representative Population Sample. *Thorax*, 61(12), 1043–1047.

Slinde, F., Gronberg, A.M. and Engstrom, C.R. (2002) Individual Dietary Intervention in Patients with COPD During Multidisciplinary Rehabilitation. *Respiratory Medicine*, 96(5), 330–336.

Stockley, R., O'Brien, C., Pye, A. *et al.* (2000) Relationship of Sputum Colour to Nature and Outpatient Management of Exacerbations of COPD. *Chest*, 117, 1638–1645.

Szafranski, W., Cukier, A., Ramirez, A. *et al.* (2003) Efficacy and Safety of Budesonide/ Formoterol in the Management of Chronic Obstructive Pulmonary Disease. *European Respiratory Journal*, 21(1), 74–81.

Thomas, M., McKinley, R.K., Mellor, S. *et al.* (2009) Breathing Exercises for Asthma: A Randomised Controlled Trial. *Thorax*, 64(1), 55–61.

Van Manen, J.G., Bindels, P.J.E., Dekker, F.W. *et al.* (2006) Risk of Depression in Patients with Chronic Obstructive Pulmonary Disease and its Determinants. *Thorax*, 57, 412–416.

Vermeeren, M.A., Creutzberg, E.C., Schols, A.M. *et al.* (2006) Prevalence of Nutrition Depletion in a Large Out Patient Population of Patients with COPD. *Respiratory Medicine*, 173, 1349–1355.

Wagena, E.J., Arrindell, W.A., Wouters, E.F.M. *et al.* (2005) Are Patients with COPD Psychologically Distressed? *European Respiratory Journal*, 26, 242–248.

White, A.R., Rampes, H. and Campbell, J. (2006) Acupuncture and Related Interventions for Smoking Cessation. *Cochrane Database of Systematic Reviews*, 1. Art. No.: CD000009. DOI: 10.1002/14651858.CD000009.pub2.

Wood-Baker, R., McGlone, S., Venn, A. *et al.* (2006) Written Action Plans in Chronic Obstructive Pulmonary Disease Increase Appropriate Treatment for Acute Exacerbations. *Respirology*, 11, 619–626.

ZuWallack, R. (2007) The Non Pharmacologic Treatment of Chronic Obstructive Pulmonary Disease: Advances in Our Understanding of Pulmonary Rehabilitation. *Proceedings of the American Thoracic Society*, 4, 549–553.

19 Older people

Carl Margereson and Irrah Sibindi

Introduction

Long-term conditions addressed in other chapters of this section are generally more common in older people, but a major focus here will be on long-term care issues relating to stroke. Falls and mental health problems in older people will also be considered as well as issues around service delivery. This will facilitate discussion around some of the key themes initially outlined in the National Service Framework for Older People (NSFOP) (Department of Health (DoH) 2001a) and elaborated on further in subsequent policy documents. These themes and many of the care principles relating to stroke are of course relevant to all groups of older people whatever the disorder. Similarly, conditions such as stroke and dementia do not only affect older people, and many of the care delivery principles explored are relevant whatever the life stage.

Policy-shaping services for older people

Based on the principles of the NHS Plan (DoH 2000), the NSFOP set standards for tackling age discrimination and promoting person-centred care, and was the first ever comprehensive strategy to ensure fair, high-quality, integrated services for older people. More recently a report by the National Director for Older People looked at progress made as a result of the NSFOP, as well as work still to be completed using three major themes: Dignity in Care; Joined-up Care; and Healthy Ageing (DoH 2006a). This report draws attention to the significant progress made in a number of key areas, not least in the development of stroke services. There have been numerous consultation and policy documents released, further shaping services with a strong emphasis on integration between independent, voluntary, health and social care sectors (DoH 2004, 2005a, 2005b, 2006b).

The NSFOP of 2001 has eight standards outlining what is expected so that health and social care agencies work toward developing effective services to support independence and promote health in older people. Standard five of the NSFOP focuses on reducing the incidence of stroke and the development of integrated stroke care services. Building on this standard, in 2007 a National Stroke Strategy (NSS) was published with a framework of 20 quality markers (QMs) for raising the quality of stroke prevention, treatment, care and support over the next decade (DoH 2007a). The National Collaborating Centre for Chronic Conditions (NCCCC) (2008) published national clinical guidelines with the major focus on acute stroke and transient ischaemic attack care. The Intercollegiate Stroke Working Party (ISWP 2008b) in their recently updated UK *National Guidelines for Stroke* cover all aspects of stroke care including long-term management following recovery as well as the recommendations of the NCCCC national guidelines.

Stroke

There are over 67,000 deaths due to stroke (Cerebrovascular Accident or CVA) each year in the UK (British Heart Foundation 2005) and it is the third largest cause of death in England and the single largest cause of adult disability, with 300,000 living with moderate to severe disability (National Audit Office 2005). The occurrence of stroke is catastrophic and can occur across all age groups with 25 per cent occurring in those under 65 years. There are two main causes of stroke but both result in interruption to the blood supply to the brain.

The most common type of stroke (80 per cent) is caused by a blockage – an ischaemic stroke which occurs when a clot of blood blocks an artery carrying blood to the brain. This may be through a cerebral thrombus (clot), cerebral embolism – where a blood clot, air bubble or fat globule (embolism) is carried in the bloodstream to the brain or through a blockage in tiny blood vessels deep within the brain (lacnar stroke). The second type of stroke occurs (20 per cent of cases) when there is bleeding (haemorrhage) into the brain. This may be caused by an intracerebral haemorrhage, where a blood vessel bursts, or a subarachnoid haemorrhage, where a blood vessel on the surface of the brain bleeds into the area between the brain and the skull (subarachnoid space) (DoH 2001a).

Early recognition and assessment of strokes

Sudden onset of numbness, weakness or paralysis, slurred speech, blurred vision, confusion and headache are common signs of stroke. Some individuals may experience a transient ischaemic attack (TIA) also known as a 'mini-stroke' where symptoms and signs resolve within 24 hours but this should be regarded as a warning sign as there is a high risk of a subsequent stroke occurring. With most people having their first symptoms outside hospital the NSS stresses the importance of the need for members of the public and health and social care staff to be able to recognise the main symptoms of stroke and for it to be treated as a medical emergency (QM1). With around 1.9 million brain cells lost for each minute a stroke goes untreated (DoH 2007a), early recognition of symptoms and immediate action is important to reduce death and disability. The Face-Arm-Speech-Test (FAST) is a pre-hospital assessment tool and can help in rapid assessment (Harbison *et al.* 2003):

- Facial weakness – Can the person smile? Is the mouth or eye drooping?
- Arm weakness – Can the person raise both arms?
- Speech problems – Can the person speak clearly and understand what is said?·
- Time to call 999.

Immediate care is required necessitating urgent hospital admission so that the chance of survival is improved and complications minimised. There is strong evidence that people are more likely to survive and to recover more function if admitted promptly to a hospital-based stroke unit where there is specialist assessment, diagnosis, management and rehabilitation (ISWP 2008a). A brain scan is essential to identify the cause, as treatment is different for ischaemic and haemorrhagic stroke. Where ischaemic stroke has occurred, 'clot-busting' drugs (thrombolytics) may be beneficial in those aged 18 to 80 years, but need to be given within three hours of symptoms starting. Thereafter, to reduce the risk of clotting, short-term aspirin is often prescribed initially with many then requiring long-term therapy with anti-clotting drugs such as warfarin.

Many organisations offer information on stroke and you will find contact details at the end of the chapter.

Early and continuing rehabilitation following stroke

Following a stroke, individuals may experience a whole range of difficulties affecting mobility, breathing, swallowing, vision, hearing and mental function. A full multidisciplinary assessment following agreed local protocols should take place within five working days (DoH 2007a). Early and ongoing rehabilitation following stroke is crucial and improvements can often be seen even after a number of years. Yet it can be a very frustrating time as basic skills associated with activities of living need to be relearned and new skills acquired, and a range of professionals and agencies need to work collaboratively if rehabilitation is to be effective. The NSS explores 'Life after Stroke' and stresses the importance of achieving a good quality of life and the maximisation of independence, well-being and choices for individuals, their relatives and carers, wherever the care setting. For those cared for in nursing homes and residential homes assessment and treatment from specialist rehabilitation services should still be available.

Despite evidence to show the benefits of stroke rehabilitation only half receive effective rehabilitation in the first six months following discharge (DoH 2007a). Depression is a problem experienced by many coping with long-term health problems but as many as one-third of individuals following stroke are affected (Hackett *et al.* 2005). It is suggested that the reader interested in rehabilitation also reads Chapter 13 which explores quality requirements outlined in the National Service Framework for Long Term Conditions (DoH 2005b). The Stroke Association offers a very useful information booklet on stroke rehabilitation which can be easily accessed on their website (www.stroke.org.uk/).

Specific problems following stroke

Limb weakness

Following a stroke the transmission of nerve impulses from the brain to limbs are affected resulting in varying degrees of weakness with arm function often affected. Where there is mild weakness on one side of the body this is called hemiparesis and, when severe, hemiplegia. Altered limb function is a common feature following stroke and if long-term problems such as deformity and pain are to be avoided, ongoing therapy is crucial. Rehabilitation of arm function is an important aim and carers should be guided by physiotherapists so that following specialist assessment appropriate exercises can be encouraged on a regular basis, thus improving dexterity and strength (Winstein *et al.* 2004). Often after some time there is increased tone to limbs and if spasticity and shortening of affected limbs are to be minimised then gentle exercise of individual joints needs to be carried out. Impaired balance increases individual risk further, particularly from falls, and steps should be taken to reduce risk by progressive balance training and the use of walking aids where appropriate. Various visual impairments can also make balance and mobility difficult following stroke. Controlling eye movement may be problematic (e.g. nystagmus), as may be the ability to recognise familiar objects (visual agnosia), and other age-related visual problems such as cataract and glaucoma need to be identified and corrected where possible (ISWP 2008a).

A physiotherapist specialising in neurological disorders will not only carry out an assessment where mobility is affected, but will guide carers in the retraining activities which will need to be practised and encouraged. Short-term goals which are realistic will increase motivation and may at first simply involve transferring from bed to chair, chair to toilet and moving around the bed (Van Peppen *et al.* 2004). Time should be taken to individualise regimens and in some instances more intensive therapy may be necessary. Limb weakness, particularly when severe, reduces the ability to correct posture and change position. Shoulder pain can also be troublesome following stroke yet can be minimised by correct and careful handling of the weak arm, avoiding excessive ranges of movement during exercises, correct positioning and support of the arm, as well as effective assessment of pain and the administration of prescribed analgesia. Recognition and assessment of pain following stroke is necessary and whether pain is neuropathic as a result of damage to nerve fibres or musculoskeletal, where optimal control is not achieved, referral to a specialist in pain management is required (see Chapter 6).

Immobility can result in skin pressure ulceration, muscle weakness, limb swelling, joint damage, contractures and pain as well as chest infections and constipation. As well as motor loss (reduced movement) there may also be sensory loss (reduced sensation) with increased risk of accidental injury. A high standard of nursing care is required and training of carers may be needed so that correct positioning of individuals is adopted in bed and chair, and correct moving and handling techniques utilised to minimise risk. Careful planning and execution of all activities of living is necessary if accidents are to be avoided.

Speech difficulty

Communication can be severely affected following stroke with an inability to form and understand words (aphasia and dysphasia) and occurs most commonly where there is damage to the left cerebral hemisphere in the brain. Dysarthria is where speech becomes slurred owing to poor muscle control and swallowing difficulties (dysphagia) can also be experienced. Speech difficulties can result in a great deal of distress and frustration, and assessment by a speech and language therapist is necessary, with problems persisting at six months often requiring specific therapy in a group setting or one to one (Hilari *et al.* 2003). It is important that an effective communication method is established and shared with the family and all carers. 'Speakability' is a UK charity which offers support to those who have a communication disability as a result of stroke or other illness (www.speakability.org.uk).

Promoting continence

Elimination problems are common following stroke and although incontinence increases with age the *National Audit of Continence Care for Older People* (Wagg *et al.*

2006) identified major deficiencies in assessment and care for older people with bladder and bowel problems. Although the NSFOP required the establishment of integrated continence services for older people by 2004, progress has been somewhat disappointing. Incontinence can result in increased risk of skin pressure ulceration, and may also have a profound impact on quality of life, dignity, body image, self-esteem and causes major stress for those affected and their carers. Following incontinence there should be strict attention to personal hygiene with clothing changed if necessary, and this should be carried out with the minimum of delay and fuss. Sensitive verbal and non-verbal communication at such times can do much to minimise the distress which is inevitably felt by individuals.

Although there are many possible causes of incontinence, research shows that improving mobility and toileting skills can result in a significant reduction in incontinence (van Houten *et al.* 2007). Overactive bladder syndrome in older people is the most common underlying cause of urinary incontinence in men and women, is associated with increased risks of falls and injuries, including fracture, and can often be treated successfully with a combination of lifestyle and pharmacological therapies (Wagg *et al.* 2007). Potter *et al.* (2007) argue that there is an urgent need to re-establish the fundamentals of continence care into the daily practice of medical and nursing staff, with action needing to be taken with regard to the establishment of truly integrated, quality services.

In promoting continence, basic assessment and care by those looking after older people and the use of assessment and management protocols is important. Wherever possible the cause of incontinence (e.g. urinary tract infection) needs to be identified and treated together with appropriate lifestyle changes, yet all too often management intervention focuses only on containment products (Dingwall and McLafferty 2006; Thomas *et al.* 2008). There should be a well-documented care plan and where possible simple treatments offered such as bladder retraining and pelvic floor exercises. Other members of the multidisciplinary team such as the physiotherapist and occupational therapist may be able to assist with mobility and toileting and only as a last resort should an indwelling catheter be used. A continence adviser will be able to assist and teach individuals and carers in the use of different continence aids and services available. Discharge home with continuing incontinence should only take place after the carer (family member) or client has developed skill and confidence and is reassured regarding arrangements for continuing supplies of continence aids and services which must be in place (ISWP 2008a). Guidelines on urinary and faecal incontinence may be accessed from the National Institute for Health and Clinical Excellence (NICE 2006a, 2007a).

Problems with eating and drinking

Age Concern (2006a) report that 14 per cent of older people aged over 65 years in the UK are malnourished, four out of ten admitted to hospital are malnourished on arrival and six out of ten are at risk of becoming malnourished, or of their situation getting worse in hospital. In the same year the Commission for Healthcare Audit and Inspection (2006) produced a report on older people services identifying nutrition as an issue of importance to older people and expressed concern about the need for improvement in this area.

Medical conditions may contribute to increased risk of malnutrition and dehydration. Following stroke, for example, swallowing difficulties are common and early assessment by a speech and language therapist is essential to avoid airway obstruction and aspiration pneumonia. The multidisciplinary team, including the dietician, need to work together to identify appropriate ways of meeting dietary and hydration needs. Until swallowing is possible, the use of a nasogastric tube may be necessary and a small number may require a gastrostomy where a tube is inserted into the stomach through an opening on the abdominal wall. Where there is difficulty in taking oral medication, a pharmacist will be able to advise and tablets should not be routinely crushed. Where there are ongoing problems with swallowing, a specialist speech and language therapist is normally involved.

There may be many reasons why eating and drinking is problematic, and in addition to swallowing impairment there may be problems with manual dexterity and cognitive ability. This can result in poor oral hygiene and regular mouth care throughout the day must be carried out by carers if necessary to ensure that teeth and the oral cavity generally remain healthy. If dentures are worn, these should be cleaned regularly and inserted each day and, where ill-fitting, damaged or perhaps lost, a dental referral made (ISWP 2008a).

Ongoing monitoring of nutritional intake is imperative and effective protocols need to be in place so that difficulties can be identified early. Communication difficulties may mean that some are not able to articulate their dietary needs effectively and it is essential that carers regularly monitor weight and body mass index (BMI) (see Chapter 5). Carers need to be aware of the importance of nutrition, not only as a basic human need but in increasing individual resilience and contributing to improved physical and mental health. Time must be taken to identify food preferences and choice should be offered. Mealtimes should be pleasurable for all, no matter how nutritional intake is achieved, and where assistance is needed this important pleasurable, social ritual should not be hurried. Guidelines on nutritional support in adults are available from NICE (2006b).

Problems with intimacy

For a number of people living with a long-term condition there may be difficulties with intimacy, and although problems may not be directly related to a medical condition sexual dysfunction is common after stroke. These issues need to be discussed sensitively by carers and if necessary referred for assessment so that identifiable causes can be treated where possible. The psychosocial and emotional impact of stroke can be devastating and many of these issues are explored in Chapter 2.

Older people and mental health

In promoting mental health in older people standard seven of the NSFOP draws attention to the importance of access to integrated mental health services to ensure effective diagnosis, treatment and support of individuals and carers. Mental health problems in later life are not an inevitable part of ageing and many disorders are often preventable and treatable. However, more than 3.5 million older people in the UK suffer with mental health problems, and Age Concern (2007) report that the extent of mental illness in older people is alarming. This includes depression, psychosis, stress and alcohol abuse, and there are currently 700,000 people in the UK with dementia of whom approximately 570,000 live in England (DoH 2009a). The number of people with dementia will double over the next 30 years to 1.4 million, costing the UK economy over £50 billion a year (Knapp *et al.* 2007).

What is dementia?

In January 2009 a National Dementia Strategy was published so that significant improvements are made to dementia services across three key areas: improved awareness; earlier diagnosis and intervention; and a high quality of life (DoH 2009a). Dementia refers to the loss of memory and other cognitive skills due to changes in the brain caused by disease or trauma and involves gradual decline of mental ability affecting intellectual and social skills to the point where life becomes difficult. Along with problems with memory function there can be disorientation problems (time, person and place) as well as personality changes (Woods 2000). Such cognitive impairment may involve poor judgement, attention and concentration, aphasia (inability to produce or comprehend language), apraxia (difficulty saying what is intended), agnosia (inability to recognise familiar objects) and disturbance in executing movements, severe enough to interfere with activities of living. The person may also have an altered sleep pattern which may place great strain on carers. Co-morbid mental health problems, such as anxiety, depression and even delusions and hallucinations, are not uncommon. The causes of dementia are not well understood but all result in structural and chemical changes in the brain leading to the death of brain tissue. Multiple environmental factors may also be implicated (Knapp *et al.* 2007) including alcohol, brain injury, drug abuse, drug side-effects and vitamin B12 deficiency.

In 1906 Alois Alzheimer, a German neurologist, first described Alzheimer's Disease (AD), as a progressive and degenerative illness which results in the development of 'plaques' and 'tangles' in the brain, leading to the death of brain cells. As a result, and over time, symptoms become worse. AD is the most common type of dementia in people who are 65 years and older but the illness can develop much earlier. The precise aetiology is not known but genetic, lifestyle factors (including smoking), head injuries and environmental factors are likely to be implicated. In vascular dementia, the blood supply to the brain becomes disrupted leading to a death of brain cells. Sometimes vascular dementia results from a stroke (called single-infarct dementia) or a series of strokes (multi-infarct dementia). Physical health problems such as high blood pressure, heart problems, high cholesterol and diabetes are implicated in the development of vascular dementia.

Dementia with Lewy bodies (DLB) was identified in the early twentieth century by Frederich Lewy in 1912. Lewy bodies are tiny spherical protein deposits found on the nerve cell and their presence interrupts the action of chemical messengers including acetylcholine and dopamine. These bodies are also found in the brains of people with Parkinson's Disease. DLB starts rapidly and acutely with decline occurring over a few months before levelling off. Like the Alzheimer type, DLB is sometimes associated with vascular dementia. Presenting features may involve symptoms similar to both Alzheimer and Parkinson's disease with problems including difficulty with attention and alertness, spatial disorientation and difficulty in planning ahead, although memory is less affected than in Alzheimer-type dementia.

Early recognition and diagnosis of dementia

Early provision of support at home can decrease institutionalisation by 22 per cent and, even where cases are complex, if there is a strong mental health team admission to a care home can be reduced by 6 per cent (Challis *et al.* 2002; Gaugler *et al.* 2005). Yet early consultation and diagnosis can be delayed not only due to the stigma associated with dementia but where increasing forgetfulness is attributed to the ageing process and therefore ignored. As a result, only one-third of people with dementia receive a formal diagnosis at any time during the illness (National Audit Office 2007).

The Mini Mental-State Examination (MMSE) (Folstein *et al.* 1975) is the most commonly used tool of cognitive function. The test lasts a maximum of 20 minutes, and has been found to be accurate in screening dementia with a sensitivity of 69 per cent and a specificity of 90 per cent. The test evaluates cognition in five areas: orientation, instant recall, attention span, computation, delay recollection and speech. The maximum score is 30 and a score of 23 or lower is suggestive of cognitive impairment. Commissioning of local services to include the establishment of memory clinics and the use of agreed assessment tools should result in early detection and referral to specialist care.

Treatment and care

Dementia results in disability, is debilitating and causes enormous distress, and, with no cure, service providers must assist individuals and their families to live well, no matter what stage of the illness (DoH 2009a). Good-quality care from diagnosis to the end of life is paramount whether this is in the community, hospital or care home setting. Margallo-Lana *et al.* (2001) found that mental health needs of older people (especially those living in care homes) are generally not met. The behavioural manifestations of dementia are very common and distressing to the individual, family and carers. Current input from the mental health services is generally on an ad-hoc basis or reactive with referrals at times of crisis. Yet symptoms such as hallucinations can be challenged and may diminish with distraction and reassurance having a positive and rewarding effect.

The Alzheimer's Society (2008) has criticised current practice regarding the use of anti-psychotic medicines for the management of behavioural and psychological symptoms in people with dementia. The use of such medication should be reviewed regularly and withdrawn quickly wherever it is clinically inappropriate. In 2007, amended guidance by the National Institute for Health and Clinical Excellence (NICE 2007b) recommended the use of the drugs donepezil (Aricept), rivastigmine (Exelon) and galantamine (Reminyl) for people with *mild to moderate* AD. These drugs should only be continued where there is demonstrable slowing of cognitive decline, and improvements in functioning and/or behaviour. Anti-Parkinson medication can also be effective if the sufferer experiences symptoms such as rigidity and stiffness, even though the medication may make symptoms such as hallucinations and confusion problematic.

A detailed and informative paper published by NICE (2006c) explores how health and social care workers can support people with dementia.

Depression

One in four people over age 65 suffer with depression or serious symptoms of depression. Prevalence of depression is greater in residential care homes compared to other care settings and the young-old are at higher risk particularly where there is severe disability. Depressed mood and severe symptoms such as wishing to be dead are particularly common in those cared for in residential care facilities (McDougall *et al.* 2007). Many older people face significant life changes and stressors that put them at risk of depression and there is also greater risk where there is a history of depression, failing health, substance misuse problems or inadequate social support. Once again there is an assumption by many that such feelings are to be expected during this particular life stage but this is not the case. As a result, co-morbid anxiety and depression are often under-treated in older people despite evidence that the benefits of treatment outway any potential risks (Heffern 2000).

Recognition of depression is complex, and there are many people with long-term conditions who present with chronic somatisation where physical symptoms are investigated without a cause being found. It is often easier for people to discuss physical symptoms than admit to being depressed. The consultation style of some professional care workers may not facilitate the exploration of feelings so that needs are unmet in this area. According to Ames (1991), causes and risk factors of depression among the older population include:

* loneliness and isolation due to living alone, death of close loved ones, relocation, decreased mobility due to physical ill-health or loss of driving privileges;
* reduced sense of purpose – feeling purposelessness, retirement, loss of identity;
* health problems – chronic severe pain, cognitive decline, illness, altered body image due to surgery/disease;
* medications – polypharmacy can trigger depression;
* fear – death, anxiety over financial problems/health issues;
* recent bereavement – family member, spouse, partner, pet.

Comprehensive holistic assessments will identify those with mood disorder and carers need to be sensitive to significant life events which have been experienced, and where there is unresolved grief and chronic sorrow. Where there is a high index of suspicion GP referral is important and, where appropriate, referral made to a community mental health team for older people. Early identification of problems and any benefit derived from intervention such as cognitive behavioural therapy will of course depend a great deal on the beliefs held by practitioners and carers who need to be aware of their own ageist assumptions (Evans 2007).

Delirium in older people

Delirium (acute confusional state) is characterised by a disturbance of fluctuating consciousness and impaired cognition developing over a short period of time as a direct consequence of a general medical condition, drug withdrawal or intoxication (Royal College of Physicians (RCP) 2006). The risk of delirium is found across a wide range of medical disorders where disturbed physiological balance contributes to delirium in older people and affects 30 per cent of those admitted to medical areas (McManus *et al.* 2007). The hyperactive type of delirium characterised by agitation with hallucinations and inappropriate behaviour is easily recognised whereas the hypoactive type with reduced activity and lethargy can be easily missed (Inouye 2004). There is greater risk of delirium in older people where there is, for example, severe illness, dementia, physical frailty and polypharmacy, and predisposing factors include:

- immobility;
- use of physical restraint;
- use of bladder catheter;
- iatrogenic events (as a result of treatment);
- malnutrition;
- psychoactive medications;
- intercurrent illness;
- dehydration.

(RCP 2006)

Information obtained from a relative or carer can often help to distinguish between delirium and dementia and it is recommended that cognitive testing be carried out on all older people admitted to hospital, with serial measurements in those at risk to detect delirium or its resolution (RCP 2006). When confusion is suspected the use of cognitive screening tools such as the Abbreviated Mental Test (AMT) (Jitapunkul *et al.* 1991) (see Table 19.1) or the Mini-Mental State Examination (MMSE) (Folstein *et al.* 1975; Anthony *et al.* 1982) may be used although these cannot distinguish between delirium and dementia. The Confusion Assessment Method (CAM) (Inouye *et al.* 1990) can help to differentiate delirium from dementia or detect its onset but appropriate health workers should be trained in its use. A full physical assessment will also be necessary along with a range of clinical investigations to identify and thus treat any underlying cause.

Unfortunately care settings can often contribute to increasing the risk of delirium particularly in hospitals where sensory overload can lead to disorientation. Individuals should be cared for in a good sensory environment with a reality orientation approach and with involvement of the multidisciplinary team (RCP 2006). Care settings can often be alien places where everything may seem unfamiliar, and supportive care where there is continuity from regular nursing staff can help. Time should be taken to improve personal orientation with the use of clocks and calendars and, where hearing aids and spectacles are normally used, then these should be readily accessible and checked regularly (Cole 2005). Relatives and carers should be encouraged to visit on a regular basis and the use of photographs and other familiar

Table 19.1 Abbreviated Mental Test score (AMT) (a score of less than 8/10 is abnormal)

1 Age
2 Time (to nearest hour)
3 Address for recall at end of test
4 Year
5 Name of hospital
6 Recognition of two people (e.g. doctor/nurse)
7 Date of birth
8 Year of First World War
9 Name of present monarch
10 Count backwards 20–1 (this also tests attention)

Source: Jitapunkul *et al.* (1991). Reproduced with permission.

items can be reassuring. Encouraging mobility where possible and engagement in various activities can also have a positive effect. Restraint during an episode of delirium does not prevent falling and may increase injury risk, and it may be preferable to nurse individuals on a low bed or a mattress on the floor (RCP 2006). Where medication is needed for agitation, the effects of this should be evaluated carefully and there should be close observation by carers. Finally, high-quality nursing care where all needs are met across all activities of living will not only reduce risk of delirium but will minimise the risk of complications where delirium is present.

Effective care planning and delivery for older people

Independent living depends on the ability of individuals to carry out a range of personal activities, but this can be difficult as a result of the ageing process and where there are specific medical conditions. Formal assessment must be undertaken by a therapist or nurse to facilitate individual safety and independence. Following stroke, for example, a range of services which are easily accessible is often necessary and should be in place to support the long-term needs of individuals and their carers (NSS QM 13). Degeling *et al.* (2006) argue that care models must recognise the rights and responsibilities of people with long-term conditions to be informed, to be consulted and involved in decision-making and to enter agreements with care providers that specify what they can expect from others and what others can expect from them.

Assessment

A comprehensive, holistic assessment is crucial if any subsequent care plan is to be effective. All activities of living can be affected and there can be wide-ranging, complex needs where dependency is increased. A case management approach is often used where one key professional is responsible for coordinating care, and ensuring that there is ongoing and periodic physical, social and psychological assessment. Degeling *et al.* (2006) use the term 'risk assessment' rather than 'needs assessment' so that an individual's view of what is at risk becomes the focus with subsequent care planning likely to be more effective.

Comprehensive assessment processes are necessary so that functional impairment, self-care deficits and actual/potential risks are identified early and effective measures taken to resolve these. Carried out effectively, assessment can often avoid the necessity for long-term residential nursing home care. To avoid duplication, health and social care sectors have developed single assessment process strategies (DoH 2007a) and protocols reflecting inter-agency working, which allow assessments to be completed by a variety of professionals across different agencies, and information technology is being developed further to facilitate sharing of data. Information on the single assessment process may be found on the Department of Health website (DoH 2007b) and also the Centre for Policy on Ageing website (CPA 2008).

There are as many as seven million informal carers in the UK providing unpaid help to relatives or neighbours with chronic illness or disability (Maher and Green 2002). Carers can experience multiple disadvantages and in those over the age of 50 there is evidence to show that the more intense the care given, the less likely they are to make use of public services (Age Concern 2006b). Carers are entitled to an assessment of their own support needs, and The Carers (Equal Opportunities) Act 2004 builds on the Carers and Disabled Children Act 2000, and requires local authorities to inform carers of their entitlement to an assessment of their needs (DoH 2005c). Such an assessment must include a consideration of whether carers work or wish to work, and whether they participate or wish to participate in any education, training or leisure activity.

There are times when comprehensive assessment across a number of areas is needed while at other times a more focused assessment in one or two specific areas is appropriate (see Chapter 5).

Care planning

Following risk assessment a care plan needs to be developed, and Degeling *et al.* (2006) argue for 'year-based pathways' that specify the cycles (daily, weekly, monthly, yearly) of sequences of activities that will be undertaken by people with a long-term condition and also their carers, service providers and support services. A comprehensive written care plan should identify the agreed risks to be addressed and the outcomes expected, as well as who will do what and when. Individuals should have their progress measured against the goals/outcomes set at regular intervals, and evaluation will identify the extent to which arranged care/services are successful at meeting risks identified in the assessment phase. The importance of client and carer involvement in all care planning activities is stressed in the NSFOP (standard two). Ongoing information, advice and support for relatives and carers throughout the care pathway and lifelong should be available, and a clear consistent point of contact identified (DoH 2007a) (QM3).

Care planning alone will not meet the long-term needs of older people, and health and social care cultures and services need to reflect the guiding principles outlined under the Department of Health's three major themes: Dignity in Care, Joined-up Care and Healthy Ageing (DoH 2006a). In the next section some of these guiding principles will be considered.

Dignity in Care

Although standard one of the NSFOP draws attention to the importance of rooting out age discrimination a large section of the NSF is devoted to the promotion of person-centred care (standard two), outlining the requirement for older people to be treated as individuals and enabled to make choices about their own care no matter where they are cared for. *Living Well in Later Life*, a joint review of the progress on the NSFOP by the Audit Commission, Healthcare Commission and Commission for Social Care Inspection (Commission for Healthcare Audit and Inspection 2006), found evidence of ageism across all services, from patronising and thoughtless treatment, to the failure of some mainstream services to take seriously the needs and aspirations of older people, and noted a failure to treat vulnerable older people with dignity. In 2006 the Department of Health launched the Dignity in Care campaign with the purpose of refocusing attention on delivering health and social care in ways which treat people with dignity and respect (DoH 2006c). Table 19.2 lists the expectations of what constitutes a service that respects dignity.

Table 19.2 Dignity in Care campaign

High-quality care services that respect people's dignity should:

1   Have a zero tolerance of all forms of abuse
2   Support people with the same respect you would want for yourself or a member of your family
3   Treat each person as an individual by offering a personalised service
4   Enable people to maintain the maximum possible level of independence, choice and control
5   Listen and support people to express their needs and wants
6   Respect people's right to privacy
7   Ensure people feel able to complain without fear of retribution
8   Engage with family members and carers as care partners
9   Assist people to maintain confidence and a positive self-esteem
10 Act to alleviate people's loneliness and isolation

Source: DoH (2006c).

The Joint Committee on Human Rights (2007) published its inquiry into the human rights of older people in healthcare, highlighting many deficiencies even though the Human Rights Act of 1998 was implemented in 2000. Yet abuses against older people's human rights continue, with many service providers failing to adopt a strategy for human rights. Age Concern (2008) have recent documented cases of malnutrition, inappropriate use of sedation, semi-naked patients being left in view of other patients and visitors, and degrading treatment of individuals involving physical, sexual and psychological abuse. In a recent UK report 2.6 per cent of people aged 66 and over living in private households reported that they had experienced mistreatment involving a family member, close friend or care worker during the past year equating to 227,000 people who were neglected or abused (O'Keeffe *et al.* 2007).

The Dignity in Care campaign requires services to have a 'zero tolerance of all forms of abuse' and carers should be mindful that older people are regarded as a vulnerable group and must be protected from harm and exploitation. The Protection of Vulnerable Adults (POVA) scheme, as set out in the Care Standards Act 2000, covers adult placement schemes, care homes and domiciliary care, and ensures that those who have harmed or mistreated vulnerable adults in their care cannot work with vulnerable adults again (DoH 2009b). Age Concern (2008) highlight the continuing abuses against older people's rights and argue that there is an inclination to rely on terms like 'dignity' and 'respect' in policy documents, without linking them to their legal underpinning, the Human Rights Act. Groups from black and ethnic minority groups are small but growing, and services need to be culturally sensitive, reflecting the diversity of the community they serve. All carers need to reflect regularly on the degree to which local culture and practices are all-inclusive preserving privacy, dignity, respect and confidentiality.

Joined-up care

Successful long-term care depends on effective communication and collaboration between all sectors. Following stroke, for instance, clients and carers should have the name of a stroke care coordinator who they can contact for advice (DoH 2001a) and the NSS (DoH 2007a) calls for a range of services to be in place and easily accessible for long-term care and support (QM13). This aspect of care is also supported by quality requirements 5, 7, 8 and 9 of the *National Service Framework for Long Term Conditions* (2005b). A wide range of community-based services are often required enabling individuals to remain independent. The *Expert Patient Programme* (DoH 2001b) provides training for people in developing the skills they need to take effective control of their lives. Similarly there is increasing recognition of the support that carer's need and *Caring with Confidence* builds on the earlier *Expert Carers Programme* offering structured training programmes for carers (DoH 2009c), empowering and enabling them with training available on a face-to-face and distance learning basis.

As well as offering everyone with a long-term condition a care plan, all primary care trusts and local authorities are establishing joint health- and social care-managed networks and teams to support individuals. Continuity is crucial, and older people and their carers need a clear, consistent point of contact with services with coordination not only between health and social care services but other sectors such as housing, transport, employment education and leisure services as well as the voluntary sector (DoH 2001a). Flexible, multidisciplinary services in the community are essential and in response to complex needs, physiotherapy, occupational therapy, speech and language therapy, podiatry, continence services and community mental health services may all be needed as part of an agreed care plan.

Often there is a lack of knowledge about what is available in local areas and professional carers, particularly case managers (e.g. community matrons) (DoH 2005d) need to be aware of all services available across different sectors and organisations. More innovative and creative ways of working are being seen and primary care trusts and local authorities are now involved in the commissioning of services to meet the needs of individuals with long-term conditions (DoH 2006b). It is required that service users are involved in the planning, development, delivery and monitoring of services and are informed how their views are influencing these services (DoH 2007a) (QM4).

With effective monitoring, problems can often be identified early and crisis avoided by speedy responses. Health losses as well as loss of confidence can occur over a very short time frame in older people, and if independence is to be restored, timely intervention is crucial. Primary care trusts and local authorities have worked together to develop rapid response services. Standard three of the NSFOP (DoH 2001a) requires that older people have access to a new range of intermediate care services at home or in designated care settings to promote their independence by providing enhanced services from the NHS and councils to prevent unnecessary hospital admission. These services facilitate early discharge from hospital and are associated with greater functional independence at six months (Green *et al.* 2005). People need to feel confident that protocols are in place to deal with any crisis and deterioration, apart from simply calling the emergency services which is often their only recourse. Where general hospital care is unavoidable, care for older people must be delivered through appropriate specialist care by hospital staff who have the right set of skills so that there is maximum benefit from being in hospital (standard four NSFOP).

Accommodation issues may need to be addressed and may involve arranging special equipment to improve safety. Information and guidance should be available on possible benefit entitlement and the *Supporting People Programme* (Department for

Communities and Local Government 2001) brought several funding streams together so that local authorities can help with housing support to aid the transition to independent living, and details may be found at www.spkweb.org.uk/. The *Supporting People* website offers a directory with a search facility so that support services can be identified in specific local areas. The Direct Payments (DoH 2003) initiative also offers further choice and personal control where payments are given to individuals so that they are able to organise and pay for social services needed. The law has changed in this area so that councils must make a direct payment to eligible individuals who are able to give consent.

Healthy ageing

The NSFOP (standard eight) promotes the health and well-being of older people so that they can live independently at home or in community settings for as long as possible. This has been repeated in a number of reports and policy documents since. Modification of risk factors for disease offers benefits even in later life in terms of levels of functional ability, disease prevention and improved sense of well-being. But with health promotion known to benefit mostly those already advantaged, the challenge is targeting those suffering social disadvantage (Quine *et al.* 2004). Similarly, health promotion activities need to take into account differences in lifestyle, cultural and religious beliefs.

Primary prevention involves reducing risk before health is compromised, while secondary prevention strategies are utilised where risk is already high. Following stroke, for example, managing risk through encouragement of lifestyle changes is important (DoH 2007a) (QM2), with people from black and minority ethnic communities as well as those experiencing economic disadvantage at greater risk. Carers need to be aware of the greater prevalence of some diseases in specific groups such as hypertension and stroke in African-Caribbeans and diabetes and heart disease among South Asians.

Although there are a number of medical conditions that can predispose to stroke (e.g. cardiovascular disease and diabetes), prevention should include smoking cessation, reduced alcohol and salt consumption, improved diet and increased physical activity. These same preventative measures along with management of high blood pressure are also valid in reducing the risk of other major health problems. Those at high risk, either due to specific medical conditions or because of adverse lifestyle factors, should be identified and attempts made to reduce risk by offering advice and making lifestyle changes. Where there are significant cardiovascular risks drugs may need to be prescribed to correct high cholesterol levels (statins) and hypertension (to keep systolic level below 130 mmHg) while some may need anticoagulants (e.g. warfarin) where there is risk of blood clotting (ISWP 2008a).

Preventing falls in older people

Falls can be a cause of major disability, social isolation, lower quality of life and early entry into residential care (Tinetti 2003) and for many older people falling is a constant worry. The aim of the NSFOP (standard six) is to reduce the number of falls resulting in serious injury. Some musculoskeletal changes are expected as part of the ageing process and there can be significant loss of muscle bulk and strength due to inactivity which, in the lower limbs, can contribute to the risk of falls complicated by fractures, particularly where there is osteoporosis. Appropriate health promotion strategies which incorporate gentle exercises into daily regimens can do much to promote mobility and prevent falls. Sensory losses including difficulties with sight and hearing can also contribute to increased risk and should be corrected where possible.

Intrinsic risk factors include mobility problems, medication, visual impairment, impaired cognition/depression and postural hypotension. Factors in the home environment include poor lighting, steep stairs, loose carpets, slippery floors, badly fitting footwear/clothing, lack of safety equipment and inaccessible lights/windows (DoH 2001a). Risk of falling rises with the number of drugs taken and the number of chronic diseases each person has (Lawlor *et al.* 2003). Polypharmacy often presents problems and it is estimated that around 30 per cent of hospital admissions involving those aged 65 and over are due to adverse drug events with most of these preventable (Cresswell *et al.* 2007). Sedating and/or blood pressure-lowering drugs are examples of drugs which may increase risk, and medication review involving pharmacists is important so that risk may be minimised whenever possible (Zermansky *et al.* 2006).

If falls are to be prevented, a specialist falls service should be available within specialist multidisciplinary and multi-agency services for older people and work with older people who are at high risk (DoH 2001a). It is crucial that a risk assessment is undertaken as part of the single assessment process. There is a particular risk of older people falling in hospital and residential care or nursing home settings and any falls should be recorded as part of a risk reduction strategy. Further guidance on falls is available from NICE (2004).

One of the major factors contributing to poor health and the ability to cope is the degree of social engagement and perceived social support. Communities will find this ever more challenging as more people live in single-person households either through choice or when partners for whatever reason are no longer around. For some individuals this may not pose a problem but for others may result in social isolation. More local initiatives are needed in helping older people make healthier choices, remain socially engaged and active and therefore live more meaningful lives. Age Concern are committed to the promotion of healthy lifestyles in older people (Age Concern 2006b) and offer an innovative health promotion programme called *Ageing Well* with a focus on coronary heart disease, stroke, accidents, cancer and mental health, and information may be accessed at www.ageconcern.org.uk/. Various settings, including local day centres, community halls, individual homes and residential care settings, are used to deliver a range of activities. The scheme is supported by coordinators and volunteers and is an example of one model where the social engagement of older people and the resulting benefits can become a reality. The importance of lay health promotion models in supporting 'life checks' is outlined in government policy (DoH 2006a) and Age Concern's *Ageing Well* projects are using trained volunteer health mentors in this initiative.

Conclusion

Perhaps we should end on a positive note. Forecasts predict that the proportion of people over age 65 years in the population will grow from 18 per cent today to 23 per cent in 2030. Ideas and images around ageing are being constantly challenged and society strongly influences our perceptions of how people should age. Yet evidence reveals that levels of health and disability in older people are falling due not only to improvements in areas such as healthcare, but to more people in middle age preparing for retirement in terms of their physical and mental health.

Successful ageing is associated not only with the absence of disease and risk factors, maintenance of physical and cognitive functioning and active engagement with life but also with psychosocial elements such as zest, resolution and fortitude, happiness, relationships between desired and achieved goals, self-concept, morale, mood and overall well-being (Rowe and Kahn 1998; Bowling and Dieppe 2005). While we of course celebrate the increasing numbers ageing successfully, in this chapter the focus has been on those who are living longer but where physical and/ or mental health are compromised. There may be greater challenges posed for this group, but comprehensive holistic assessments, joint care planning, integration of services, collaborative working and, not least, respect for older people can do much to improve quality of life.

Table 19.3 Useful contacts (including helpline support)

Age Concern Charity providing a range of services including day care and information. Campaigns on issues like age discrimination and pensions working to influence public opinion and government policy	www.ageconcern.org.uk/ National Age Concerns: www.ageconcern.org.uk/ AgeConcern/National_Age_ Concerns.asp Age Concern England Astral House 1268 London Road London SW16 4ER Tel: 0800 009966 (free helpline)
Alzheimers Society A membership organisation which works to improve the quality of life of people affected by dementia by providing help and information	www.alzheimers.org.uk/site/ Alzheimer's Society Devon House 58 St Katharine's Way London E1W 1JX Tel: 020 7423 3500 Email: enquiries@alzheimers.org.uk
The Stroke Association UK-wide charity funding research into prevention, treatment and better rehabilitation. Helps those following stroke and their families directly through its rehabilitation and support services	www.stroke.org.uk/ Stroke Information Service The Stroke Association 240 City Road London EC1V 2PR Tel: 0845 3033 100 E-mail: info@stroke.org.uk
Carers UK Member-led charity of carers fighting to end the injustices associated with caring	www.carersuk.org/ Carers UK 20 Great Dover Street London SE1 4LX Tel: 02073784999 Email: info@carersUK.org

Table 19.3 continued

Speakability National charity supporting and empowering people with aphasia and their carers	www.speakability.org.uk/ Speakability 1 Royal Street London SE1 7LL Tel: 020 7261 9572 Email: speakability@speakability.org.uk
Commission for Social Care Inspection (CSCI) Set up by the government but independent to improve social care and stamp out bad practice	www.csci.org.uk/ Commission for Social Care Inspection 33 Greycoat Street London SW1P 2QF Tel: 08450150120 Email:enquiries@csci.gsi.gov.uk
Action on Elder Abuse Charity which works to protect and prevent the abuse of vulnerable older adults. Provides advice and guidance to older people and others	www.elderabuse.org.uk/ Action on Elder Abuse Astral House 1268 London Road London SW16 4ER Tel: 020 8765 7000 (UK helpline 0808 8088141) Email: enquiries@elderabuse.org.uk
Voice UK National charity supporting people with learning disabilities and other vulnerable people who have experienced crime and abuse. Also supports families, carers and professional workers	www.voiceuk.org.uk/ VOICE UK Rooms 100–106 Kelvin House RTC Business Centre London Road Derby DE24 8UP Tel: 01332 291042 (Helpline 0845 1228695) Email: voice@voiceuk.org.uk
Office of the Public Guardian Court of Protection Helps protect people who lack capacity. Court of protection makes decisions in relation to property and affairs and healthcare and personal welfare of adults who lack capacity	www.publicguardian.gov.uk/about/court-of-protection.htm Customer Services – The Office of the Public Guardian and the Court of Protection Archway Tower 2 Junction Road London N19 5SZ Tel: 0845 330 2900 Email: customerservices@publicguardian.gsi.gov.uk

References

Age Concern (2006a) *Hungry to be Heard*. London: Age Concern Reports. Online. Available at: www.ageconcern.org.uk/AgeConcern/Documents/Hungry_to_be_Heard_August_2006.pdf (accessed 9 March 2009).

Age Concern (2006b) *As Fit as Butchers' Dogs? A Report on Healthy Lifestyle Choice and Older People*. London: Age Concern Reports. Online. Available at: www.ageconcern.org.uk/AgeConcern/Documents/494_0206_HealthyChoices.pdf (accessed 9 March 2009).

Age Concern (2006c) *Older Carers. Policy Position Papers.* London: London Policy Unit, Age Concern.

Age Concern (2007) *Improving Services and Support for Older People with Mental Health Problems.* Online. Available at: www.ageconcern.org.uk/AgeConcern/Documents/full_report.pdf (accessed 10 March 2009).

Age Concern (2008) *On the Right Track? A Progress Review of the Human Rights of Older People in Health and Social Care.* London: Age Concern Reports. Online. Available at: www.ageconcern.org.uk/AgeConcern/Documents/On_the_right_track_FINAL.pdf (accessed 9 March 2009).

Age Concern (2009) Ageing Well Programme. Online. Available at: www.ageconcern.org.uk/AgeConcern/44D65A10F661464DAB9E71AFBE7683C9.asp (accessed 9 March 2009).

Alzheimer's Society (2008) *Dementia: Out of the Shadows.* London: Alzheimer's Society.

Ames, D. (1991) Epidemiological Studies of Depression Among the Elderly in Residential and Nursing Homes. *International Journal of Geriatric Psychiatry*, 6, 347–354.

Anthony, J.C., LeResche, L., Niaz, U. *et al.* (1982) Limits of the 'Mini-Mental State' as a Screening Test for Dementia and Delirium Among Hospital Patients. *Psychological Medicine*, 12, 397–408.

Bowling, A. and Dieppe, P. (2005) What is Successful Ageing and Who Should Define it? *British Medical Journal*, 331, 1548–1551.

British Heart Foundation (2005) *Coronary Heart Disease Statistics.* London: British Heart Foundation.

Centre for Policy on Ageing (CPA) (2008) *Single Assessment Process.* London: CPA. Online. Available at: www.cpa.org.uk/sap/sap_about.html (accessed 28 March 2009).

Challis, D., von Abendorff, R., Brown, P. *et al.* (2002) Care Management, Dementia Care and Specialist Mental Health Services: An Evaluation. *International Journal of Geriatric Psychiatry*, 17, 315–325.

Cole, M.G. (2005) Delirium in Elderly Patients. *Focus*, 3, 320–332.

Commission for Healthcare Audit and Inspection (2006) *Living Well in Later Life. A Review of Progress Against the National Service Framework for Older People.* London: Healthcare Commission.

Cresswell, K.M., Fernando, B., McKinstry, B. *et al.* (2007) Adverse Drug Events in the Elderly. *British Medical Bulletin*, 83, 259–274.

Degeling, P., Close, H. and Degeling, D. (2006) *Re-thinking Long Term Conditions. A Report on the Development and Implementation of Co-produced, Year-based Integrated Care Pathways to Improve Service Provision to People with Long Term Conditions.* United Kingdom: The Centre for Clinical Management Development, Durham University.

Department for Communities and Local Government (2001) *Supporting People, Communities and Local Government.* Online. Available at: www.spkweb.org.uk/ (accessed 9 March 2009).

Department of Health (DoH) (2000) *The NHS Plan: A Plan for Investment, A Plan for Reform.* London: DoH.

Department of Health (DoH) (2001a) *Older People. National Service Framework for Older People.* London: The London Stationery Office. Online. Available at: www.dh.gov.uk/en/Publicationsandstatistics/Publications/PublicationsPolicyAndGuidance/DH_4003066 (accessed 9 March 2009).

Department of Health (DoH) (2001b) *The Expert Patient. A New Approach to Chronic Disease Management for the 21st Century.* London: The Stationery Office. Online. Available at: www.dh.gov.uk/en/Publicationsandstatistics/Publications/PublicationsPolicyAndGuidance/DH_4006801 (accessed 9 March 2009).

Department of Health (DoH) (2003) Direct Payments Guidance: Community Care, Services for Carers and Children's Services (Direct Payments) Guidance England 2003. London: DoH. Online. Available at: www.dh.gov.uk/en/Publicationsandstatistics/Publications/PublicationsPolicyAndGuidance/DH_4096246 (accessed 9 March 2009).

Department of Health (DoH) (2004) *Choosing Health: Making Healthy Choices Easier.* London: DoH.

Department of Health (DoH) (2005a) *Supporting People with Long Term Conditions. An NHS and Social Care Model to Support Local Innovation and Integration.* London: The Stationery Office. Online. Available at: www.dh.gov.uk/en/Publicationsandstatistics/Publications/PublicationsPolicyAndGuidance/DH_4100252 (accessed 9 March 2009).

Department of Health (DoH) (2005b) *The National Service Framework for Long Term Conditions.* London: The Stationery Office.

Department of Health (DoH) (2005c) *Carers and Disabled Children Act 2000 and Carer (Equal Opportunities) Act 2004 Combined Policy Guidance.* London: The Stationery Office.

Department of Health (DoH) (2005d) *Supporting People with Long Term Conditions – Liberating the Talents of Nurses Who Care for People with Long Term Conditions.* London: DoH.

Department of Health (DoH) (2006a) *A New Ambition for Old Age – Next Steps in Implementing the National Service Framework for Older People.* Norwich: The Stationery Office.

Department of Health (DoH) (2006b) *Commissioning Framework for Health and Well Being.* London: The Stationery Office.

Department of Health (DoH) (2006c) *About the Dignity in Care Campaign.* Online. Available at: www.dh.gov.uk/en/SocialCare/Socialcarereform/Dignityincare/DH_065407 (accessed 10 March 2009).

Department of Health (DoH) (2006d) *Our Health, Our Care, Our Say: A New Direction for Community Health Services.* London: The Stationery Office.

Department of Health (DoH) (2007a) *National Stroke Strategy.* Norwich: The Stationery Office. Online. Available at: www.dh.gov.uk/en/Publicationsandstatistics/Publications/PublicationsPolicyAndGuidance/DH_081062 (accessed 9 March 2009).

Department of Health (DoH) (2007b) Single Assessment Process. Guidance and Resources. Online. Available at: www.dh.gov.uk/en/SocialCare/Chargingandassessment/SingleAssessmentProcess/DH_079509 (accessed 9 March 2009).

Department of Health (DoH) (2009a) *Living Well with Dementia. A National Strategy. Putting People First.* London: The Stationery Office.

Department of Health (DoH) (2009b) Protection of Vulnerable Adults (POVA) Scheme in England and Wales for Adult Placement Schemes, Domiciliary Care Agencies and Care Homes: A Practical Guide. London: DoH Online. Available at: www.dh.gov.uk/en/Publicationsandstatistics/Publications/PublicationsPolicyAndGuidance/DH_093299 (accessed 9 March 2009).

Department of Health (DoH) (2009c) *Caring with Confidence.* London: DoH Online. Available at: www.dh.gov.uk/en/SocialCare/Deliveringadultsocialcare/Carers/NewDealforCarers/DH_075475 (accessed 9 March 2009).

Dingwall, L. and McLafferty, E. (2006) Do Nurses Promote Urinary Continence in Hospitalised Older People? An Exploratory Study. *Journal of Clinical Nursing,* 15, 1276–1286.

Folstein, M.F., Folstein, S.E. and McHugh, P.R. (1975) Mini-Mental State. A Practical Method for Grading the Cognitive State of Patients for the Clinician. *Journal of Psychiatric Research,* 12, 189–198.

Gaugler, J.E., Kane, R.L., Kane, R.A. *et al.* (2005) Early Community-based Service Utilization and Its Effects on Institutionalization in Dementia Caregiving. *The Gerontologist,* 45, 177–185.

Green, J., Young, J., Forster, A. *et al.* (2005) Effects of Locality Based Community Hospital Care on Independence in Older People Needing Rehabilitation: Randomised Controlled Trial. *British Medical Journal,* 331, 317–322.

Hackett, M.L., Yapa, C., Parag, V. *et al.* (2005) Frequency of Depression After Stroke: A Systematic Review of Observational Studies. *Stroke,* 36, 1330–1340.

Harbison, J., Hossian, O., Jenkinson, D. *et al.* (2003) Diagnostic Accuracy of Stroke Referrals from Primary Care, Emergency Room Physicians, and Ambulance Staff Using the Face Arm Speech Test. *Stroke,* 35, 71–76.

Heffern, W. (2000) Psychopharmacological and Electroconvulsive Treatment of Anxiety and Depression in the Elderly. *Journal of Psychiatric and Mental Health Nursing*, 7(93), 199–204.

Hilari, K., Wiggins, R., Roy, P. *et al.* (2003) Predictors of Health Related Quality of Life (HRQL) in People with Chronic Aphasia. *Aphasiology*, 17, 365–381.

Inouye, S.K. (2004) A Practical Program for Preventing Delirium in Hospitalized Elderly Patients. *Cleveland Clinic Journal of Medicine*, 71, 890–896.

Inouye, S.K., van Dyck, C.H., Alessi, C.A. *et al.* (1990) Clarifying Confusion: The Confusion Assessment Method. A New Method for Detection of Delirium. *Annals of International Medicine*, 113, 941–948.

Intercollegiate Stroke Working Party (ISWP) (2008a) *Care After Stroke or Transient Ischaemic Attack*. London: Royal College of Physicians.

Intercollegiate Stroke Working Party (ISWP) (2008b) *National Guidelines for Stroke* (3rd edn). London: Royal College of Physicians.

Jitapunkul, S., Pillay, I. and Ebrahim, S. (1991) The Abbreviated Mental Test: Its Use And Validity. *Age and Ageing*, 20, 332–336.

Joint Committee on Human Rights (2007) *The Human Rights of Older People in Healthcare* (Rep. No. Eighteenth report of session 2006–2007). London: The Stationery Office.

Knapp, M., Prince, M., Albanese, E. *et al.* (2007) *Dementia UK: The Full Report*. London: Alzheimer's Society.

Lawlor, D.A., Patel, R. and Ebrahim, S. (2003) Association Between Falls in Elderly Women and Chronic Diseases and Drug Use: Cross Sectional Study. *British Medical Journal*, 327, 712–717.

Maher, J. and Green, H. (2002) *Carers 2000*. London: The Stationery Office.

Margallo-Lana, M., Reichelt, K., Hayes, P. *et al.* (2001) Longitudinal Comparison of Depression, Coping, and Turnover Among NHS and Private Sector Staff Caring for People with Dementia. *British Medical Journal*, 322, 769–770.

McDougall, F.A., Mathews, F.E., Kvaal, K. *et al.* (2007) Prevalence and Symptomatology of Depression in Older People Living in Institutions in England and Wales. *Age and Ageing*, 36, 562–568.

McManus, J., Pathansali, R., Stewart, R. *et al.* (2007) Delirium Post-stroke. *Age and Ageing*, 36, 613–618.

National Audit Office (NAO) (2005) *Reducing Brain Damage: Faster Access to Better Stroke Care*. London: NAO.

National Audit Office (NAO) (2007) *Improving Services and Support for People with Dementia*. London: NAO.

National Collaborating Centre for Chronic Conditions (NCCC) (2008) *Stroke: National Clinical Guideline for Diagnosis and Initial Management of Acute and Transient Ischaemic Attack (TIA)*. London: Royal College of Physicians.

National Institute for Health and Clinical Excellence (NICE) (2004) *CG21 Falls: Quick Reference Guide*. Online. Available at: www.nice.org.uk/Guidance/CG21/QuickRefGuide/pdf/English (accessed 9 March 2009).

National Institute for Health and Clinical Excellence (NICE) (2006a) *CG40 Urinary Incontinence. Quick Reference Guide*. Online. Available at: www.nice.org.uk/guidance/index.jsp?action=download&o=30279 (accessed 9 March 2009).

National Institute for Health and Clinical Excellence (NICE) (2006b) *Nutrition Support in Adults: Quick Reference Guide*. Online. Available at: www.nice.org.uk/guidance/index.jsp?action=download&o=29978 (accessed 9 March 2009).

National Institute for Health and Clinical Excellence (NICE) (2006c) *Supporting People with Dementia and their Carers in Health and Social Care*. Online. Available at: www.nice.org.uk/nicemedia/pdf/CG042NICEGuideline.pdf (accessed 9 March 2009).

National Institute for Health and Clinical Excellence (NICE) (2007a) *CG49 Faecal Incontinence: Quick Reference Guide*. Online. Available at: http://www.nice.org.uk/Guidance/CG49/QuickRefGuide/pdf/English (accessed 9 March 2009).

National Institute for Health and Clinical Excellence (NICE) (2007b) *Alzheimer's Disease: Donepezil, Galantamine, Rivastigmine (Review) and Memantine.* Online. Available at: www.nice. org.uk/Guidance/TA111 (accessed 10 March 2009).

O'Keeffe, M., Hills, A., Doyle, M. *et al.* (2007) *UK Study of Abuse and Neglect of Older People. Prevalence Survey Report.* London: National Centre for Social Research (NatCen)/King's College.

Potter, J., Peel, P., Mian, S. *et al.* (2007) National Audit of Continence Care for Older People: Management of Faecal Incontinence. *Age and Ageing*, 36, 268–273.

Rowe, J.W. and Kahn, R.L. (1998) *Successful Ageing.* New York: Pantheon Books.

Royal College of Physicians (RCP) (2006) Concise Guidance to Good Practice. Number 6. The Prevention, Diagnosis and Management of Delirium in Older People. London: Royal College of Physicians. Online. Available at: www.rcplondon.ac.uk/pubs/contents/6be09b43–4f53–46ad-aa11–9bac401f3164.pdf (accessed 10 March 2009).

Quine, S., Kendig, H., Russell, C. *et al.* (2004) Health Promotion for Socially Disadvantaged Groups: The Case of Homeless Older Men in Australia. *Health Promotion International*, 19, 157–165.

Thomas, L., Cross, S., Barrett, J. *et al.* (2008) *Treatment of Urinary Incontinence After Stroke in Adults* (Rep. No. CD004462). Cochrane Database of Systematic Reviews.

Tinetti, M.E. (2003) Clinical Practice: Preventing Falls in Elderly Persons. *New England Journal of Medicine*, 348, 42–49.

van Houten, P., Achterberg, W. and Ribbe, M. (2007) Urinary Incontinence in Disabled Elderly Women: A Randomized Clinical Trial on the Effect of Training Mobility and Toileting Skills to Achieve Independent Toileting. *Gerontology*, 53, 205–210.

Van Peppen, R.P.S., Kwakkel, G., Wood-Dauphinee, S. *et al.* (2004) The Impact of Physical Therapy on Functional Outcomes After Stroke: What's the Evidence? *Clinical Rehabilitation*, 18, 833–862.

Wagg, A., Peel, P. and Potter, J. (2006) *National Audit of Continence Care for Older People.* London: Royal College of Physicians.

Wagg, A.S., Cardozo, L., Chappel, C. *et al.* (2007) Overactive Bladder Syndrome in Older People. *BJU International*, 99, 502–509.

Winstein, C.J., Rose, D.K., Tan, S.M. *et al.* (2004) A Randomised Controlled Comparison of Upper-extremity Rehabilitation Strategies in Acute Stroke: A Pilot Study of Immediate and Long term Outcomes. *Archives of Physical Medicine and Rehabilitation*, 85, 620–628.

Woods, R.T. (2001) Discovering the Person with AD: Cognitive, Emotional and Behavioral Aspects. *Aging and Mental Health*, 5 (suppl. 1), S7–S16.

Zermansky, A.G., Alldred, D.P., Petty, D.R. *et al.* (2006) Clinical Medication Review by a Pharmacist of Elderly People Living in Care Homes – Randomised Controlled Trial. *Age and Ageing*, 35, 586–591.

20 Long-term renal conditions

Swapna Williamson and Breeda McManus

Introduction

Chronic kidney disease (CKD) is a progressive, irreversible and long-term condition, and involves an abnormality in one or both kidneys and a loss of renal function which may or may not include kidney damage. Kidney damage is caused by disease of the kidney itself, glomerulonephritis (that is, inflammation of the nephron, the unit structure of the kidneys) or by diseases that affect multiple organs, such as in diabetes (Redmond and McClelland 2006). As kidney function deteriorates, the risk of complications increases, i.e. anaemia and renal bone disease. In the early stages, CKD can be almost undetectable; however, in some people it will progress to established renal failure (ERF), which is when the kidneys no longer function and the patient needs renal replacement therapy (RRT).

CKD is increasingly recognised as a public health problem as the majority of people with this condition are asymptomatic and may not be aware that they have any form of kidney problem (Holcomb 2005; Royal College Physicians (RCP) 2008). The incidence of people with ERF in the United Kingdom (UK) is also increasing (The Renal Association, UK Renal Registry 2003). CKD affects approximately 10 per cent of the population (Coresh *et al.* 2003). Worldwide, it is estimated that over 1.1 million patients with ERF currently require maintenance dialysis, which is increasing at a rate of 7 per cent per year (Lysaght 2002). If the trend continues, by 2010 the number will exceed two million (Xue *et al.* 2001). In the UK at the end of 2006, 43,901 patients were receiving RRT (The Renal Association, UK Renal Registry 2007).

Pathophysiology and related signs and symptoms of CKD

The functional unit of the kidney is the nephron. Each kidney contains about one million nephrons (Marieb 2004). The kidneys regulate the volume and composition of body fluids through filtration, secretion and reabsorption (Field *et al.* 2001; Thomas 2002). The glomerular filtration rate (GFR) measures the rate at which fluid is filtered by the kidneys and specifically the ability of the glomerulus (a network of blood capillaries that are encapsulated in the Bowman's capsule) to filter plasma. The glomerular filtration membrane allows filtration of blood components except blood cells and plasma proteins. The glomerular filtrate passes through the nephrons and becomes urine. The GFR is related to the perfusion pressure (the pressure arising from the passage of fluid) in the kidneys and to renal blood flow.

Table 20.1 Symptoms of reduced kidney function

1 Fatigue and general weakness
2 Headache
3 Nausea and vomiting
4 Low energy and poor physical function
5 Muscle cramps
6 Pruritus (itching)
7 Bad taste in mouth/loss of appetite
8 Hiccoughs
9 Pedal oedema (accumulation of fluid in the feet)
10 Oliguria (reduced volume/absence of urine)
11 Poorer psychosocial functioning: anxiety, distress, decreased sense of well-being, depression and difficulties with memory and concentration

During systemic hypotension (low blood pressure) the sympathetic nervous system responds by stimulating vasoconstriction, which decreases renal blood flow and reduces the GFR. The retention of fluid and sodium by the kidney increases blood volume and thus increases blood pressure.

Hypertension is one of the main causes of CKD. In systemic hypertension (high blood pressure) small blood vessels supplying the nephrons constrict and restrict glomerular blood flow and filtration pressure. As the GFR decreases, kidney function is progressively impaired with associated signs and symptoms (see Table 20.1). However, hypertension may either cause CKD or be a consequence of it. High blood pressure is associated with faster progression of CKD, which increases the risk of developing CVD and may lead to death (DoH 2005; RCP 2008). The associated complications due to impaired kidney function may lead to anaemia, imbalances of calcium and phosphate resulting in renal bone disease and calcification of the blood vessels.

Chronic kidney disease (CKD)

CKD is a long-term and often progressive condition (DoH 2005) when there is reduction in the estimated glomerular filtration rate (eGFR) due to structural or functional impairment of the kidney. Technically, CKD is defined as either kidney damage causing proteinuria or haematuria (protein and blood cells excreted in the urine respectively), or GFR of less than $60\,\mathrm{ml/min/1.73\,m^2}$ present on at least two occasions for over three months (see Table 20.2) (RCP 2008). At its mildest, it can remain undetected and for the majority of people with CKD the main risk is cardiovascular disease. A minority of people develop ERF, which requires treatment by dialysis and kidney transplant.

The stages of CKD

Identification of the stages is crucial to understand the extent of kidney damage in order to initiate appropriate intervention for patients with CKD. Traditionally, serum creatinine level (creatinine is a waste product produced by muscles) has been used to identify kidney function but its level is dependent on muscle mass and its excretion, which is variable (Thomas *et al.* 2006). Presently the estimated glomeru-

Table 20.2 Stages of chronic kidney disease (National Kidney Foundation – Kidney Disease Outcomes Quality Initiative)

Stage	Description	GFR (ml/min/1.73 m²)
1	Kidney damage with normal or increased GFR	≥90
2	Kidney damage with mild reduction in GFR	60–89
3	Moderate reduction in GFR	30–59
4	Severe reduction in GFR	15–29
5	Kidney failure	≤15 (or dialysis)

lar filtration (eGFR) is considered to be a more accurate measure of kidney function than with serum creatinine only (Thomas 2007) and the glomerular function rate (GFR) is the best index of overall kidney functions (RCP 2008). The GFR in healthy adults is approximately 100 ml/min/1.73 m².

The universally accepted National Kidney Foundation–Kidney Disease Outcomes Quality Initiative (NKF–KDOQI) USA (2002) classification of CKD divides CKD into five stages based on evidence of kidney damage and the level of renal function as measured by GFR. Staging of CKD is based on internationally recognised classification and is shown in Table 20.2.

Causes and risk factors of CKD

The main causes of CKD are in descending order of risk (USRDS 2001):

- diabetic nephropathy (see Chapter 14);
- glomerulonephritis;
- reflux nephropathy (a progressive lesion caused by repeated infections in either or both kidneys);
- renovascular disease (blood vessels within the kidneys);
- hypertension;
- polycystic kidney disease (fluid-filled cysts in the kidneys).

Risk factors of CKD are cardiovascular disease, proteinuria, hypertension, diabetes, smoking, ethnicity, chronic use of non-steroid anti-inflammatory drugs (NSAID) (such as ibuprofen) and urinary outflow obstruction due to kidney stones or an enlarged prostate (see below) (NICE 2008). However, old age, a family medical history of CKD and recovery from acute renal failure are risk factors for progression of CKD (DoH 2005). Diabetes mellitus can increase the risk of CKD (Levy *et al.* 2006; NICE 2008) (see Chapter 14).

Hypertension

Hypertension has been reported in 74 per cent of patients with newly diagnosed ERF making it one of the commonest complicating co-morbidities (USRDS 2001). There are many causes of hypertension, from essential hypertension with no specific cause established, to secondary hypertension associated with CKD and endocrine abnormalities (Dosh 2001). Essential hypertension is related to several abnormal physiologic characteristics, including genetic predisposition and environmental factors such as obesity and high sodium and/or alcohol intake (Brown and Haydock 2000; Dosh 2001). The complex interaction of these factors leads to changes in the reninangiotensin system (the system which plays a central role in salt and water homeostasis, and blood pressure control) and increased peripheral vascular resistance (resulting from constriction of small arteries and helps in maintaining perfusion to the vital organs by sustaining blood pressure) (Dosh 2001). Ultimately, untreated hypertension can lead to increased risk of stroke, myocardial infarction, heart failure, peripheral vascular disease and renal impairment (Brown and Haydock 2000; McCarley and Salai 2005).

Smoking

While there may not be direct links with kidney disease, smoking 'furs up' arteries and is clearly linked to heart disease and cancer. It is also known to reduce one's general level of fitness and contributes to the development of long-term health problems including CKD and cardiovascular disease.

Black or Asian ethnicity

The risk of developing CKD increases with South Asian and African ethnicity. People of South Asian origin are particularly at risk of CKD linked to diabetes; whereas people of African Caribbean origin have an increased risk of CKD linked to hypertension (DoH 2005).

Chronic use of NSAID

Long-term use of NSAID can cause both acute renal failure (ARF) and CKD and can also result in further impairment of kidney function in the presence of pre-existing CKD (The Renal Association 2007).

Bladder outflow obstruction (kidney stone or an enlarged prostate gland)

Bladder outflow obstruction resulting in high blood pressure and chronic urinary retention can cause acute or chronic kidney failure (The RCP and Renal Association 2006). A recurrent obstruction following a previous transurethral resection of prostate (an operation to remove some of the enlarged prostate gland so that urine can flow more freely) may also result in bladder outflow obstruction. Rule *et al.* (2005), in a community-based study, found a clear association between benign prostatic hyperplasia (a condition in which the prostate gland becomes enlarged) and CKD.

Assessment of CKD

Assessment of patients with CKD and patients at risk of developing CKD is vital for initiating and maintaining appropriate management strategies for prevention and reduction of disease progression. Primary care nurses and doctors are important in identifying high-risk CKD patients, and in advising new and existing patients of lifestyle changes to reduce the progression of the condition (NICE 2008). The general assessment of patients with chronic conditions has been detailed in Chapter 5.

However, the following specific assessment of either suspected or established CKD will be useful for planning appropriate care management.

Subjective data

It is important to seek relevant subjective data from the patient, spouse and family members in order to understand the causation of CKD and to plan for further investigation and treatment modalities:

- **Past medical history**: A detailed history of multi-organ diseases such as SLE (systematic lupus erythematosus), diabetes, hypertension, cardiovascular disease, ARF (acute renal failure) and lower urinary tract conditions.
- **Family history**: CKD or polycystic kidney disease.
- **Medication management review**: NSAID treatment history.
- **Lifestyles**: Exercise, diet, smoking and alcohol intake.

Objective data

- **Blood pressure**: One of the main functions of the kidney is to control blood pressure. Monitoring blood pressure is crucial, as high blood pressure causes further damage to the kidney. Patients with kidney disease may develop cardiovascular disease.
- **Urinalysis**: A routine analysis of urine using a dipstick can identify the presence of infection, protein loss and haematuria. Proteinuria is a significant indicator of kidney disease. Haematuria of renal origin indicates renal inflammation (glomerulitis, nephritis), tumour or stones in the kidneys. Protein and blood can be detected on urine dipstick testing, and laboratory tests, such as blood tests, should be carried out if significant results are found (see below).
- **Lab tests**: A full blood test can reveal much about the functioning of the body's systems and general level of health. Specific blood tests such as protein–creatinine ratio (PCR), the albumin–creatinine ratio (ACR) and eGFR should be carried out in suspected CKD. Other tests, such as urine microscopy, culture and sensitivity and urine cytology may also be required.
- **Renal ultrasound/scan**: This is a non-invasive technique of determining kidney obstruction, measurement of kidney size, screening for polycystic disease or neoplasm. Doppler ultrasonography (US) may be used to evaluate venous and arterial blood flow.
- **Renal biopsy**: This is an invasive procedure of obtaining kidney tissue for histological analysis. Indications for renal biopsy include unexplained acute/chronic kidney disease with normal renal size, histology likely to influence treatment, histology likely to offer prognosis. For this procedure an evaluation of risk–benefit ratio should be considered.

Early detection and prevention of CKD

Part two of the National Service Framework for Renal Services (DoH 2005; RCP 2008) states that a majority of people with CKD have a greater risk of developing cardiovascular disease and death than progression to established renal failure

(ERF). The risk of developing CKD increases with age and some conditions, such as diabetes and hypertension, often coexist with CKD (NICE 2008). At present, in the UK, renal replacement therapy (RRT) is costing over 2 per cent of the total NHS budget (The Renal Association 2007; RCP 2008).

Early detection of patients at high risk of developing CKD and appropriate management is crucial to prevent or delay the progression and to reduce or prevent the development of complications. However, owing to a lack of specific symptoms, people with CKD are often not diagnosed or diagnosed late when CKD is at an advanced stage. Once the patient reaches stage 5 of CRF (eGFR of <15) they are identified as having ERF (see Table 20.2). It occurs when a person's kidneys are no longer functioning or when a person has 10 per cent, or less, of normal renal function remaining (Gabriel 1990).

Generally, it is believed that once CKD has advanced to a certain point, it usually progresses to ERF. This point seems to vary with the disease and the individual. According to Obrador *et al.* (1999) and the United States Department of Health and Human Services (USDHHS) (2000) optimal care for patients prior to development of ERF includes strategies to slow the progression of renal failure, appropriate management of uremic complications, prevention or attenuation of co-morbid conditions such as reducing cardiovascular risk factors and treating anaemia, sufficient preparation for ERF therapy and expedient initiation of dialysis.

At its early stage CKD can be asymptomatic and almost undetectable (DoH 2005; RCP 2008). However, simple and freely available diagnostic tests are available for identification of patients for referral to specialists' services (NICE 2008). This will allow timely referral to secondary care for lifestyle and appropriate medical intervention to combat cardiovascular disease. CKD can progress to ERF either rapidly or slowly (Stein *et al.* 2004). The measures to prevent progression of CKD include monitoring eGFR, advice to patients on smoking, weight, exercise, salt and alcohol intake, regular blood pressure monitoring and blood pressure control (a target of less than 130/80 mmHg).

Early detection of CKD is crucial for those with diabetes, hypertension and acute kidney disorders. Hypertension, cardiovascular disease and diabetes are the high-risk factors in the development of CKD (Holcomb 2005); however, CKD can contribute in the development of CVD and hypertension. Thus, CKD, diabetes, hypertension and cardiovascular disease tend to interact in a complex way (DoH 2005; RCP 2008). Figure 20.1 shows the various interactions between disease conditions in the causation of CKD.

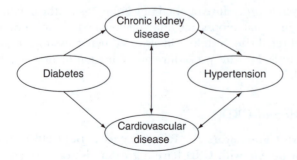

Figure 20.1 Interaction of disease conditions causing CKD.

Table 20.3 People at high-risk conditions requiring renal function test

---

People with the diagnosis of:

---

1 Diabetes
2 Hypertension
3 Bladder outflow obstruction
4 Cardiovascular disease (coronary heart disease, stroke, peripheral vascular disease)
5 Heart failure
6 Recurrent urinary tract infections
7 Metabolic disorders causing recurrent kidney stones
8 Systemic disease – systemic lupus erythematosus
9 A family history of stage 5 CKD/genetic risk of kidney disease
10 Patients on angiotensin-converting enzyme inhibitors (ACE inhibitors) or angiotensin II receptor blockers (ARBs)
11 Neurogenic bladder and patients with surgical urinary diversion
12 Patients maintained on long-term NSAIDs (>12 months)

For early detection of CKD, the people in a high-risk category of developing CKD require a regular renal function test (Table 20.3).

Principles of care of patient with CKD

CKD is progressive; however, with good management the progression can be slowed down. This implies mainly focusing on blood pressure, lipid and glycaemic control, smoking cessation and avoiding nephrotoxic drugs. Interventions to minimise progression of CKD include lifestyle changes and reduction of blood pressure irrespective of the diagnosis of hypertension or diabetes. The use of medication, such as angiotensin-converting enzyme (ACE) inhibitors and angiotensin receptor blockers (ARBs), are effective at reducing progression when there is concurrent proteinuria (NICE 2008). Early treatment with both is effective in order to preserve kidney function and also to become as cost effective as possible.

Diabetic people need, regular monitoring and care management in order to slow progression and improve outcomes (Burrows-Hudson 2005). Diabetics with albuminuria or low eGFR should be managed in conjunction with the local diabetic team. They should be under close attention for glycaemic and blood pressure control (see Chapter 14), aiming for a target of 130/80 mmHg. Many studies over the years have shown the benefits of early intervention and treatment of diabetic nephropathy at the microalbuminuria stage (this is signified when the urine dipstick is negative but the urine albumin:creatine ratio is raised) by using ACE inhibitors or ARBs.

The national and local guidelines enable progressive CKD and associated complications such as cardiovascular risk and anaemia to be managed in the community prior to referral to renal services. Otherwise, referral of all people with CKD would overwhelm renal services. This requires collaboration and partnership between primary care and renal teams that will result in reducing the numbers of patients referred late for RRT involving dialysis or kidney transplant. However, timely investigation, appropriate and effective treatment and follow-up will minimise the risk of progression and complications (DoH 2005). The measures that will help in reducing the risk of progression and complications are indicated in Table 20.4.

Table 20.4 Minimising the risk of progression of CKD

Measures to reduce CKD progression and to prevent complications:

1 Early detection and timely medical intervention
2 Modification of lifestyles
3 Reducing blood pressure whether or not hypertensive or diabetic
4 Maintaining blood pressure at low level in patients with proteinuria
5 Identification and treatment of micro vascular complications
6 Prompt management of urinary tract conditions, especially infection
7 Management of anaemia (CKD-related)
8 Management of bone disease (CKD-related)
9 Referral from primary care to the specialist renal service at appropriate stages to optimise outcomes

Table 20.5 Advice for the patient with CKD

1   Take adequate rest and exercise
2   Regular skin care
3   Cessation of smoking
4   Monitoring weight loss
5   Limit alcohol intake
6   Low salt intake
7   Healthy eating
8   Medications – Lipid-lowering, antihypertensive drugs
9   Glycaemic control
10 Regular medical check-up
11 Compliance with the treatment regimen

Chronic renal failure generally progresses on to ERF. Although incurable, its progression can be slowed down and symptoms effectively managed. It is important that primary renal teams collaborate with secondary teams to raise awareness about kidney disease, highlighting the need for changing lifestyles to reduce the risk of developing CKD (Table 20.5).

Care and management of patients with ERF

Established renal failure (ERF) is CKD stage 5 when the GFR is less than 15 ml/minute requiring RRT (see Table 20.2), which involves dialysis therapy (haemodialysis/peritoneal dialysis) or kidney transplantation based on the advice from a kidney specialist. Deciding on which form of dialysis to choose is complex because it involves major changes in lifestyle and dependence on a treatment without which the patient's life will be at risk.

Haemodialysis

Haemodialysis removes extra fluid, salts and wastes from the bloodstream by filtering the blood through an artificial kidney (dialyser) (Terrill 2002). Blood is pumped through a machine where it comes into contact with a purified dialysis solution (dialysate), which allows wastes to move from blood into the dialysate. This occurs across a special filtering unit called the dialyser or artificial kidney, which then returns purified blood to the body (Terrill 2002). Haemodialysis sessions occur three times per week with each session lasting four or five hours normally in a dialysis centre either within the hospital setting (in-centre dialysis), or in a satellite unit. Haemodialysis renders the patient completely dependent upon a machine for survival. Chronic dialysis is well known to impose a considerable burden on patients and families. In addition to regular attendance for dialysis, the successful treatment of patients with ERF requires strict control of dietary, fluid and medication intake (Morduchowicz *et al.* 1993).

The dietary restrictions on dialysis include low potassium, sodium and phosphate and fluid restriction. All dialysis patients are advised to adhere to a renal diet. Phosphates are not completely removed by dialysis and are found in many foods. Patients should take medication to help reduce phosphate absorption. Keeping the right balance of fluid in their bodies is also essential for good health when on dialysis. For haemodialysis, a patient's fluid intake is determined considering the amount of their urinary output; in most cases fluid intake is restricted to 1000 to 1500 ml per day. Accurate measuring of fluid intake and output is required.

Self-care/home haemodialysis

Home haemodialysis offers a number of potential advantages. People do not have to travel to hospital or wait for treatment once there. There is also more flexibility at home to tailor the dialysis regimen by changing the timing or length of sessions making it easier to lead a normal life and also to be employed. However, over the years the development of satellite dialysis units has brought a decline in home haemodialysis and a decline in the number of people learning to do their own dialysis. By taking a more active role in their own care, people can regain control over their life that is so often lost when living with a long-term condition. The National Institute for Health and Clinical Excellence (NICE 2008) have recommended that all patients who are suitable for home haemodialysis should be offered the choice of having haemodialysis in the home or in a renal unit. Before it is decided whether home haemodialysis is a suitable option for an individual, there should be a full assessment of the patient's healthcare needs and social and home circumstances. If the home environment is not suitable for home dialysis most dialysis units now offer independent dialysis facilities where people can carry out their own treatment within an existing dialysis unit close to work or home; this offers flexibility and saves on waiting times.

Peritoneal dialysis

This treatment uses peritoneal membrane as a semi-permeable membrane. A peritoneal dialysis (PD) catheter is inserted into the peritoneal cavity through the anterior abdominal wall. PD fluid (dialysate) is infused into the peritoneal cavity. Solutes cross from the blood into the dialysate through the peritoneal membrane by diffusion and convection. Excess fluid is removed by osmotic pressure within the dialysate. After the fluid remains in the peritoneal cavity for a few hours it is drained out and the process is repeated (manually four bags per day). Automated peritoneal dialysis (APD) uses a machine to complete the dialysis fluid exchange. This treatment is done overnight while the person is sleeping. Most people need to spend eight to ten hours attached to the machine every night (Kelley 2004; Redmond and Doherty 2005). There are several complications of peritoneal dialysis, including infections and peritonitis. The common signs and symptoms of peritonitis are cloudy effluent in dialysis bag, abdominal pain and tenderness, high temperature, nausea and vomiting. It is essential to regularly monitor those undergoing peritoneal dialysis in order to prevent its complications. Regular cleansing of the catheter exit site is essential to prevent infection. People should avoid baths and swimming pools and when showering should cover the exit site with protective dressings. Hands should be washed thoroughly before and after exit site care (Henrich 1999).

Transplantation

Transplantation is another form of RRT and is the treatment of choice for most people with ERF. Kidneys for transplants are mainly harvested from people who have been diagnosed as having irreversible brain stem damage but it is also possible to transplant and obtain a kidney from a living donor. Pre-emptive transplantation (where a kidney transplant is planned prior to having to initiate renal replacement therapy) is seen as the 'gold standard' treatment for patients approaching ERF. Currently the number of pre-emptive transplantations is still very low and people should be encouraged to determine if their family members would be interested in donating prior to them commencing RRT. The blood group is important in transplantation because the donor's blood must be compatible with that of the recipient. Before transplantation an attempt is made to match the tissue types of the donor and the recipient. Deceased donor kidneys are allocated primarily by blood group and tissue type match. Long-term graft survival rates improve with better matching,

Although a transplant is an excellent treatment for most people, some may encounter problems post-surgery. One of the most common problems is the possibility of rejection. The body system responsible for the rejection process is the immune system. The normal process of the body's own immune system is to fight off foreign bodies, i.e. viruses and bacteria. However, the immune system can fight against the transplanted organ. During this process the immune system sends lymphocytes to attack the foreign body (the transplanted kidney) causing acute rejection. To prevent the rejection the person is given immuno-suppressants that reduce the immune system's effectiveness thus helping to prevent and treat the rejection process. In some cases a kidney biopsy is necessary to confirm the rejection. If positive for rejection the person is given a high dose of steroids to suppress the rejection process.

Education on immuno-suppressant treatment is vital in order to prevent both acute/chronic rejection. A healthy diet is encouraged as excessive weight gain can be a problem after transplants, partly due to the effect of steroid medicines that can increase appetite, but also possibly due to feeling so much better and wanting to eat things that were restricted previously. A renal dietician can assist with dietary advice. People are also encouraged to undertake exercise and activity. Those travelling abroad are warned about the extra risks of infection but are advised not to travel for a year post-transplantation. All transplant patients should avoid live vaccines. Immuno-suppression increases the risks of skin cancer; transplant patients should avoid direct sun exposure and should use high-factor sun block to protect their skin.

Psychosocial aspects of care of CKD

Psychosocial care, especially those who are undergoing dialysis or renal transplantation, is being given more significant importance in the current health and social care environment. A loss of renal function requiring haemodialysis leads to dramatic life changes and may result in modifications to their status in a variety of marital, familial, occupational, financial and social contexts affecting patients' perception of social support and leading to depression (Cukor *et al.* 2007). People with CKD, and receiving dialysis, often undergo a series of tests and medical procedures which can lead to fear, anxiety, confusion, irritation and negative feelings. Lopes *et al.* (2002) found a greater prevalence of depression in patients being treated for end-stage renal disease, which is associated with increased frequency and duration of hospitalisation. In turn, this can affect the medical outcomes of these people through increased stress and a reduction in compliance with, or access to, dialysis and medical regimens (Kimmel and Peterson 2005; Cukor *et al.* 2006). The contemporary care of people with CKD and ERF often includes biopsychosocial perspectives through a multidisciplinary team approach which also involves patients, their carers, relatives and significant others (DoH 2005). Formerly, people were only managed by secondary care by renal physicians and teams of specialist nurses in renal units (Griffith 2007). However, today greater collaboration between primary and secondary services has been identified as necessary in order to provide quality and holistic care to these people.

Chronically ill people encounter various physical, social, psychological, occupational and financial challenges affecting their overall quality of life. Those with CKD and ERF experience a number of illness-induced stressors that exert lifestyle-disrupting effects. The need for long-term dialysis, for example, has significant consequences for patients and their households. Major changes to lifestyle are necessary to accommodate treatment, which may have an impact on his or her ability to work or attend school or college. Among the most common of these are physical disability and incapacitation, decreased strength and stamina, chronic pain, complex medical regimes, the significant amount of time required for the treatment, especially RRT, and its associated economic burdens. These are believed to compromise psychosocial well-being and to contribute to emotional distress (Devins *et al.* 1997). Fixed dialysis schedules and the cost of treatment can also interfere with paid employment or active recreational pursuits causing alterations in mood, anxiety and dependency, which in turn may affect other family members adversely. For some, the impact of illness is so profound that the illness comes to dominate their self-concept and they begin to see themselves solely in terms of the disease. As such, it is likely that both the illness trajectory and the patients' self-concept shape psychosocial responses to the chronic disease (Siegler 1989), such as negative comparisons with others and withdrawal from social roles. They perceive themselves to be stigmatised and damaged by the illness, and may feel that they are dependent on others, and they experience a sense of loss of the pre-illness self (McCay 1994).

It is crucial that healthcare professionals work in collaboration to identify the psychosocial problems that CKD and ERF patients are encountering (National Kidney Foundation 2002; DoH 2005). Appropriate and timely information with regard to treatment options, as well as support and reassurance to those with CKD and their families, will help them to cope effectively with the illness and treatment. An established counselling programme for these people may be helpful in order to support them in their treatment process and to help them develop their coping mechanisms. Effective social support, a social network provision of psychological and material resources will benefit end-stage renal disease patients and help them cope with stress (Kimmel 2001). This will also help these people in dealing with uncomfortable feelings, generating hope, enhancing self-esteem, maintaining relationships with others and retaining a sense of well-being.

In general, people receiving home haemodialysis report a better quality of life than those who have haemodialysis in hospital (NICE 2002). This is because in some patients' and carers' experience home haemodialysis offers a number of potential advantages over hospital dialysis as they do not have to travel to hospital or wait for treatment. It is also empowering in that it affords the person some degree of control over their own care and treatment. There is also more flexibility at home to tailor for the dialysis regimen by changing the timing or duration of dialysis, making it easier for patients to lead a normal life and also to be employed. Further, evidence suggests that home haemodialysis is as clinically effective as hospital haemodialysis (NICE 2002). People receiving dialysis supported by fully trained carers at home in their family environment find it less distressing. Cohen *et al.* (2007) and Kimmel and Patel (2006) found that haemodialysis patients' perception of good family and social support is associated with increased compliance.

People with CKD may have a negative self-perception of their illness because it requires modification or elimination of various lifestyle behaviours. Low self-esteem, and external locus of control, a lack of perceived support and severity of impairment all influence individuals' perception of their illness/condition. There is evidence that ERF can also affect self-esteem and adherence to treatment regimens. The experience of living with a chronic illness like CKD or RRT is unique to each person and their family (Jablonski 2004). Gregory *et al.* (1998) identified that as these patients continue to live with regular medical intervention and its associated stress, they quite often question the meaning of illness and life. This can result in body image distortion, low self-esteem, helplessness, dependency on healthcare professionals, carers and family members, and can alter relationships with their significant others (White and Grenyer 1999). Consequently, adjustment and adaptation to the treatment modalities become major issues (Tanyi and Werner 2008). The way people perceive their ability to change or control their lives has a major impact on their willingness or ability to comply with treatment (Poll and Kaplan De-Nour 1980). However, professional carers play a key role in providing integrated person-centred care to patients with ERF receiving haemodialysis and in meeting their bio-psychosocial, spiritual needs and support requirements, thus facilitating a better quality of care and potentially improved overall quality of life (Tanyi and Werner 2008).

End-of-life care

The numbers of people with ERF are growing, with a disproportionate increase among those who are older, dependent and with multiple co-morbidities. For a number of reasons some people with ERF may decide not to have dialysis treatment, or choose to stop having it after a period of time. For some, the burden of frequent dialysis is felt to outweigh likely survival and quality-of-life benefits (a complex and difficult decision likely to apply more often to those with poorer prognoses). Others, owing to complications arising from coexisting illnesses such as cardiac disease, may be coming to the end of their lives while still on dialysis. Those who choose not to have dialysis usually have multiple co-morbidities and require a service that continues to provide specialist care in the community, enabling them to live well to the end of their lives and die in a preferred place of care. The aim of end-of-life care is to keep people with ERF comfortable and independent for as long as possible.

Palliative provision within UK renal services is limited, but the recent *National Service Framework for Renal Services* (DoH 2005) has promoted service development. End-of-life care has been defined by the National Council for Palliative Care as the care that helps all those with advanced, progressive, incurable illness to live as well as possible until they die. Part 2 of the *National Service Framework for Renal Services* (DoH 2005) states the key quality requirements for end-of-life care are designed to support people with ERF both to live out the remainder of their lives as fully as possible and to die with dignity. This necessitates a coordinated strategy between primary and secondary care involving the patients and their relatives and is essential

Table 20.6 Useful contacts (including helpline support)

NHS Direct
Offers telephone support for people with long-term conditions

Tel: 0845 4647

National Kidney Federation
National UK charity run by patients with kidney disease. Aims to promote both the best renal medical practice and treatment, and the health of persons suffering from chronic kidney disease (CKD) or established renal failure (ERF)

www.kidney.org.uk
National Kidney Federation
The Point
Coach Road
Shireoaks
Worksop
Notts S81 8BW

Tel: 01909 544999
Helpline: 0845 6010209
Email: nkf@kidney.org.uk

Kidney Research UK
UK charity funding research that focuses on the prevention and management of kidney disease. Also dedicated to improving patients' care and raising awareness of kidney disease

www.kidneyresearchuk.org
Kidney Research UK
Registered Office
Kings Chambers
Priestgate
Peterborough PE1 1FG

Tel: 0845 300 1499
Email: kidneyhealth@kidneyresearchuk.org

The British Kidney Patient Association (BKPA)
Organisation offering support, advice and financial help for those with kidney disease and their families

www.britishkidney-pa.co.uk
The British Kidney Patient Association
(BKPA)
Bordon
Hants GU35 9JZ

Tel: 01420 472021/2
Email: info@britishkidney-pa.co.uk

in order to provide effective and culturally sensitive palliative care through a multi-disciplinary team care approach (DoH 2005). People should receive a timely evaluation of their prognosis and information about the choices available to them, as well as to ensure that those near the end of their lives receive a care plan, jointly agreed with their renal team, which is built around their individual needs and wishes. End-of-life issues should be discussed and planned involving patients, family and friends. The person should be allowed to die with dignity and their wishes met wherever practical, such as in their choice of place of death, and respect for religious and cultural beliefs. Sensitive bereavement support may be suggested for family, friends, partners, carers and staff.

Conclusion

The incidence of CKD has become a major health concern worldwide. The identification of people with CKD and their management of the disease in its early stages by the primary healthcare team can greatly reduce the progression and consequences of CKD. Effective collaboration of primary and secondary health services will facilitate better care for those needing complex investigations and those with ERF by having access to a specialist renal team.

A coordinated and collaborative healthcare approach will be useful for integrating the care pathways for diabetes, cardiovascular disease and CKD in order to manage and minimise the impact of these interacting long-term conditions (DoH 2005). This involves timely identification of those who are at high risk of developing CKD and appropriate treatment modalities including end-of-life care, which will help enhance the quality of life of people with CKD.

References

Brown, M.J. and Haydock, S. (2000) Pathoaetiology, Epidemiology and Diagnosis of Hypertension. *Drugs*, 59 (suppl. 2), 1–12.

Burrows-Hudson, S. (2005) Chronic Kidney Disease: An Overview. *American Journal of Nursing*, 105(2), 40–49.

Cohen, S.D., Sharma, T., Acquaviva, K. *et al.* (2007) Social Support and Chronic Kidney Disease: An Update. *Advance Chronic Kidney Disease*, 14, 335–344.

Coresh, J., Astor, B.C., Greene, T. *et al.* (2003) Prevalence of Chronic Kidney Disease and Decreased Kidney Function in the Adult US Population: Third National Health and Nutrition Survey. *American Journal of Kidney Disease*, 41(1), 1–12.

Cukor, D., Paterson, R.A., Cohen, S.D. *et al.* (2006) Depression in End-stage Renal Disease and Haemodialysis Patients. *Nature Clinical Practice Nephrology*, 2, 678–687.

Cukor, D., Cohen, S.D., Paterson, R.A. *et al.* (2007) Psychosocial Aspects of Chronic Disease: ESRD as a Paradigmatic Illness. *Journal of American Society of Nephrology*, 18, 3042–3055.

Department of Health (DoH) (2005) *The National Service Framework for Renal Services Part Two: Chronic Kidney Disease, Acute Renal Failure and End of Life Care*. London: DoH Publications.

Devins, G., Beanlands, H., Mandin, H. *et al.* (1997) Psychosocial Impact of Illness Intrusiveness Moderated by Self-concept and Age in End-stage Renal Disease. *Health Psychology*, 16, 529–553.

Dosh, S. (2001) The Diagnosis of Essential and Secondary Hypertension in Adults. *Journal of Family Practice*, 50(8), 707–712.

Field, M., Pollock, C. and Harris, D. (2001) *The Renal System: Basic Science and Clinical Conditions*. Edinburgh: Churchill Livingstone.

Gabriel, R. (1990) *Causes and Symptoms of Kidney Failure*. London: Kluwer Academic Press.

Gregory, D.M., Way, C.Y., Hutchinson, T.A. *et al.* (1998) Patients' Perceptions of their Experiences with ESRD and Haemodialysis Treatment. *Qualitative Health Research*, 8, 764–783.

Griffith, K.E. (2007) Using the Quality Outcome Framework (QOF) to Help Chronic Renal Patients. *Practice Nursing*, 18(7), 356–360.

Henrich, W.L. (1999) *Principles and Practice of Dialysis* (2nd edn). Philadelphia, PA: Lippincott, Williams & Wilkins.

Holcomb, S.S. (2005) Evaluating Chronic Kidney Disease Risk. *The Nurse Practitioner*, 30(4), 12–25.

Jablonski, A. (2004) The Illness Trajectory of End-stage Renal Disease Dialysis Patients. *Research and Theory for Nursing Practice: An International Journal*, 18(1), 51–72.

Kelley, K.T. (2004) How Peritoneal Dialysis Works. *Nephrology Nursing Journal*, 31(5), 481–487.

Kimmel, P. (2001a) *Management of Patients with Chronic Renal Disease*. In Greenberg, A. (ed.) *Primer on Kidney Diseases*. London: Academic Press.

Kimmel, P.L. (2001b) Psychosocial Factors in Dialysis Patients. *Kidney International*, 59, 1599–1613.

Kimmel, P.L. and Peterson, R.O. (2005) Depression in End-stage Renal Disease Patients Treated with Dialysis: Tools, Correlates, Outcomes and Needs. *Seminar in Dialysis*, 8, 91–97.

Kimmel, P.L. and Patel, S.S. (2006) Quality of Life in Patients with Chronic Kidney Disease: Focus on End-stage Renal Disease Treated with Haemodialysis. *Seminar in Nephrology*, 26(1), 68–79.

Levy, J., Morgan, J. and Brown, E. (2001) *Oxford Handbook of Dialysis*. Oxford: Oxford University Press.

Levy, J., Pusey, C. and Singh, A. (2006) *Fast Facts: Renal Disorders*. Oxford: Health Press.

Lopes, A.A., Bragg, J., Young, E. *et al.* (2002) Depression as a Predictor of Mortality and Hospitalisation Among Haemodialysis Patients in the United States and Europe. *Kidney International*, 62, 199–207.

Lysaght, M.J. (2002) Maintenance Dialysis Population Dynamics: Current Trends and Long-term Implications. *Journal of American Soc. Nephrology*, 13, 37–40.

Marieb, E. (2004) *Human Anatomy and Physiology*. San Francisco, CA: Pearson Education.

McCarley, P.B. and Salai, P.B. (2005) Cardiovascular Disease in Chronic Kidney Disease: Recognising and Reducing the Risk of a Common CKD Comorbidity. *American Journal of Nursing*, 105(4), 40–52.

McCay, E. (1994) Recovering from the Impact of Illness. *Journal of Psychosocial Nursing*, 34(11), 40–44.

Morduchowicz, G., Sulkes, J., Aizic, S. *et al.* (1993) Compliance in Haemodialysis Patients: A Multivariate Regression Analysis. *Nephron*, 64(3), 365–368.

National Institute for Clinical Excellence (2002) *Guidance on Home Compared with Hospital Haemodialysis for Patients with End-stage Renal Failure*. London: NICE.

National Institute for Health and Clinical Excellence (2008) *Identifying and Treating Long-term Kidney Problems (Chronic Kidney Disease) Nice Clinical Guideline 73*. London: NICE.

National Kidney Foundation (2002) *Clinical Practice Guidelines for Chronic Kidney Disease: Evaluation, Classification and Stratification*. New York: National Kidney Foundation.

Obrador, G.T., Ruthazerm, R., Arora, P. *et al.* (1999) Prevalence of and Factors Associated with Suboptimal Care before Initiation of Dialysis in the United States. *Journal of the American Society of Nephrology*, 10, 1793–1800.

Poll, I.B. and Kaplan De-Nour, A. (1980) Locus of Control and Adjustment to Chronic Haemodialysis. *Psychological Medicine*, 10, 153–157.

Redmond, A. and Doherty, E. (2005) Peritoneal Dialysis. *Nursing Standard*, 19(40), 55–65.

Redmond, A. and McDevitt, M. (2004) Acute Renal Failure: Recognition and Treatment in Ward Patients. *Nursing Standard*, 18(22), 46–51.

Redmond, A. and McClelland, H. (2006) Chronic Kidney Disease: Risk Factors, Assessment and Nursing Care. *Nursing Standard,* 20(10), 48–58.

Royal College of Physicians of London and the Renal Association (2006) *Chronic Kidney Disease in adults: UK Guidelines for Identification, Management and Referral.* London: The Renal Association.

Royal College of Physicians (2008) *Chronic Kidney Disease: National Clinical Guideline for Early Identification and Management in Primary and Secondary Care.* London: Royal College of Physicians.

Rule, A.D., Jacobson, D.J., Roberts, R.O. *et al.* (2005) The Association Between Benign Prostatic Hyperplasia and Chronic Kidney Disease in Community-Dwelling Men. *Kidney International,* 67, 2376–2382.

Siegler, I.C. (1989) *Development Health Psychology, The Adult Years: Continuity and Change.* Washington, DC: American Psychological Association.

Stein, A., Wild, J. and Cook, P. (2004) *Vital Nephrology.* London: Class Health.

Tanyi, R.A. and Werner, J.S. (2008) Women's Experience of Spirituality within End-stage Renal Disease and Haemodialysis. *Clinical Nursing Research,* 17(32), 32–49.

Terrill, B. (2002) *Renal Nursing: A Guide to Practice.* Oxfordshire: Radcliffe Medical Press.

The Renal Association. UK Renal Registry (2003) The Sixth Annual Report. Online. Available at: www.renalreg.com/reports/renal-registry-reports/2003/ (accessed 9 April 2009).

The Renal Association. UK Renal Registry (2007) The 10th Annual Report. Online. Available at: www.renalreg.com/reports/renal-registry-reports/2007 (accessed on 9 April 2009).

Thomas, N. (ed.) (2002) *Renal Nursing* (2nd edn). London: Bailliere Tindall.

Thomas, N. (2007) Recent Development in the Care and Management of Chronic Kidney Disease (CKD). *Primary Health Care,* 17(6), 41–45.

Thomas, N. and Gallagher, H. (2007) The Diagnosis and Management of Chronic Kidney Disease. *Practice Nurse,* 33(1), 12–16.

Thomas, N., Coldstream, F. and Cox, S. (2006) Managing Chronic Kidney Disease in the Community. *British Journal of Renal Medicine,* 11(1), 26–28.

United States Department of Health and Human Services (USDHHS) (2000) *Healthy People 2010* (2nd edn). Washington, DC: US Government Printing Office.

United States Renal Data System (USRDS) (2001) Annual Data Report: Incidence and Prevalence of ESRD. Online. Available at: www.usrds.org/adr.htm. (accessed 9 April 2009).

White, Y. and Grenyer, B.F.S. (1999) The Biopsychosocial Impact of End-stage Renal Disease: The Experience of Dialysis Patients and Their Partners. *Journal of Advanced Nursing,* 30, 1312–1320.

Xue, J.L., Ma, J.Z., Louis, T.A. *et al.* (2001) Forecast of the Number of Patients with End-stage Renal Disease in the United States to the Year 2010. *Journal of American Society of Nephrology,* 2(12), 2753–2758.

21 The immuno-compromised client

Robert Pratt and Simon Jones

Introduction

For almost everyone, happiness and well-being are related to the attainment and preservation of good health or the restoration of health following acute episodes of illness. A variety of factors influence the potential of each person to achieve these goals, including social, political, economic and occupational circumstances and inherited attributes. Freedom from infectious diseases is an additional critical influence underpinning both individual and community health. Throughout the world, and especially in resource-poor regions, acute and chronic infections account for a substantial and preventable amount of misery, ill-health, disability and premature deaths.

Having an effective immune system for preventing or containing and minimising the consequences of inevitable incidents of infection during life is an essential prerequisite for good health. However, for many, individual genetic characteristics, life events, external circumstances and infections and diseases can temporarily or permanently impair the ability of their immune system to provide this protection. Immunosuppression is relatively common in many populations throughout the world, significantly increasing the global burden of infectious diseases.

In order to facilitate an understanding of the causes of immunosuppression, this chapter begins with a brief review of the salient features of the immune system, followed by a brief account of the range of immunodeficiency disorders. The remainder of the chapter will focus on the care and support of persons who are immuno-compromised as a result of chronic infection with the human immunodeficiency virus (HIV), the most prevalent and challenging cause of progressive immunosuppression in people throughout today's world. Following an exploration of the pathophysiology of HIV disease, essential elements of the care and support of clients will be discussed, including clinical monitoring, anti-retroviral therapy and infection control. A principal goal of clients with chronic disease is to manage their condition effectively. Using the experience gained over many years in London with the HIV Positive Self-Management Programme (PSMP), this chapter will conclude with a detailed consideration of the role of community-centred programmes led by 'expert patients' in supporting clients to develop knowledge, skills and attitudes to help them better manage their chronic condition and improve the quality of their lives.

Immune system

Immunity (that is, the body's physiological ability to resist infectious diseases) has evolved in humans over many millennia and affords crucial protection without which survival would be impossible. An understanding of normal immune mechanisms is necessary to appreciate the underlying pathophysiology and clinical consequences of disorders of immunity and to develop appropriate and relevant individualised care and support strategies for immuno-compromised persons.

The immune system is composed of a network of organs, tissues, cells and molecules which respond to and interact with each other in the recognition and containment and/or destruction of invading disease-causing (pathogenic) micro-organisms or other antigens, i.e. any foreign (non-self) material. These coordinated responses are derived from both innate (non-specific) and adaptive (acquired) immune mechanisms.

Innate immunity is inborn and consists of physical barriers (intact skin, mucous membranes and ciliated cells), chemical secretions (gastric acid, digestive enzymes, other bactericidal lysozymes and bacteriostatic fatty acids of the skin), the complement system and natural killer (NK) and phagocytic cells. Although many cells in the body engage in phagocytosis, the principal phagocytes are specialised white blood cells: granulocytes (neutrophils, eosinophils) and monocytes and their progeny, circulating macrophages. Other macrophages are fixed in tissues strategically located throughout the body (e.g., lungs, liver, spleen). NK cells especially target and destroy virus-infected and tumour cells.

Phagocytic cells engulf antigens, such as pathogenic micro-organisms, digest them and then project minute fragments of these antigens (epitopes) on their cell surface. This process transforms phagocytic cells into antigen-presenting cells (APC) which circulate throughout the lymphatic system and bloodstream, 'presenting' the antigen to the lymphocytes. When these cells recognise a specific antigen, they rapidly increase in numbers and initiate the antibody and cell-mediated responses described below.

Innate immune mechanisms are non-specific, i.e. they attempt to prevent the invasion of pathogens or neutralise and/or destroy any invading material they recognise as foreign. These mechanisms do not need to differentiate between the different types of pathogens that may infect persons; they just need to recognise self from non-self. Consequently, the development of immunological memory is not a facet of innate immunity. That important role is reserved for enhanced immune mechanism we acquire in the process of adapting to our changing environment and circumstances, i.e. adaptive immunity.

Adaptive immunity is gained after birth and is highly specific, targeting a specific micro-organism or groups of micro-organisms which are closely related. This type of immunity is governed by the actions of a group of white blood cells known as lymphocytes. These originate as stem cells in the bone marrow and mature as either B-lymphocytes or T-lymphocytes. These two types of lymphocytes govern antibody-mediated (B-lymphocytes) or cell-mediated immune responses (T-lymphocytes).

Antibody-mediated immunity

B-lymphocytes are transformed into antibody-secreting plasma cells when they are presented with and recognise a specific antigen. These 'y-shaped' antibodies (also known as immunoglobulins, abbreviated 'Ig') are protein molecules that are designed to be equally specific (e.g. antibodies to hepatitis A virus will only combine with that virus, and will not bind to hepatitis B virus). When combining with a specific antigen, an immune complex is formed which activates a system of plasma proteins known as complement (because they complement the activity of antibodies). Activated complement attach to immune complexes causing the cell membrane to rupture (lysis) and provoking an inflammatory response that leads to their destruction.

There are five classes of antibodies which are sequentially secreted by plasma cells. During primary infection (i.e. the initial few weeks following infection), the first antibody, known as IgM, is produced by plasma cells but recedes after a few months and then disappears as the plasma cells stop producing it and change to producing the second antibody, IgG. Unlike IgM, this antibody is long-lasting and a profile of IgG produced in response to previous infections can be identified in all individuals. Consequently, the presence of IgG is generally used in testing for previous exposure to infections and/or existing chronic productive infections (e.g. Hepatitis C, HIV disease).

Cell-mediated immunity

When presented with an antigen they recognise, T-lymphocytes differentiate into two different types of helper cells (CD4$^+$ T-lymphocytes): helper cell 1 (TH1) and helper cell 2 (TH2). These two activated immune cells deliver their help by secreting a distinct profile of cytokines, soluble protein molecules that act as cell-to-cell messengers to stimulate or inhibit the growth of immune cells and amplify or depress immune responses. Examples of cytokines include interferons and interleukins. Cytokines secreted by TH1 cells provoke the activation of cytotoxic T-lymphocytes (CD8$^+$ cells) that, like NK cells, hunt down and kill virus-infected cells. TH2 cells secrete a collection of cytokines that provide programming instructions to plasma cells, facilitating the production of specific and highly effective antibodies. When the pathogen has been destroyed or the infection has been contained, suppressor T-lymphocytes will down-regulate the activation and return adaptive immune responses to their normal steady-state of vigilance.

Working together, innate and adaptive immune responses provide all persons with an impressive armoury of weapons needed to protect them from the constant threat of infection by pathogenic micro-organisms. However, not everyone has or retains an effective immune system and, without this immuno-competence, their health and well-being will be in peril.

Immunodeficiency disorders

Temporary or permanent immunosuppression, regardless of the cause, greatly increases individual vulnerability to infectious diseases. There are many different types of immunodeficiency disorders which are classified as being either primary or secondary.

Primary (congenital) immunodeficiency disorders are genetically determined and are almost always seen in male infants and children. Over 200 different primary immunodeficiency disorders are recognised, some with complex aetiologies. Many

Table 21.1 Secondary causes of immunodeficiency

Renal disease – e.g. nephrotic syndrome, renal insufficiency
Endocrine diseases – e.g. diabetes mellitus
Liver disease – e.g. chronic hepatitis
Neoplastic disease – e.g. leukaemia, end-stage cancer
Infections – e.g. Epstein–Barr virus, measles virus, varicella-zoster virus, human immunodeficiency virus, *Mycobacterium tuberculosis*
Rheumatologic diseases – e.g. rheumatoid arthritis, systematic lupus erythematosus (SLE)
Malnutrition (and alcoholism)
Burns
Radiation
Splenectomy
Chemotherapeutic drugs – e.g. corticosteroids, immunosuppressants, anti-cancer drugs

of these are extremely serious, if not life-threatening (e.g. infants with 'severe combined immunodeficiency' (SCID)). Some primary immunodeficiency disorders can be treated by transplanting bone marrow stem cells donated by a sibling with an identical human leucocyte antigen (HLA) genetic match, or, in some cases, by a parent. If transplantation is not an option, other treatments, such as anti-microbial drugs (for prophylaxis and treatment for infections) and intravenous human normal immunoglobulin (HNIG), may be used. Experimental gene therapy for treating some types of primary immunodeficiency disorders shows some promise but is currently not in widespread use due to adverse events in those treated with this technique.

Fortunately most people are born with a competent immune system but later in life some acquire an immunodeficiency disorder as a result of another medical condition or life circumstances and events (see Table 21.1). These are known as secondary immunodeficiency disorders and although many resolve, others progress to chronic immunodeficiency.

One of the most common global causes of chronic immunodeficiency is malnutrition. Most of the enzyme systems involved in immune responses are protein-based and people who are severely malnourished are, by definition, chronically immunosuppressed. However, because HIV disease has become perhaps the most defining and enduring pandemic disease of our times, and arguably the most frequent cause of chronic immunodeficiency throughout the world, it will feature as the main focus of the remainder of this chapter.

HIV infection and AIDS

Since its recognition as a new communicable disease in the early 1980s, the global pandemic of HIV infection and AIDS expanded rapidly in many regions throughout the world. In some countries, particularly in sub-Saharan Africa, progress made in previous decades in reducing infant mortality, increasing maternal and child health and extending life expectancy has been eradicated by national epidemics of HIV infection. During the past quarter of a century there has been an annual global increase in the estimated number of people living with HIV infection (Figure 21.1) (UNAIDS 2007). However, there are, perhaps, some encouraging changes now being observed in the epidemiological direction of this maturing pandemic.

Epidemiology

During 2007, an estimated 33.2 million people in the world were living with HIV (67 per cent of them in sub-Saharan Africa), both men and women being equally affected. Add to this the 25 to 30 million people who have already died from AIDS and the magnitude of the pandemic becomes startling. Each day during 2007 over 6800 persons became infected with HIV, 50 per cent of these being under the age of 25. Every day during 2007, more than 5700 people died from AIDS (see Table 21.2) (UNAIDS 2007).

Although the percentage of people in the world who are infected with HIV (the global prevalence) has stabilised since 2001, the actual number of persons living with HIV is increasing each year owing to the accumulation of continuing new infections in people with longer survival times in a continuously growing general world population. This has resulted in an annual global increase in the estimated number of people living with HIV (Figure 21.1) (UNAIDS 2007). However, more encouragingly, during 2007 there have been localised reductions in prevalence in specific countries and a reduction in both HIV-associated deaths (due to better availability of and access to anti-retroviral treatment) and in the number of annual new HIV infections globally (UNAIDS 2007).

An analysis of epidemiological trends by UNAIDS (2007) has indicated that this maturing global pandemic has developed into two broad patterns. Generalised epidemics that are sustained in general populations is the pattern seen in many sub-Saharan African countries, especially in the southern part of the continent, and in some countries outside of Africa (e.g. Haiti and Papua New Guinea). In the rest of the world, epidemics are mainly concentrated among populations most at risk of exposure and infection (e.g. men who have sex with other men, injecting drug users, sex workers and their sexual partners).

Sub-Saharan Africa, with an estimated 22.5 million adults and children living with HIV in 2007, has been the most severely affected region in the world, where AIDS remains the leading cause of death. More than two out of every three persons (and 90 per cent of children) infected with HIV live in this region where more than three in four (76 per cent) of AIDS-associated deaths occurred. Other regions with large

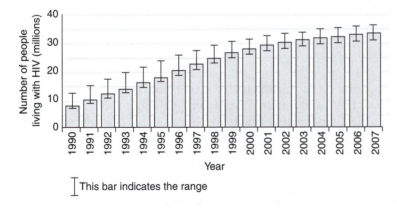

Figure 21.1 Estimated number of people living with HIV globally (1990–2007) (source: courtesy of UNAIDS/WHO. Reproduced with permission).

Table 21.2 Global summary of the AIDS epidemic, December 2007

Number of people living with HIV in 2007	Total	33.2 million [30.6–36.1 million]
	Adults	30.8 million [28.2–33.6 million]
	Women	15.4 million [13.9–16.6 million]
	Children under 15 years	2.1 million [1.9–2.4 million]
People newly infected with HIV in 2007	Total	2.5 million [1.8–4.1 million]
	Adults	2.1 million [1.4–3.6 million]
	Children under 15 years	420,000 [350,000–540,000]
AIDS deaths in 2007	Total	2.1 million [1.0–2.4 million]
	Adults	1.7 million [1.6–2.1 million]
	Children under 15 years	290,000 [270,000–320,000]

Source: Courtesy of UNAIDS/WHO.

numbers of persons living with HIV are South and South-East Asia (4.0 million), Latin America (1.6 million), Eastern Europe and Central Asia (1.6 million) and North America (1.3 million) (UNAIDS 2007). In a current global population of approximately six and a half billion people, it is salutary to remember that China and India together are home to almost one-third of all the people in the world. As relatively new national epidemics continue to expand in these two countries, it is disturbing to contemplate the impact this will have on the future course of the global pandemic.

The prevalence of adults and children living with HIV in Western and Central Europe is estimated to be 760,000 (UNAIDS 2007). The countries with the largest number of cases are the United Kingdom (UK), France, Italy and Spain (UNAIDS 2008). In the UK, the annual number of newly diagnosed HIV infections has more than doubled from 4154 in 2001 to 8925 in 2006. The UK has one of the highest rates of new HIV diagnoses in Western and Central Europe (149 per one million population) in 2006, which is exceeded only by Portugal's 205 per one million population (EuroHIV 2007; UNAIDS 2008). There were an estimated 73,000 persons living with HIV in the UK in 2006 (121 persons living with HIV per 100,000 population) (Health Protection Agency 2007). Although London continues to be the epicentre, accounting for 41 per cent of new HIV diagnoses in 2006, significant increases in new HIV diagnoses have occurred in the East Midlands, Northern Ireland and Wales (Health Protection Agency 2007).

Transmission

Early in the pandemic, the means by which HIV is transmitted from one person to another became clear. HIV is transmitted by blood (including menstrual blood), semen and pre-ejaculate fluid, vaginal fluids and breast milk. It is not spread by tears, sweat or saliva.

Sexual transmission

Unprotected, penetrative sexual intercourse remains the usual means by which most people are exposed to this virus. Worldwide, heterosexual transmission is the principal way people become infected and is the predominant transmission pattern in generalised epidemics in general populations, such as national epidemics in Africa. Although vaginal intercourse is the most frequent type of sexual activity, unprotected anal intercourse can also transmit HIV, whether it occurs between heterosexual men and women or between men who have sex with other men. Oral sex may transmit HIV but it is generally considered a lower risk activity than vaginal or anal intercourse. However, repeated exposure to semen and pre-ejaculate fluid or to vaginal fluids (and menstrual blood) may increase the risk to the person performing oral sex (Public Health Agency of Canada 2004).

The presence of another sexually transmitted infection, either an inflammatory condition, such as gonorrhoea or an ulcerative disease (e.g. primary syphilis or genital herpes), significantly facilitates both the transmission and acquisition of HIV. There is extensive high-quality research to show that male circumcision protects against the sexual transmission of HIV from women to men (WHO 2007). This is because the penile shaft and outer surface of the foreskin is covered by a tough keratinised, stratified squamous epithelium which provides a barrier against HIV transmission. However, the inner mucosal surface of the foreskin is not keratinised (Barreto *et al.* 1997) and is richly supplied with Langerhans' cells which are susceptible to HIV infection (Hussain and Lehner 1995). During vaginal intercourse, the foreskin is pulled back down the penile shaft and the whole inner surface of the foreskin is then exposed to vaginal secretions, providing a large area where HIV transmission can take place (Szabo and Short 2000). Results of three randomised controlled trials have shown that male circumcision performed by well-trained medical professionals was safe and reduced the risk of acquiring HIV infection by approximately 60 per cent (WHO 2007).

Finally, patterns of sexual behaviour influence vulnerability to infection. In Africa, it is not unusual for people to be members of a network of concurrent partners, i.e. simultaneous long-term sexual relationships with more than one partner at one time. Referred to as concurrent relationships (Epstein 2007), this may be more risky than sequential monogamy (a more common pattern in Europe and North America) as friendship and trust within the network may lessen the consistent use of condoms and a single person's infection can spread rapidly through a group. Where concurrent relationships are the rule rather than the exception, networks can efficiently accelerate the sexual transmission of HIV throughout a society.

Mother-to-child transmission

Throughout the world, and especially in resource-poor regions, mother-to-child transmission (MTCT) is the second most frequent means of person-to-person transmission. HIV can be transmitted by an HIV-infected woman to her infant during pregnancy, during birth when the newborn infant comes into contact with infected maternal birth fluids, and shortly after birth or during the early months and years of life while being breastfed. Most children become infected during the peripartum period, i.e. during or shortly after delivery (Pratt and Pellowe 2006). There is a wealth of good-quality research evidence to show that antenatal screening for HIV infection and a combination of interventions for women found to be infected can significantly reduce the risk of MTCT. These interventions include: anti-retroviral treatment for the pregnant women (if indicated) or anti-retroviral chemoprophylaxis, elective caesarean section delivery and modifications in infant feeding practices (Pratt and Pellowe 2006).

Injecting drug use

HIV is efficiently transmitted by sharing blood-contaminated needles, syringes and injection paraphernalia, a common phenomenon among injecting drug users (IDUs). In Europe and North America, IDUs account for a significant number of persons living with HIV. However, drug users are, by and large, sexually active individuals and are often sex workers. Consequently, they may also acquire HIV infection as a result of sexual exposure (Pratt 2003). Needle and syringe exchange programmes can reduce the transmission of syringe-borne viruses without increasing illicit drug use and are effectively used in many countries as part of a wider harm-reduction strategy (Heimer 1998; Allgeier 2006). It is worth noting that some non-injectable drugs, such as alcohol, crack cocaine and more notoriously, fluni-trazepam (Rohypnol™) or GHB (gamma-hydroxybutryate), the so-called 'date rape drugs', can render a person incapable of making responsible and safe judgements and result in increasing their risk of sexual exposure to HIV.

Healthcare transmission

HIV has been transmitted to patients from healthcare interventions and from infected patients to healthcare workers. In many parts of the world, patients are at considerable risk of being infected with HIV (and other blood-borne viruses) as a result of unscreened transfusions of contaminated human blood and blood components, transplantation of infected donor organs, tissues and semen, the use of unsterilised HIV-contaminated needles and syringes and other equipment used for invasive procedures. Healthcare workers are at risk of potential exposure to blood-borne viruses if they come into contact with the blood, other body fluids or the moist mucous membranes of their patients. The risk of accidental transmission of HIV to patients or healthcare workers is greatest in resource-impoverished regions of the world where healthcare infrastructures are weak, healthcare practice is poor, and safe, affordable and effective healthcare provision is not easily available.

Standard infection prevention and control precautions, an essential element of strategies designed to protect healthcare workers and patients from blood-borne viruses, have been developed and are in wide use in the UK and other countries in the industrialised world (Pratt 2003; Pratt *et al.* 2007). The consistent incorporation of these precautions into everyday clinical practice provides the best available protection against occupational exposure to HIV and other blood-borne viruses during healthcare practice.

Diagnosis of HIV infection

There are two major variants of HIV, known as HIV-1 and HIV-2. The former is the dominant AIDS-causing virus in the world whereas HIV-2 is fairly restricted to the west coast of Africa. However, both types of infection are seen in the UK.

The standard diagnostic test for HIV infection throughout the world is the HIV antibody test. This uses a laboratory technique known as enzyme immunoassay (EIA) to detect HIV-specific antibody G (IgG) in an infected person's blood, saliva or urine. This test is very accurate, having a high degree of both sensitivity and specificity. Most people will develop detectable IgG antibodies (i.e. seroconvert) within two to eight weeks (average 25 days) following infection, and virtually all newly infected persons will seroconvert by 12 weeks. In the UK, all antibody tests test simultaneously for HIV-1 and HIV-2 IgG.

Testing for viral proteins is more frequently being done to detect early infection as this protein is present in the blood before IgG appears. Antibody tests are not used to identify infection in newborn infants (as they would only detect passively transferred maternal antibodies); rather a nucleic-acid amplification test (NAT) is used, known as PCR DNA (polymerase chain reaction DNA). A variety of 'rapid' tests are available in clinics where results can be available within 20 minutes and, in the USA and other countries, government-approved self-testing kits for use at home and Internet testing are available.

Pathogenesis

During the first few months following infection (primary infection), some people will develop a generally self-limiting seroconversion syndrome, commonly experiencing fatigue, fever, rash, lymphadenopathy, diarrhoea, candidiasis and other diverse symptoms. During primary infection, increasing viral replication provokes an antibody and cell-mediated immune response, and the level of virus in the blood (viral load) is suppressed (see Figure 21.2). Towards the end of primary infection, IgG antibodies to HIV can be detected in the blood, i.e. seroconversion has taken place.

Following this, a productive infection is established and the infected person enters a long asymptomatic period (clinical latency) of generally many years. However, the virus continues to replicate at an approximate rate of ten billion new copies every day, and, although waning immune responses steadfastly continue to suppress viral replication, it cannot keep up with the relentless rate of replication, and over time there develops a steady increase in viral load corresponding to a progressive loss of immune function as measured by the numbers of CD4$^+$ T-lymphocytes in the peripheral blood (see Figure 21.2).

Towards the end of clinical latency, infected persons will start to feel unwell with various constitutional systems (e.g. weight loss, fevers, night sweats, diarrhoea), and are classified as having early symptomatic disease. Without specific anti-retroviral treatment, these persons will quickly progress to late symptomatic disease (i.e. the acquired immunodeficiency syndrome (AIDS)) where they will experience a variety of opportunistic infections and cancers and associated multi-system pathology, and die. Globally, tuberculosis is the most frequent opportunistic infection people with AIDS develop.

Anti-retroviral therapy

Unrelenting viral replication will eventually cause fatal damage to the immune system and this can be measured by monitoring the level of specialised immune system cells, the CD4$^+$ helper T-lymphocytes. A normal CD4$^+$ T-cell count in an adult in the UK is generally around 1000 cells per cubic millimetre (cells/mm^3). As the CD4$^+$ cell count decreases over time with a corresponding increase in the amount of HIV in the blood (viral load), anti-retroviral therapy (ART) is eventually required.

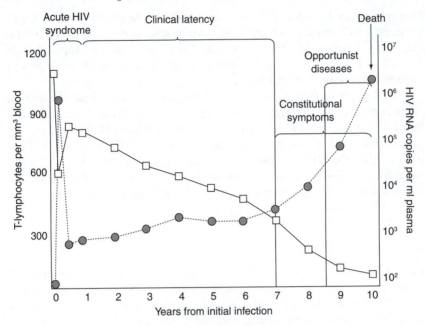

Figure 21.2 The clinical course of HIV infection and disease in relation to the CD4⁺ T-lymphocyte cell count [□] and the viral load [●] (source: Pratt *et al.* (2005)).

Current guidelines in both the UK and the USA recommend starting ART in all persons with a CD4⁺ cell count of 350 cells/mm³ (or lower) (British HIV Association 2008).

Effective ART has been available in the UK since the early 1990s and consists of a regimen of a combination of different anti-retroviral drugs that either inhibits viral enzymes used by HIV to replicate, or block cell-surface receptors which HIV uses to attach to and enter cells it has targeted for infection. These drugs inhibit HIV from replicating; they do not eliminate the virus from the body and once these drugs are stopped (or the patient becomes resistant to them), the viral load will rebound to pre-treatment high levels with consequent new damage to an already compromised immune system.

Newly introduced anti-retroviral drugs, such as the integrase and entry inhibitors, offer an increasingly powerful and effective armoury of anti-retroviral agents to depress replication and drive down the viral load below the level of detection. This has the effect of increasing or, more usually, restoring the patient's health and well-being, and decreasing (but not eliminating) their level of infectiousness to other people.

Self-management

Managing chronic conditions such as HIV can be a complex, time-consuming and challenging process. However, due to the nature of long-term illness it is often the patients, rather than healthcare professionals, who are responsible for the routine management of their day-to-day physical, psychological and emotional health. This 'self-management' will often involve:

[all] the tasks that individuals must undertake to live well with one or more chronic conditions. These tasks include having the confidence to deal with medical management, role management, and emotional management of their conditions.

(Adams *et al.* 2004)

Many tasks will be specific to the patient's illness, but there is also a core of common tasks that all patients with long-term chronic conditions will be asked to perform. These include:

- closely monitoring their symptoms and responding with appropriate actions;
- dealing with acute attacks or exacerbations of the disease;
- making major lifestyle changes;
- dealing with fatigue;
- adhering to intricate medication and treatment regimens;
- attending clinical visits for tests, physical examinations and consultations;
- managing work;
- developing strategies to deal with the social and psychological consequences of the illness (DoH 2001).

The positive self-management programme for people living with HIV

Since its first UK pilot in 2002, there is no doubt that the EPP has proven extremely successful in giving 'people the confidence to take more responsibility and self-manage their health, while encouraging them to work collaboratively with health and social care professionals' (EPP 2008). It does, however, take an extremely generic approach to self-management and does not provide any specific health information; nor does it address clinical needs. Such an approach is wholly sufficient for many people living with a long-term chronic condition; and for those who do not have complex disease-related issues, the EPP is extremely beneficial. However, for people living with a complex chronic disease (CCD), conditions such as HIV that involve immuno-compromisation, multiple morbidities and complicated treatment regimens, and require the attention of multiple healthcare professionals, the EPP is not enough (Sevick *et al.* 2007). They require bespoke self-management programmes that address their condition-specific needs as well as those shared by others with less demanding long-term illnesses.

For this reason, in addition to the CDSMP, Stanford University has created a number of disease-specific courses, one of which is the Positive Self-management Program (PSMP), a self-management programme designed specifically for people living with HIV. Also first piloted in the UK in 2002, the PSMP is very similar in structure, content and delivery to the EPP but, importantly, it is one week longer than the EPP and this extra time is specifically designed to address the needs of people living with HIV. It aims to give participants greater confidence in coping with HIV and enables them to gain the skills and techniques to improve their quality of life and maintain their physical, psychological and mental health and well-being. The PSMP does not conflict with existing programmes or treatment. It is designed to enhance regular treatment and HIV-specific education (Stanford University 2008) and has proven extremely effective at improving the lives of immuno-compromised clients.

Self-management and beyond

The experience gained in the UK suggests that self-management programmes do achieve their goal of making life better for people living with chronic disease by supporting self-care and providing participants with the tools they need to move beyond their illness; enabling them to more effectively manage their condition. Empowering people with knowledge, skills and advice, self-management programmes are successful at enhancing the lives of participants by boosting their confidence, widening their horizons, and encouraging them to build supportive social networks. The success of community-based self-care programmes such as the EPP and the PSMP continues to provide compelling evidence of the value of peer-led patient self-management programmes for people living with chronic conditions. However, one of the most important aspects of all these self-management programmes is that they are peer-led initiatives facilitated by trained lay facilitators. Many of the facilitators have completed the programmes themselves and for participants, knowing that is extremely inspirational. Not only does it provide them with 'positive role-models' but it also shows participants that the techniques they are learning can work. For example, on completion of the PSMP many participants say they leave with 'a real belief that there is life beyond HIV' (Jones 2009). Life beyond a compromised immune system.

Conclusion

HIV infection is present in all countries and the long-term consequences of this pandemic will over time impact, one way or another, on every country. This is an evolving pandemic, likely to be with us for generations to come, threatening global public health and healthcare provision, and political and economic stability. Although maturing and stabilising in the UK and in other countries in the Western world, it continues to expand in other regions, notably Asia, Africa and Eastern Europe. The impact of this expansion on individuals, communities, health services and nations will be severe and is yet to be fully realised.

The increasing numbers of HIV-infected persons becoming progressively immunosuppressed will require more than just nursing and medical support. Community-based programmes led by 'experts' who are themselves living with this condition can provide invaluable practical support to enable affected persons to develop skills, knowledge and effective 'self-management' strategies to maximise their health and quality of life.

For further information on:

The immune system
National Institutes of Health – National Institute of Allergy and Infectious Diseases. *Understanding the Immune System*: http://www3.niaid.nih.gov/topics/immuneSystem/default.htm.

Information on HIV infection and AIDS
The National AIDS Manual (NAM): www.aidsmap.com.
i-Base HIV Treatment Information: www.i-Base.info.

The Positive Self-management Program (PSMP)
Stanford University: http://patienteducation.stanford.edu/programs/cdsmp.html.

The Expert Patients Programme (EPP)

Expert Patients Programme Community Interest Company: www.expertpatients.co.uk/public/default.aspx.

The Positive Self-management Programme (PSMP) in the UK

Living Well: www.livingwelluk.com.

References

Adams, K.G., Greiner, A.C. and Corrigan, J.M. (eds) (2004) Report of a Summit. The 1st Annual Crossing the Quality Chasm Summit: A Focus on Communities. 6–7 January. Washington, DC: National Academies Press.

Agency for Healthcare Research and Quality (AHRQ) (2007) *Patient Self-management Support Programs: An Evaluation.* Final Contract Report. AHRQ Publication No. 08–0011, November. Online. Available at: www.ahrq.gov/qual/ptmgmt/ptmgmt.pdf (accessed 27 November 2008).

Allgeier, R. (2006) *A Report on the Effectiveness of Needle and Syringe Exchange.* Cardiff: National Public Health Service for Wales. Online. Available at: www2.nphs.wales.nhs.uk:8080/VulnerableAdultsDocs.nsf/Public/16B044272B5B529F8025718E005704BE/$File/NXConwy-2005Final(3).doc (accessed 13 June 2008).

Barreto, J., Caballero, C. and Cubilla, A. (1997) Penis. In: Sternberg, S.S. (ed.) *Histology for Pathologists* (2nd edn). Philadelphia, PA: Lippincott-Raven.

British HIV Association (2008) British HIV Association Guidelines for the Treatment of HIV-1 Infected Adults with Antiretroviral Therapy (draft for consultation). Online. Available at: www.bhiva.org/files/file1030835.pdf (accessed 13 June 2008).

Department of Health (DoH) (2001) *The Expert Patient: A New Approach to Chronic Disease Management for the 21st Century.* Nottingham: HMSO Crown Copyright.

Department of Health (DoH) (2009a) Expert Patients' and Self-management – What is Self-management? Online. Available at: www.dh.gov.uk/en/Aboutus/MinistersandDepartmentLeaders/ChiefMedicalOfficer/ProgressOnPolicy/ProgressBrowsableDocument/DH_5380856 (accessed 3 April 2009).

Department of Health (DoH) (2009b) What is the Expert Patients Programme? Online. Available at: www.dh.gov.uk/en/Aboutus/MinistersandDepartmentLeaders/ChiefMedicalOfficer/ProgressOnPolicy/ProgressBrowsableDocument/DH_5380860 (accessed 3 April 2009).

Epstein, H. (2007) *The Invisible Cure: Africa, the West and the Fight against AIDS.* New York: Farrar, Strauss & Giroux.

EuroHIV (2007) *HIV/AIDS Surveillance in Europe: End-year Report 2006 No. 76.* Saint-Maurice : Institut de Veille Sanitaire. Online. Available at: www.eurohiv.org (accessed 13 June 2008).

Expert Patients Programme (EPP) (2008) About Expert Patients – What is EPP. Online. Available at: www.expertpatients.co.uk/public/default.aspx?load=ArticleViewer&ArticleId=500 (accessed 27 November 2008).

Health Protection Agency (UK Collaborative Group for HIV and STI Surveillance) (2007) *Testing Times. HIV and Other Sexually Transmitted Infections in the United Kingdom.* London: Health Protection Agency, Centre for Infections. Online. Available at: www.hpa.org.uk/web/HPAweb&HPAwebStandard/HPAweb_C/1203084355941 (accessed 13 June 2008).

Heimer, R. (1998) Syringe Exchange Programs: Lowering the Transmission of Syringe-borne Diseases and Beyond. *Public Health Reports,* 113 (suppl. 1), 67–74. Online. Available at: www.pubmedcentral.nih.gov/picrender.fcgi?artid=1307728&blobtype=pdf (accessed 13 June 2008).

Hussain, L.A. and Lehner, T. (1995) Comparative Investigation of Langerhans Cells and Potential Receptors for HIV in Oral, Genitourinary and Rectal Epithelia. *Immunology,* 85, 475–483. Online. Available at: www.pubmedcentral.nih.gov/picrender.fcgi?artid=1383923&blobtype=pdf (accessed 13 June 2008).

Jones, S. (2009) Living Well's Positive Self-management Programme for People Living with HIV. *AIDS & Hepatitis Digest*, 130 (March), 1–5.

NHS Expert Patients Programme (NHS EPP) (2002) *Self-management of Long-term Health Conditions: A Handbook for People with Chronic Disease*. Boulder, CO: Bull Publishing.

Pratt, R.J. (2003) *HIV & AIDS: A Foundation for Nursing and Healthcare Practice* (5th edn). London: Arnold – Hodder Headline Group.

Pratt, R.J. and Pellowe, C.M. (2006) Preventing Perinatal and Infant HIV Infection. *Infant*, 2(3), 58–61. Online. Available at: www.richardwellsresearch.com/richardwells/pdfs%20and%20 documents/Infant%20-%20Preventing%20Perinatal%20Infection%20April%202006.pdf.

Pratt, R.J., Pellowe, C.M., Wilson, J.A. *et al.* (2007) epic2: National Evidence-Based Guidelines for Preventing Healthcare-associated Infections in NHS Hospitals in England. *Journal of Hospital Infection*, 65S, S1–S64. Online. Available at: www.richardwellsresearch.com/richardwells/ pdfs%20and%20documents/epic2-final%20glines.pdf.

Public Health Agency of Canada (2004) Oral Sex and the Risk of HIV Transmission; *HIV/AIDS Epi Update*, May. Online. Available at: www.phac-aspc.gc.ca/publicat/epiu-aepi/epi_update_ may_04/13_e.html (accessed 13 June 2008).

Sevick, M.A., Trauth, J.M., Ling, B.S. *et al.* (2007) Patients with Complex Chronic Diseases: Perspectives on Supporting Self-Management. *Journal of General International Medicine*, 22 (suppl. 3), 438–444.

Stanford University (2008) Chronic Disease Self-Management Program. Online. Available at: http://patienteducation.stanford.edu/programs/cdsmp.html (accessed 27 November 2008).

Szabo, R. and Short, R.V. (2000) How Does Male Circumcision Protect Against HIV Infection? *British Medical Journal*, 320, 1592–1594. Online. Available at: http://bmj.bmjjournals.com/cgi/ content/full/320/7249/1592?ck=nck (accessed 13 June 2008).

UNAIDS (2007) *AIDS Epidemic Update*. UNAIDS/07/27E/J1322E. Geneva: Joint United Nationals Programme on HIV/AIDS (UNAIDS) and World Health Organisation (WHO). Online. Available at: www.unaids.org/en/KnowledgeCentre/HIVData/EpiUpdate/EpiUp- dArchive/2007/default.asp (accessed 13 June 2008).

UNAIDS (2008) *AIDS Epidemic Update – Regional Summary: North America, Western and Central Europe*. UNAIDS/08/14E/J1532E. Geneva: Joint United Nationals Programme on HIV/AIDS (UNAIDS) and World Health Organisation (WHO). Online. Available at: www.unaids.org/ en/KnowledgeCentre/HIVData/EpiUpdate/EpiUpdArchive/2007/default.asp (accessed 13 June 2008).

WHO (2007) New Data on Male Circumcision and HIV Prevention: Policy and Programme Implications. WHO/UNAIDS Technical Consultation. Online. Available at: http://data. unaids.org/pub/Report/2007/mc_recommendations_en.pdf (accessed 13 June 2008).

22 End-of-life issues

Deebs Canning

Introduction

Over the past four decades, since the establishment of the 'Modern Hospice Movement', palliative care in the United Kingdom has become recognised as a medical speciality with an ever-growing body of knowledge and expertise. Further, government policy and practice frameworks have been developed, particularly over the past decade which has seen the mainstreaming of palliative care expertise into general healthcare (Clark *et al.* 1997; Robbins 1997).

This chapter will discuss palliative care, which seeks to ease the suffering of people whose illness cannot be cured, and its current relationship with long-term conditions and the challenge of illness trajectories in long-term conditions, including the incidence of suicide in this population. Strategies for success will be outlined touching on collaborative partnerships and capacity building through workforce development across the specialities. Such strategies can work to minimise fragmentation of care and facilitate collaboration between healthcare professionals in all settings to best meet the multidimensional needs of individuals and carers.

Definitions

Palliative care is defined by the World Health Organisation (WHO) as

> an approach that improves the quality of life of patients and their families facing the problem associated with life-threatening illness, through the prevention and relief of suffering by means of early identification and impeccable assessment and treatment of pain and other problems, physical, psychosocial and spiritual.
>
> (World Health Organisation 2002, 84)

While some have argued that this early definition is more 'cancer focused', key principles and core values outlined have been used to underpin other descriptions found in the literature and have been adapted by related professional bodies. For the purposes of this chapter the terms 'palliative care' and 'end-of-life care' will be used interchangeably.

What do patients say they want with regard to their end-of-life care?

Any discussion regarding the appropriate end-of-life care for those living with a long-term condition requires some consideration of what they themselves need and desire from service providers. Palliative care and hospices have been seen by some as synonymous with 'a good death'. While there is a considerable amount of discourse regarding 'a good death' and what that might be, there are only a small number of studies that have specifically asked individuals for their own views on this important, albeit sensitive topic, with the majority of those involved being diagnosed with cancer. This is ultimately a very subjective perspective and a 'template' criterion may work against ensuring that patient-centred care is delivered by all healthcare workers (Canning *et al.* 2005). Further, it has been argued that the needs of those with co-morbidity where there is mental illness have had even less of a voice with regard to their wishes regarding end-of-life care (National Council for Hospice and Specialist Palliative Care Services (NCHSPCS) 2000; France 2007).

The issue of individual control over changing circumstances is significant and the role of care providers in enabling and supporting individual autonomy while recognising and responding to both impeding and facilitating circumstances is crucial (Proot *et al.* 2004). This works to develop a therapeutic and trusting relationship between practitioner and patient, which has been identified as fundamental to ensure the facilitation of a mutual autonomy (Mok and Chiu 2004; Canning *et al.* 2005). Palliative care patients have individual needs regarding their end-of-life care which may be summarised as:

- information-sharing (sensitive and timely);
- empowerment;
- advocacy;
- choice;
- continuity of care;
- physical, psychological, social, economic and spiritual needs met.

Such needs are brought about not solely by the disease process and its physical impact but also by the existential reality of the individual's anticipated death and their reactions to such an event. These reactions are typically diverse and multidimensional, requiring sensitive and timely responses from knowledgeable and skilled healthcare workers (Canning *et al.* 2005) in all care settings.

In terms of preferred place of death, the majority of people diagnosed with a long-term condition do not wish to die in hospital, but rather in their own home or a hospice. However, the NHS and social care support services available are often lacking so that many patients die in hospital 'when there is no clinical reason for them to be there' (National Audit Office 2008, 7).

Cultural competence is also a significant responsibility of healthcare professionals involved in end-of-life care, where a comprehensive understanding of the diverse cultural nuances of communication, family dynamics, decision-making and spiritual issues is essential in caring for each individual with a long-term condition. Ethnically sensitive care needs to recognise both the patient's and carer's individual worldview along with their location in the context of the wider community (NCHSPCS 2001; NCPC 2006a).

In recent years, however, it has been identified that while comprehensive hospice and palliative care services and expertise are available for those diagnosed with cancer, a growing number of individuals with life-limiting illnesses other than cancer and their carers, struggle not only to access these services but to receive optimal care from primary providers (National Audit Office 2005; Fitzsimons *et al.* 2007; DoH 2008).

Policy frameworks and end-of-life care

A number of initiatives have recently been introduced to help address these inequities regarding patients with long-term conditions. In 2007, the House of Lords passed the Palliative Care Bill introduced by Baroness Finlay, a well-known practising palliative care medical consultant, to help address this hiatus of progress through strategic responsibility. Specifically the Bill was designed to make it a statutory obligation for local commissioners and service providers to 'develop and report against an annual strategy to improve palliative care provision in their area' (NCPC 2007, 16).

The National Service Frameworks (NSFs) for coronary heart disease, renal services, long-term conditions, mental health, diabetes and older persons, explored in other chapters of this final section, acknowledge the importance of palliative care provision to individuals with cancer and other conditions. These NSFs all contain specific standards on end-of-life care and, while this is to be applauded, gaps remain where specific groups are not addressed.

In 2004 the National Institute for Health and Clinical Excellence (NICE) released the long-awaited palliative and supportive care guidelines. These complimented previously released NICE guidelines focusing on haematological cancers (NICE 2003). While they are only specific to adults with cancer (NICE 2004) they do outline separate standards on 'general palliative care' (a palliative approach) and 'specialist palliative care'. These guidelines have been used to form the framework for other palliative care guidelines for long-term diseases other than cancer such as heart failure.

End-of-life care frameworks and tools

One of the arguments regarding the introduction of palliative care services and the commencement of a palliative care approach, particularly for those individuals with non-malignant illness, relates to the difficulty in predicting when individuals are approaching the end of life. For example, the reality of 'sudden death' for some, particularly those with heart failure, makes this a more complex issue, especially when trying to honour the wishes of the patient in terms of their end-of-life care. Various prototypal death trajectories have been put forward for chronic progressive illnesses other than cancer (Lynn *et al.* 1997; Glare and Christakis 2005; Murray *et al.* 2005).

More recent government initiatives such as the *NHS End of Life programme* (DoH 2006) have been introduced with increased allocated funding, in an attempt to extend the boundaries of palliative care access to all patients regardless of diagnosis, and to enable them to live and die in the place of their choice as outlined in the NSFs. Specifically the three key end-of-life care (EoLC) tools, endorsed by the previously mentioned NICE cancer guidelines, have been rolled out across the country.

They include the Gold Standards Framework (GSF) and the Liverpool Care Pathway and Preferred Priorities of Care, the latter a form of Advance Care Planning and closely linked to the Mental Capacity Act (2005) enacted in 2007.

Gold Standards Framework (GSF)

GSF is a framework of multiple tools, tasks and resources which may be adapted within general practices and community nursing teams to improve end-of-life care for those with any end-stage illness. It promotes seven key tasks enabling those approaching the end of life to be identified, their care needs assessed, and a plan of care with all relevant agencies put in place. GSF focuses on optimising continuity of care, teamwork, advanced planning (including out of hours), symptom control and patient, carer and staff support. Although developed for use in primary care it is also being used in care homes and for all disease groups.

The GSF outlines helpful prognostic indicators which, when combined with clinical experience and open communication with patients and the multidisciplinary team, aims to guide clinicians in identifying those individuals whose prognosis is poor and who would benefit from palliative care services.

Liverpool Care Pathway (LCP)

The Liverpool Care Pathway for the Dying provides an evidence-based framework for the delivery of appropriate care for dying patients and their relatives. It affirms the vision of transferring the model of excellence for the care of the dying from hospices into other healthcare settings, such as acute hospitals, the community and care homes, and empowering generic healthcare workers to deliver optimal care to dying patients wherever they may be practising.

Advance Care Planning (ACP)

ACP is a process involving discussion between an individual with a long-term condition and their care providers irrespective of discipline. If the patient wishes, their family and friends may be included. With the individual's agreement, this discussion is documented, regularly reviewed and communicated to key persons involved in their care. An ACP might include the individual's concerns, understanding of their illness and prognosis, and preferences for types of care or treatment that may be beneficial in the future. Collaborative national guidelines on ACP have recently been released involving the Royal College of Physicians, the National Council for Palliative Care, the Alzheimer's Society and the Royal College of Nursing (Royal College of Physicians 2009).

Preferred Priorities of Care (PPC)

PPC is an example of ACP and is a patient-held document designed to facilitate patient choice in relation to end-of-life issues, by providing the opportunity to discuss difficult issues that may not otherwise be addressed to the detriment of patient care.

Initiating difficult discussions regarding end-of-life care

Continuity of care is one of the key strands of the EoLC strategy which is underpinned by effective communication, not only between the patient, carer and the healthcare professionals, but between different levels of care (primary and secondary), and between the various services which may all be involved. While the EoLC tools already discussed are helpful, especially for generalists, they require effective communication between the patient, carer and clinician. Individuals with advanced disease who verbalise feelings of hopelessness are often greatly reassured by health professionals who are prepared to discuss with them what they might expect or want in the future and how their symptoms might be relieved and other needs met. This ensures that the clinician can ascertain the patient's own views and wishes regarding their ongoing care and the illness experience which is central to the preferred priorities of care and the principles of palliative care.

Unfortunately, many healthcare professionals avoid such conversations. For example, despite more than one-third of patients with heart failure dying within 12 months of diagnosis (Aldred *et al.* 2005), discussions regarding prognosis and options for supportive care are not always forthcoming, with some having to work out for themselves that they are dying (McCarthy *et al.* 1997). Professional development in this area is therefore crucial for all healthcare professionals if skills and confidence in this area are to be improved.

Patients with severe mental illness have also been found to be very concerned about end-of-life issues, wanting to be involved in discussions regarding future treatment options (Foti *et al.* 2005). However, presumptions of both incompetence and emotional instability are common, fuelled by long-standing stigmatisation and discrimination, and treatment decisions may take place with other members of their family, health advocates, or not at all (Foti *et al.* 2005). As many individuals with serious mental illness die at a younger age than the general population, it has been suggested that discussions regarding advanced care planning should be introduced earlier in their illness, along with clear documentation of preferences in all appropriate records across all sectors of care. This ensures that individual wishes can be made known even when people may no longer be able to communicate these themselves.

Not all individuals may wish to discuss their preferences when first broached, but initiating what is clearly a sensitive and difficult discussion will help to build a trusting and open relationship. It may be that when raised again at a later time, the patient will be 'ready' to explore possible options.

Mental health issues in end of life

It is estimated that between 10 and 20 per cent of palliative care patients will develop some type of psychiatric disorder requiring skilled assessment and management (e.g. depression, anxiety, delirium) (Lloyd-Williams 2006). In terms of end-of-life care, mental health problems can be addressed from two perspectives – those individuals diagnosed with a pre-existing mental health issue (e.g. bipolar disorder, schizophrenia), among the most disadvantaged and unrepresented group in society (Davie 2006; France 2007) and those who may develop mental illness as a consequence of their long-term or life-threatening illness (e.g. advanced cancer, dementia, degenerative neurological disease).

Given the higher risk of those with pre-existing mental health problems developing long-term conditions such as cardiovascular, respiratory and liver disease, and higher rates of mortality and morbidity (Dembling *et al.* 1999; Casey 2005; McCasland 2007), it would be reasonable to expect that a greater number of this population might benefit from palliative care services. Problems may be further exacerbated by social exclusion including homelessness, and long-term use of neuroleptic medication as well as non-compliance (Phair 2007). Despite these difficulties, this population has been found to experience problems in accessing palliative care services. This can often be made worse by negative public attitudes to mental illness and subsequent stigma contributing to delays in appropriate referral and treatment.

Recent literature reviews looking into the palliative care needs of individuals with a pre-existing mental illness have found that although there is ample evidence regarding the relationship between mental health issues and poor physical health, there is a dearth of empirical literature examining the challenges of managing those with co-morbidity, specifically their palliative care needs or guidelines for healthcare professionals (France 2007).

Addressing mental health issues in palliative care

A need for improved psychological assessment and intervention within palliative care services has been highlighted in recent years (Hackett and Gaitan 2007). The NICE guidelines (2004) outline specifically that healthcare professionals should provide regular and systematic psychological assessments to this group and continually monitor their mental health. However, concerns have been raised regarding what is the most appropriate assessment tool to identify such mental health issues in this population. Also needing to be considered is whether the clinical staff working in palliative care have the ability to assess mental health issues appropriately (Hackett and Gaitan 2007).

Several 'assessment blockers' have been identified which can be barriers to healthcare professionals providing optimal support and appropriate treatment to patients with long-term conditions and mental health issues (Hackett and Gaitan 2007, 277):

- Difficulties around differentiation between adaptive and non-adaptive coping.
- Difficulties around the differentiation between physical and psychological symptoms.
- Fear of mental health issues.
- A lack of knowledge about how to communicate with people who have mental health issues.

Problems have been identified in the ability of both mental health and palliative care professionals to work effectively together often due to having differing goals of care for the patient (McCormack and Sharp 2006). Furthermore, healthcare professionals practising in settings other than mental health, may also find the management of this group far more challenging, especially if there is violent or aggressive behaviour as this can impact negatively on the professional's ability to form a 'therapeutic relationship' (McCormack and Sharp 2006). Collaboration with mental health specialists in areas such as assertiveness training and dealing with psychiatric emergencies can increase confidence and reduce anxiety, empowering healthcare professionals to deliver more effective care (McCasland 2007).

Cutcliffe *et al.* (2001a, 2001b) suggest that both palliative care and mental health nurses share common values and practice principles, including patient-centred approaches and advanced assessment skills. Where there are differences, for example, in counselling approaches and knowledge of physical and technical skills, then greater professional collaboration has the potential to contribute to meeting individual need more effectively with greater satisfaction for all parties. Recognising the overlap in roles between that of palliative care nurse and mental health nurse and working towards greater collaboration can avoid the polarisation which often occurs in practice when attempting to address physical and mental healthcare needs. This can be enhanced by establishing mental health specialist links to palliative care teams as well as by joint professional learning (McCormack and Sharp 2006), and these developments have included cardiac, neurology and corrective specialist services.

Long-term conditions: specific issues for specific populations

Many complex issues will often need to be addressed in individuals with long-term conditions and difficulties may intensify when the trajectory is punctuated by crisis, instability and downward deterioration. Carers will need to assist with the reality of deteriorating health status, decreased independence, social isolation, limited resources, poor access to community services, feelings of being a burden to loved ones, acceptance and depression, as well as concerns about the future (Fitzsimons *et al.* 2007).

Heart failure

Cardiac failure accounts for approximately 60,000 deaths in the UK annually (Paes 2004) and studies show that symptom severity along with psychological problems are comparable to patients with cancer and sometimes greater (Anderson *et al.* 2001; Gibbs *et al.* 2002). Even so, the NSF for coronary heart disease (CHD) identified that few patients with heart disease were generally seen by palliative care services.

Those with heart failure are much more likely to die in hospital than are patients with cancer and this is often due to difficulties in estimating prognosis or reluctance on the part of the health professional to discuss possibilities with patients (Johnson 2006). They are also more likely to receive invasive interventions in the last three days of life such as cardiopulmonary resuscitation, tube feeding and ventilation (Lynn *et al.* 1997) which may result in further distress for patients and family members.

Prevalence of anxiety and depression in people with a wide range of different medical conditions has been found to be greater than the general population with major depression in patients with heart failure estimated to be 36.5 per cent and with minor depression 25.5 per cent (Koenig 1998). Appropriate support including information is crucial for optimal end-of-life care in helping those with heart failure to cope with distressing emotions and resulting powerlessness (Murray *et al.* 2002). This is in keeping with the observations of John Hinton in the early 1960s who described the physical and mental distress of those dying with heart and renal failure as often being more explicit than of those dying with cancer (Gibbs *et al.* 2002; Johnson 2006).

Depression has been observed to increase readmission rates to hospital in those with heart failure as well as an increase in mortality at key points along the trajectory. Emotional distress experienced by depressed individuals with heart failure can activate neurohormonal pathways which can further compromise cardiopulmonary status, resulting in worsening symptoms where heart failure exists. Indeed, as we saw in Chapter 17 where depression and heart disease coexist, the risk for complications and death is increased.

Informal carers of those with heart failure are prone to social isolation and also need significant support from healthcare professionals (Aldred *et al.* 2005), particularly from primary care. These carers tend to be women over 60 years of age, who may themselves have two or more health conditions, the most common being arthritis (Barnes *et al.* 2006). If needs of both patient and carer are to be met effectively, multidisciplinary support in the community for those with established heart failure is important and should include home-based interventions with access to social care and the local palliative care team for ongoing support and palliative care advice as needed (NSF CHD).

Chronic obstructive pulmonary disease (COPD)

Despite being the fifth most common cause of death in England and Wales, patients diagnosed with COPD are not often referred to specialist palliative care services and also tend to die in hospital in the end stages. People living with COPD experience a continuous state of poor health with intermittent exacerbations which tend to lead to hospital admissions and a further decline in their function. There can be a higher symptom burden including breathlessness, fatigue and decreased mobility with poorer quality of life and there are often unmet psychological and social needs (Elkington *et al.* 2005; Goodridge 2006).

Ongoing stress experienced by informal carers in supporting loved ones with COPD can cause significant mental health issues due to the strain of taking on multiple roles over a prolonged period of time (Seamark *et al.* 2004). In particular, wives report a lack of support from healthcare providers and a desire for more support and information about their husbands' disease. Many experience unremitting fear about their partner's sudden death and can result in constant vigilance (Bergs 2002), contributing to their fatigue and exhaustion.

Loved ones can feel isolated and helpless where end-stage symptoms seem to become increasingly challenging to relieve. Breathlessness can be a distressing and profoundly disabling symptom requiring skilled use of oxygen, bronchodilators and, where appropriate, opiates such as morphine. Where symptom relief is maximised in the late stages, relatives still often require ongoing reassurance that the apparent breathing difficulties witnessed are not necessarily causing the distress often imagined. Symptoms are experienced on a number of levels and this is where enhanced collaboration between specialist physiotherapists, respiratory and specialist palliative care health professionals across primary and secondary settings is vital if needs are to be met effectively. This will help facilitate a timely, patient-centred approach to advance care planning and joint working between services has the potential to improve care, decision-making and quality of life (Goodridge 2006).

Renal failure

The NSF for renal conditions has outlined that greater support is required for those with end stage renal disease with regard to appropriate and effective palliative care. The journey from diagnosis to end-stage disease may take many years, with the latter a particularly difficult time when patients are faced with the difficult decision of discontinuing active treatment such as dialysis (Noble and Kelly 2006).

Despite modern improvements in dialysis the grind of ongoing treatment may be difficult, especially where there is co-morbidity contributing to symptom experience and disability, and patients may be too ill and infirm to contemplate when this is offered as part of ongoing care (Kurella *et al.* 2005; Nobel *et al.* 2007). In addition, while dialysis is able to keep the patient alive, the underlying chronic disease continues to progress and ultimately this can have a significantly negative impact on quality of life.

Therefore it is imperative, in keeping with the aims and objectives of the EoLC Strategy, that patients with end-stage renal failure (ESRF) and carers are empowered to make informed choices about preferred priorities of care, including treatments to be continued and how and where dying should take place, and this needs to be supported by holistic assessment which recognises the multidimensional experience of advanced illness (McKeown *et al.* 2008). Possibilities exist here for specialist palliative care clinicians to work alongside renal specialists to meet the needs of the patients and to capacity-build both specialist and generalist healthcare professionals involved across the various sectors.

Withdrawal of life-saving treatment interventions does not mean that holistic care is discontinued; on the contrary it is imperative that the team outline explicitly to patient and family how the physical, emotional, spiritual and social dimensions of care will continue to be addressed. Palliative care is not synonymous with abandoning care nor the withdrawal of holistic care, and not every patient wishes to cease their dialysis. Even so, a patient who decides not to continue with treatment may present significant and complex issues where ethics and psychiatry shadow each other closely (Nobel *et al.* 2007). For example, is a patient's decision to withdraw from dialysis the same as suicide? Most would agree that this is not the case but individuals need support from appropriate professionals so that any decision is carefully thought through and based on all available information. No one has the monopoly on ethical decision-making and patients, carers and professionals must all act within the law.

Degenerative neurological conditions

Conditions discussed in this section do not include all the various types of rapidly progressing and advanced long-term neurological problems, but end-of-life principles can be applied across this diverse range of disorders. As in previous groups care needs must include sensitive information-giving, advanced care planning and holistic support. Unfortunately there are documented instances where these needs are not always identified and addressed, including some patients with multiple sclerosis and Parkinson's disease. Work has recently been undertaken by the National Council of Palliative Care to identify the needs of these groups more specifically while mapping current service provision and highlighting best practice (NCPC 2007).

Professionals working in neurology, rehabilitation and palliative care need to work closely with primary care staff and care providers, including non-NHS care staff (social care, domiciliary and home care staff) combining expertise to support people in the advanced stages of long-term neurological conditions. Specialist palliative care teams working alongside specialist neurology and neuro-rehabilitation teams (for example, in joint clinics) promote more consistent shared practice.

Dementia

The nature and characteristics of older people and their palliative care needs has led to a call for a greater focus on this group, who tend to be the most vulnerable and in need of advocacy. Palliative care needs may arise from a variety of specific clinical illnesses, a combination of these, or generally the cumulative effect of the ageing process together with other social and emotional issues (NCPC 2005).

At any one time in the UK, 700,000 individuals are affected by dementia (NCPC 2008) with 200,000 new cases diagnosed each year. The number of individuals expected to be diagnosed with dementia by 2010 will be 870,000 and by 2050 over 1.8 million (DoH 2009). Specific differences regarding the planning of care for this group are that individuals diagnosed with dementia may also have multiple chronic medical problems and tend to be older than those who are dying from cancer.

The average time from diagnosis to death for those patients with Alzheimer's or vascular dementia is 3.3 years (Amella 2003). Most individuals with end-stage dementia live and are cared for in nursing homes or dementia-specific units. Even so, professionals practising in a variety of specialties and settings who may be involved in any stage of their journey need to be equipped to collaborate and deliver appropriate palliative care using an appropriate model of care and skills. The use of a palliative approach by all healthcare professionals should be a central focus of care delivery in care home facilities (Hockley and Clark 2002). Once again, partnerships with palliative care specialist services can ensure that appropriate workforce capacity-building is achieved and is endorsed in the recently released *National Dementia Strategy* (DoH 2009).

Stroke

The long-term prognosis of individuals following a stroke is relatively poor, although research shows that early diagnosis and treatment with clot-busting drugs where appropriate can improve survival significantly and reduce disability. Currently there is a national campaign promoting early recognition of stroke in the UK population. However, approximately 20 per cent of patients die within one month of the onset of the disease with a further 10 per cent within a year (Rogers 2003). Studies have shown that approximately 8 per cent of hospital inpatients have palliative care needs arising from their cerebrovascular disease (Rogers 2003), although there is again some reluctance on the health professional's part to initiate palliative care rather than rehabilitation due to uncertainty about prognosis. The Department of Health National Stroke Strategy released in 2007 highlights key actions designed to ensure that this population has optimal palliative care, including appropriate health and social care services and a smooth interface across healthcare settings. The use of the end-of-life tools discussed earlier is also endorsed (DoH 2007).

Advanced cancer

There are varying rates of mental health conditions affecting those with cancer, particularly at the advanced stage of their disease (Brown *et al.* 2000). This also depends upon the staging and severity of the cancer itself, along with the screening process. Organic disorders, for example, rate highly at 85 per cent in terminally ill patients (Durkin *et al.* 2003). Identification of mental health problems in cancer patients, however, has been fraught with difficulties and such problems are often misdiagnosed (Bryan and Scott 2008), or assumptions are made by healthcare professionals that individuals are simply 'sad', an expected emotion when facing one's mortality and the many losses involved. This is also made more complex due to various cultural notions of death and dying and the impact on individuals. Patients with advanced cancer may also experience a variety of physical symptoms and behaviours common to those with anxiety and depression (RCP 2007).

One study undertaken in a palliative care unit found that a majority of inpatients had a co-morbid mental illness, although it was not made clear if these pre-existed the primary illness resulting in palliative care. Even so, only a minority of these patients had received any treatment for their mental illness prior to admission (Durkin *et al.* 2003).

Patients with advanced cancer generally have a more predictable trajectory compared to other non-malignant long-term conditions. Even so, it is important for primary and secondary care healthcare professionals to be diligent in their assessment and planning in close collaboration with all other service providers in attempts to meet the needs of patients and their carers. This ensures that any predictable problems are anticipated and risk managed to avoid any undue stress or unwanted admission to hospital should the patient be at home. The use of the GSF is a valuable tool for general practitioners and district nurses, who may or may not be supported by a team of palliative care specialists. This is also the case for care homes, where residents may no longer be under the care of oncology specialists.

The primary care team has a number of key specialist services available to support when caring for patients with cancer at home, such as the Macmillan Cancer Relief and other specialist palliative care community teams operating from local hospices. GP facilitator posts have also been funded by Macmillan to help build the capacity of other primary care providers and to forge stronger links between primary and secondary care (Barnett 2002). Marie Curie Cancer Care (MCCC) is another cancer charity providing both daytime and out-of-hours care for patients in their own homes, and works in collaboration with other members of the community team. The *Delivering Choice Project* is a project recently developed by MCCC (2009) which is currently being piloted in various locations across the country. The aim is to provide timely and comprehensive home services to patients with advanced disease who wish to die at home.

Suicide

Suicide remains a significant cause of death and not surprisingly is closely associated with those living with life-limiting diseases. These include conditions such as cancer (Rodin *et al.* 2007), AIDS (Starace and Sherr 1998), ESRF (Kurella *et al.* 2005) and pulmonary disease (Goodwin *et al.* 2003). Stroke (Kishi *et al.* 2001) and degenerative neurological disorders such as Huntington's disease and multiple sclerosis (Cina *et al.* 1996) may also result in mental and cognitive disorders which are associated with an increased risk of suicidal behaviour (Stenager *et al.* 1998), although empirical evidence is limited. Death pacts between patient and carer are well documented (Brown *et al.* 1995) with 'physician-assisted suicide' and euthanasia continuing to be emotive and controversial issues within the community and among healthcare professionals. The impact of suicide upon carers and healthcare professionals involved is significant and therefore strategies are required to assist all those involved to appropriately risk-manage and recognise early signs so as to avoid such distressing outcomes.

Suicide is associated with those who suffer depression in later life. Although it is suggested that there is greater risk among patients with physical illness than the general population (Kishi *et al.* 2001), the role of somatic illness is less clear than that of mental health disorders (Waern *et al.* 2002). In primary care, patients with functional impairment, psychiatric co-morbidities, increased health service use and subjective distress have also been identified as high risk (Goodwin *et al.* 2003).

The risk of suicide increases with age and the added stress of coping with chronic life-limiting diseases. One recent study found that impaired vision, neurological disorder, stroke and malignant disease were risk factors for suicide, as was serious physical illness or disability in any organ category, especially for men (Waern *et al.* 2002). In relation to suicide pacts it has been found that when there is a history of past or present mental illness in both partners, entwined with a serious medical condition and significant social isolation, there is a need for a joint suicide risk assessment (Brown *et al.* 1995).

The vast majority of terminally ill patients with suicidal thoughts or who had attempted suicide were found to have had depressive disorders, highlighting the importance of a thorough assessment and identification of suicide risk in all settings, particularly in primary care (Goodwin *et al.* 2003). While it is known that elderly patients consult their doctor shortly before their suicide, they do not share with them their true distress. Furthermore, doctors have been found to be less likely to discuss the possibility of suicidal feelings with patients with chronic illness (Waern *et al.* 2002).

This is once again significant with regard to the assessment of all patients with long-term conditions and also those with a history of mental illness. Many of these individuals will not be cared for in specialist settings, and are therefore at risk of falling through the net. Whether in outpatient, primary or secondary care, there needs to be a greater focus on assessing this high-risk group in terms of their spiritual, psychological, social and mental health as a result of their physical impairment, and a link with specialists who can help generalist clinicians to best plan and deliver care.

The experience of 'suffering' which transcends physical pain alone for those individuals with chronic and terminal illness is overwhelming (Cassell 2003). This has led to many requests from members of the community with life-limiting disease such as motor neurone disease and multiple sclerosis to seek physician-assisted suicide, due to their inability to physically carry out the act themselves. Physician-assisted suicide and euthanasia, however, remain illegal under British law. Authors have, however, highlighted that the inspiration of hope is fundamental to effective patient care and is communicated through the therapeutic relationship between healthcare professionals and patients. This relationship can be significant in reducing the risk of suicide due to the positive influence such partnerships can have on the individual's sense of themselves and their future (Hewitt and Edwards 2006).

In May 2006, Lord Joffe's Assisted Dying for the Terminally Ill Bill was defeated in the House of Lords by 148 votes to 100 on its second reading outlining the House's opposition to assisted dying 'as a matter of principle' (NCPC 2006b, 20). Even so, this continues to be an issue that polarises opinion, particularly for healthcare professionals working in palliative care. The tenets of palliative care which include patient-centred choice and decision-making may for some appear insincere if the patient's competent choice is to seek euthanasia.

End-of-life care in the prison system

There is a growing number of older inmates across the globe dying from a number of chronic and life-limiting diseases (e.g. hepatitis, AIDS, tuberculosis) (Weiskopf 2005). Indeed, it has been proposed that in recent years these facilities have become new domains of acute, chronic and end-of-life care with numbers of inmates serving life sentences growing significantly over recent decades (Wood 2007). This does not include those who due to significantly lengthy sentences die within the facility of old age (Fowler-Kerry 2003). It is suggested that this group is often diagnosed with chronic illnesses that are associated with older people in the non-prison population often with co-morbidity (Colleran and O'Siorain 2006). As outlined in the *NSF for Older People*, at any one time the number of individuals in prison over the age of 60 is around 700. Furthermore, more than 1000 of the same age cohort leave prison each year, all having some chronic health condition (DoH 2001). This is made more complex by the high incidence of a diagnosed mental disorder among this population.

There has, however, been a significant change taking place with regard to prison healthcare in the UK including the development of palliative care services. Indeed, the *End of Life Care Strategy* has identified prisons and secure hospitals as key places of care. Outlined are those individuals detained in prisons, or sectioned under the Mental Health Act in secure hospitals who 'should be treated with dignity and respect and given as much choice as is possible about the care they receive as they approach the end of their lives' (DoH 2008, 103).

There is a dearth of literature exploring the experience of palliative care in secure environments, particularly with regard to the role of the nurse or other healthcare workers (Weiskopf 2005; Colleran and O'Siorain 2006). Not unlike other settings, developing sound and appropriate palliative care programmes within forensic facilities comes with its own unique challenges (Weiskopf 2005), with the aims of both services almost diametrically opposed. This poses the question of whether such patients are being offered appropriate and timely access to palliative care specialist services, and how forensic nurses and other health professionals are being supported by trained staff and formalised education and training to meet this very challenging role. Health professionals caring for inmates with long-term conditions need to reconcile with the facility's priorities of security, segregation and punishment while being able to provide individual, respectful and sensitive healthcare (Weiskopf 2005). Knowledge of environmental safety, skills in emergency, medical/surgical and geriatric care, effective communication and team work are vital for there to be optimal management of each inmate (Chow 2002).

Rehabilitation in end-of-life care

This may seem a rather paradoxical title; however, as outlined in the NICE palliative care guidelines, rehabilitation plays a vital and appropriate role in the care of patients with cancer and other advanced disease (NICE 2004). While depending on resources available in specific geographical and clinical areas, there are a number of rehabilitation options that may be accessed by palliative care patients. These include hospice-specific gyms, and rehabilitation outpatient clinics at large acute care facilities working in collaboration with palliative care specialist teams. The role of rehabilitation in end-of-life care obviously has different goals compared to those care units designed to help individuals meet their potential to return to employment and other life activities following significant events such as an accident or acute illness.

Palliative care services

Prior to the 1950s, there was little published research on the experiences of dying patients, and professional bodies such as the National Council of Palliative Care did not exist to profile and advocate for this population (Clark 2007). In the next few decades, however, a number of key studies began to be noted both in the United Kingdom and the United States showing clear evidence of care either being inappropriate and poor or simply being omitted altogether (Clark 2007). The 'modern hospice movement' arose in the 1960s and spread internationally to reclaim what was thought to be a more fitting approach to caring holistically for those individuals and their families struggling with the multidimensional issues of dealing with an incurable illness such as cancer.

In recent years, however, it has been identified that while comprehensive hospice and palliative care services and expertise are available for those diagnosed with cancer, a growing number of individuals with life-limiting illnesses other than cancer, and their carers, struggle to access these services, or to receive optimal care from their primary providers (National Audit Office 2005; Fitzsimons et al. 2007). Such inequities have led to this group being referred to as the 'disadvantaged dying' (Kinghorn and Gamlin 2001). Furthermore, a large majority of those who die annually in England (85 per cent) are 65 years or over and this trend is expected to increase over the next decade (Age Concern 2005). Nearly 50 per cent of this group now die from long-term conditions other than cancer such as heart disease, respiratory disease, strokes and related disorders (National Audit Office 2005), many with multiple co-morbidity. Individuals living with both a severe mental illness and a chronic life-limiting disease have been found to be further disadvantaged. Unlike palliative care, mental healthcare has not for the most part been mainstreamed into the general healthcare system. Appropriate and timely referral to palliative care is poor with care services lacking the quality of coordination often associated with the care of individuals with cancer (France 2007).

Despite the recent mainstreaming and growth of palliative care services in the NHS there are still significant gaps which relate specifically to the holistic end-of-life care for patients with long-term conditions, where evidence shows that palliative care provision in England has continued to be dependent upon diagnosis rather than need (Seymour et al. 2002). This was highlighted in the House of Commons Health Committee's 2004 report on palliative care, which identified inequalities across diagnosis, patient demographics (e.g. age and ethnicity) and geographical location (RCP 2007).

Table 22.1 Useful contacts

Help the Hospices Offers services to support hospice and palliative care professionals. Hospice information service for professionals and the public.	www.helpthehospices.org.uk Help the Hospices Hospice House 34–44 Britannia Street London WC1X 9JG Tel: 020 7520 8200 Email: info@helpthehospices.org.uk
National Council of Palliative Care Umbrella organisation for all those involved in providing, commissioning and using palliative care and hospice services in England, Wales and Northern Ireland	www.ncpc.org.uk The National Council of Palliative Care The Fitzpatrick Building 188–194 York Way London N7 9AS Tel: 020 7697 1520 Email: enquiries@ncpc.org.uk
Liverpool Care Pathway Central Team UK, The Marie Curie Palliative Care Institute, Liverpool Team working on the adaptation of the LCP for heart and renal failure. A four-phase approach is to be used to demonstrate the LCP's transferability to non-cancer cohorts	www.mcpcil.org.uk Marie Curie Palliative Care Institute (MCPCIL) Satellite Unit c/o Directorate of Specialist Palliative Care 1st Floor, Linda McCartney Centre Royal Liverpool University Hospital Prescot Street Liverpool L7 8XP Tel: 151 706 2274 Email: lcp.enquiries@rlbuht.nhs.uk
European Association for Palliative Care Aims to promote palliative care in Europe and to act as a focus for all those who work in or have an interest in the field of palliative care at the scientific, clinical and social levels	www.eapcnet.org European Association for Palliative Care Head Office National Cancer Institute Milano Via Venezian 1 20133 Milano, Italy Tel: +39 02 2390 3390 Email: info@carersUK.org
Sue Ryder Care UK charity providing compassionate care to people living with long-term and end-of-life conditions	www.sueryder.org 114–118 Southampton Row London WC1B 5AA Tel: 0845 050 1953 Email: info@suerydercare.org
Cruse Bereavement Care Promotes the well-being of bereaved people and enables anyone bereaved by death to understand their grief and cope with their loss. Services are free to bereaved people	www.crusebereavementcare.org.uk Central Office: Cruse Bereavement Care PO Box 800 Richmond Surrey TW9 1RG Tel: 020 8939 9530 Email: info@cruse.org.uk Day-by-day helpline: 0844 477 9400

Palliative care is practised in partnership between patient and professional carers, using a team model or an integrated multidisciplinary approach where typical barriers between disciplines are minimised (Clark and Seymour 1999; Faull *et al.* 2005). This enables the shared expertise to optimally address the holistic needs of patient and their carers which includes the physical, emotional, social, spiritual and psychological dimensions of each individual.

In August 2008 the first *End of Life Care Strategy* (DoH 2008) was released as part of Lord Darsi's comprehensive NHS healthcare review which clearly outlines the government's desire to ensure that palliative care is accessible to all, including those individuals diagnosed with long-term conditions, no matter what the setting in which they may be cared for. This includes acute hospitals, the community, hospices, care homes and other less prominent facilities such as prisons. The strategy also acknowledges the importance of all healthcarers working in generalist roles as being just as significant as those in specialist roles and the importance of workforce education to ensuring that this strategy meets the targets laid down.

Conclusion

This is a dynamic time in the development of palliative and end-of-life care and, although there have been enormous improvements across many areas, the evidence is clear that much more needs to be done. This is particularly vital to ensure that all individuals are able to access and experience optimal patient-centred end-of-life care, no matter what their diagnosis, economic or social circumstances. The challenges are not new but there is now a growing number of helpful tools, guidelines and collaborations between various specialist groups across various sectors which will help this to be achieved.

As outlined in the most recent government policy document on end-of-life care,

> How we care for the dying is an indicator of how we care for all sick and vulnerable people. It is a measure of society as a whole and it is a litmus test for health and social care services.
>
> (DoH 2008, 10)

Only time will tell how society has been able to demonstrate the degree of importance that has been afforded to this profoundly important measure of our care.

References

Age Concern (2005) *Dying and Death*. London: Age Concern.

Aldred, H., Gott, M. and Gariballa, S. (2005) Advanced Heart Failure: Impact on Older Patients and Informal Carers. *Journal of Advanced Nursing*, 49(2), 116–124.

Amella, E. (2003) Geriatrics and Palliative Care. Collaboration for Quality of Life Until Death. *Journal of Hospice and Palliative Nursing*, 5(1), 40–48.

Anderson, H., Ward, C., Eardley, A. *et al.* (2001) The Concerns of Patients Under Palliative Care and a Heart Failure Clinic are not Met. *Palliative Medicine*, 15, 279–286.

Barnes, S., Gott, M., Payne, S. *et al.* (2006) Characteristics and Views of Family Carers of Older People with Heart Failure. *International Journal of Palliative Nursing*, 12(8), 380–389.

Barnett, M. (2002) The Development of Palliative Care Within Primary Care. In Charlton, R.

(ed.) *Primary Palliative Care. Dying, Death and Bereavement in the Community.* Oxford: Radcliffe Medical Press.

Bergs, D. (2002) The Hidden Client – Women Caring for Husbands with COPD: Their Experience of Quality of Life. *Journal of Clinical Nursing*, 14, 805–812.

Bolger, M. (2005) Dying in Prison: Providing Palliative Care in Challenging Environments. *International Journal of Palliative Nursing*, 11(12), 619–621.

Brown, M., King, E. and Barraclough, B. (1995) Nine Suicide Pacts: A Clinical Study of a Consecutive Series 1974–93. *British Journal of Psychiatry*, 167(4), 448–451.

Brown, S., Inskip, K. and Barraclough, B. (2000) Causes of the Excess Mortality of Schizophrenia. *British Journal of Psychiatry*, 177, 212–217.

Bryan, L. and Scott, S. (2008) The Assessment of Mental State in Advanced Stage of Disease. *End of Life Care*, 2(1), 15–22.

Canning, D., Rosenberg, J.P. and Yates, P. (2005) *The Development of a Framework of Competency Standards for Specialist Palliative Care Nursing Practice.* Queensland: Queensland Nursing Council.

Casey, D. (2005) Metabolic Issues and Cardiovascular Disease in Patients with Psychiatric Disorders. *American Journal of Medicine Supplement*, 118, 15–22.

Cassell, E.J. (2003) *The Nature of Suffering* (2nd edn). Oxford: Oxford University Press.

Chow, R. (2002) Initiating a Long-term Care Nursing Service for Aging Inmates. *Geriatric Nursing*, 23(1), 24–27.

Cina, S., Smith, M., Collins, K. *et al.* (1996) Dyadic Deaths involving Huntington's Disease: A Case Study Report. *American Journal of Forensic Medicine and Pathology*, 17(1), 49–52.

Clark, D. (2007) From Margins to Centre: A Review of the History of Palliative Care in Cancer. *Lancet Oncology*, 8, 430–438.

Clark, D. and Seymour, J. (1999) *Reflections on Palliative Care. Sociological and Policy Perspectives.* Buckingham: Open University Press.

Clark, D., Hockley, J. and Ahmedzai, S. (eds) (1997) *New Themes in Palliative Care.* Buckingham: Open University Press.

Colleran, M. and O'Siorain, L. (2006) Providing Palliative Care for Prisoners. *European Journal of Palliative Care*, 13(6), 257–260.

Cutcliffe, J.R., Black, C., Hanson, E. *et al.* (2001a) The Commonality and Synchronicity of Mental Health Nurses and Palliative Care Nurses: Closer Than You Think? Part One. *Journal of Psychiatric and Mental Health Nursing*, 8, 53–59.

Cutcliffe, J.R., Black, C., Hanson, E. *et al.* (2001b) The Commonality and Synchronicity of Mental Health Nurses and Palliative Care Nurses: Closer Than You Think? Part Two. *Journal of Psychiatric and Mental Health Nursing*, 8, 61–66.

Davie, E. (2006) A Social Work Perspective on Palliative Care for People with Mental Health Problems. *European Journal of Palliative Care*, 13(1), 26–28.

Dembling, B., Chen, D. and Vachon, L. (1999) Life Expectancy and Causes of Death in a Population Treated for Serious Mental Illness. *Psychiatric Services*, 50(8), 1036–1042.

Department of Health (DoH) (2001) *National Service Framework for Older People.* London: DoH.

Department of Health (DoH) (2006) *NHS End of Life Care Progress Report.* Leicester: DoH.

Department of Health (DoH) (2007) *National Stroke Strategy.* London: DoH.

Department of Health (DoH) (2008) *End of Life Care Strategy: Promoting High Quality Care for all Adults at the End of Life.* London: DoH.

Department of Health (DoH) (2009) *Living Well with Dementia. A National Dementia Strategy.* London: DoH.

Durkin, I., Kearney, M. and O'Siorain, L. (2003) Psychiatric Disorder in a Palliative Unit. *Palliative Medicine*, 17, 21–218.

Elkington, H., White, P., Addington-Hall, J. *et al.* (2005) The Healthcare Needs of Chronic Obstructive Pulmonary Disease Patients in the Last Year of Life. *Palliative Medicine*, 19, 485–491.

Ellison, N. (2008) *Mental Health and Palliative Care Literature Review.* London: Mental Health Foundation.

Faull, C., Carter, Y. and Daniels, L. (eds) (2005) *Handbook of Palliative Care* (2nd edn). Oxford: Blackwell Publishing.

Fitzsimons, D., Mullan, D., Wilson, J.S. *et al.* (2007) The Challenge of Patients' Unmet Palliative Care Needs in the Final Stages of Chronic Illness. *Palliative Medicine,* 21, 313–322.

Foti, M.E., Bartels, S., Van Citters, A. *et al.* (2005) End-of-life Treatment Preferences of Persons with Serious Mental Illness. *Psychiatric Services,* 56(5), 585–591.

Fowler-Kerry, S. (2003) Palliative Care Within Secure Forensic Environments. *Journal of Psychiatric and Mental Health Nursing,* 10, 367–369.

France, K. (2007) *How Can a Community Palliative Care Nurse Meet the Needs of Patients with Mental Illness.* Unpublished dissertation. London: Thames Valley University.

Gibbs, J., McCoy, A., Gibbs, L. *et al.* (2002) Living With and Dying from Heart Failure: The Role of Palliative Care. *Heart,* 88 (suppl. II), 36–69.

Glare, P. and Christakis, N. (2005) Predicting Survival in Patients with Advanced Disease. In Doyle, D., Hanks, G.W., Cherny, N. and Calman, K. (eds) *The Oxford Textbook of Palliative Medicine* (3rd edn). Oxford: Oxford University Press.

Goodridge, D. (2006) People with Chronic Obstructive Pulmonary Disease at the End of Life: A Review of the Literature. *International Journal of Palliative Nursing,* 12(8), 390–396.

Goodwin, R., Kroenke, K., Hoven, C. *et al.* (2003) Major Depression, Physical Illness, and Suicidal Ideation in Primary Care. *Psychosomatic Medicine,* 65, 501–505.

Hackett, A. and Gaitan, A. (2007) A Qualitative Study Assessing Mental Health Issues in Two Hospices in the UK. *International Journal of Palliative Nursing,* 13(6), 273–281.

Hewitt, J.L. and Edwards, S.D. (2006) Moral Perspectives on the Prevention of Suicide in Mental Health Settings. *Journal of Psychiatric and Mental Health Nursing,* 13, 665–672.

Hockley, J. and Clark, D. (2002) *Palliative Care for Older People in Care Homes.* Buckingham: Open University Press.

Johnson, M.J. (2006) Palliative Care for Patients with Heart Failure: Description of a Service. *Palliative Medicine,* 20, 211–214.

Kinghorn, S. and Gamlin, R. (2001) *Palliative Nursing: Bringing Comfort and Hope.* London: Baillière Tindall.

Kishi, Y., Robinson, R. and Kosier, J. (2001) Suicidal Ideation among Patients with Acute Life-threatening Physical Illness. Patients with Stroke, Traumatic Brain Injury, Myocardial Infarction, and Spinal Cord Injury. *Psychosomatics,* 42, 382–390.

Koenig, H.G. (1998) Depression in Hospitalized Older Patients with Congestive Heart Failure. *General Hospital Psychiatry,* 20, 29–43.

Kurella, M., Kimmel, P., Young, B. *et al.* (2005) Suicide in the United States End-stage Renal Disease Program. *Journal of the American Society of Nephrology,* 16, 774–781.

Lloyd-Williams, M. (2006) Depression, Anxiety and Confusion. In Fallon, M. and Hanks, G. (eds) *ABC of Palliative Care.* Oxford: Blackwell Publishing.

Lynn, J., Harrell, F., Cohen, F. *et al.* (1997) Prognoses of Seriously Ill Hospitalized Patients on the Days Before Death: Implications for Patient Care and Public Policy. *New Horizons,* 5, 56–61.

Marie Curie Cancer Care (2009) *About the Marie Curie Delivering Choice Programme.* Online. Available at: http://deliveringchoice.mariecurie.org.uk/about_the_delivering_choice_programme/ (accessed 9 April 2009).

McCarthy, M., Addington-Hall, J. and Ley, M. (1997) Communication and Choice in Dying from Heart Disease. *Journal of the Royal Society of Medicine,* 90(3), 128–131.

McCasland, L. (2007) Providing Hospice and Palliative Care to the Seriously and Persistently Mentally Ill. *Journal of Hospice and Palliative Nursing,* 9(6), 305–313.

McCormack, P. and Sharp, D. (2006) Palliative Care for People with Mental Health Problems. *European Journal of Palliative Care,* 13(5), 198–2001.

McKeown, A., Agar, R., Gambles, M. *et al.* (2008) Renal Failure and Specialist Palliative Care: An Assessment of Current Referral Practice. *International Journal of Palliative Nursing,* 14(9), 454–458.

Mok, E. and Chiu, P. (2004) Nurse–Patient Relationships in Palliative Care. *Journal of Advanced Nursing,* 48(5), 475–483.

Murray, S.A., Boyd, K., Kendall, M. *et al.* (2002) Dying of Lung Cancer or Cardiac Failure: Prospective Qualitative Interview Study of Patients and their Carers in the Community. *British Medical Journal,* 325, 929.

Murray, S.A., Kendall, M., Boyd, K. *et al.* (2005) Illness Trajectories and Palliative Care. *British Medical Journal,* 330, 107–1011.

National Audit Office (2005) *The NHS Cancer Plan: A Progress Report.* London: The Stationery Office.

National Audit Office (2008) *End of Life Care.* London: The Stationery Office.

National Council for Hospice and Specialist Palliative Care Services (NCHSPCS) (2000) *Positive Partnerships. Palliative Care for Adults with Severe Mental Health Problems.* Occasional Paper 17. London: NCHSPCS.

National Council for Hospice and Specialist Palliative Care Services (NCHSPCS) (2001) *Palliative Care Services for Different Ethnic Groups.* London: NCHSPCS.

National Council for Palliative Care (NCPC) (2005) *Briefing Bulletin No. 14.* London: NCPC.

National Council for Palliative Care (NCPC) (2006a) *Ethnicity, Older People and Palliative Care.* London: NCPC.

National Council for Palliative Care (NCPC) (2006b) The Assisted Dying for the Terminally Ill Bill 2005. London: NCPC.

National Council for Palliative Care (NCPC) (2007) Palliative Care Bill Unopposed in the House of Lords. *Information Exchange.* London: NCPC.

National Council for Palliative Care (NCPC) (2008) *Inside Palliative Care,* 5, 17–18.

National Institute for Health and Clinical Excellence (NICE) (2003) *Guidance on Cancer Services. Improving Outcomes in Haematological Cancers.* London: NICE.

National Institute for Health and Clinical Excellence (NICE) (2004) *Guidance on Cancer Services. Improving Supportive and Palliative Care for Adults with Cancer. The Manual.* London: NICE.

Noble, H., Meyer, J. and Bridges, J. (2007) Decision-making for Renal Patients at the End of Life. *European Journal of Palliative Care,* 14(5), 204–207.

Noble, H. and Kelly, D. (2006) Supportive and Palliative Care in End Stage Renal Failure: The Need for Further Research. *International Journal of Palliative Nursing,* 12(8), 362–376.

Paes, P. (2004) Breathlessness and Fatigue in Cardiac Failure. *European Journal of Palliative Care,* 11(1), 9–11.

Phair, L. (2007) Palliative and End-of-life Care. In Neno, R., Aveyard, B. and Heath, H. (eds) *Older People and Mental Health Nursing.* Oxford: Blackwell Publishing.

Proot, I.M., Abu-Saad, H.H., Muelen, R.H. *et al.* (2004) The Needs of Terminally Ill Patients at Home: Directing One's Life, Health and Things Related to Beloved Others. *Palliative Medicine,* 18, 53–61.

Robbins, M. (1997) Assessing Needs and Effectiveness: Is Palliative Care a Special Case? In Clark, D., Hockley, J. and Ahmedzai, S. (eds) *New Themes in Palliative Care.* Buckingham: Open University Press.

Rodin, G., Zimmermann, C., Rydall, A. *et al.* (2007) The Desire for Hastened Death in Patients with Metastatic Cancer. *Journal of Pain and Symptom Management,* 33(6), 661–675.

Rogers, A. (2003) The Interface Between Acute and Palliative Care: Acute Stroke. *European Journal of Palliative Care,* 10(6), 236–238.

Royal College of Physicians (RCP) (2007) *Palliative Care Services. Meeting the Needs of Patients. Report of a Working Party.* London: RCP.

Royal College of Physicians (RCP) (2009) *Concise Guidance to Good Practice. Number 12. Advance Care Planning. National Guidelines.* London. Online. Available at: www.rcplondon.ac.uk/pubs/contents/9c95f6ea-c57e-4db8-bd98-fc12ba31c8fe.pdf (accessed 9 April 2009).

Seamark, D., Blake., S., Seamark, C. *et al.* (2004) Living with Severe Chronic Obstructive Pulmonary Disease (COPD): Perceptions of Patients and Their Carers. An Interpretative Phenomenological Analysis. *Palliative Medicine*, 18, 619–625.

Seymour, J., Clark, D. and Marples, R. (2002) Palliative Care and Policy in England: A Review of Health Improvement Plans for 1999–2003. *Palliative Medicine*, 16, 5–11.

Shah, S. (2005) The Liverpool Care Pathway: Its Impact on Improving the Care of the Dying. *Age and Ageing*, 34(2), 197.

Starace, F. and Sherr, L. (1998) Suicidal Behaviours, Euthanasia and AIDS. *AIDS*, 12, 339–347.

Stenager, E., Madsen, C., Stenager, E. *et al.* (1998) Suicide in Patients with Stroke: Epidemiological Study. *British Medical Journal*, 316(7139), 1206.

Waern, M., Rubenowitz, E., Runeson, B. *et al.* (2002) Burden of Illness and Suicide in Elderly People: Case-control Study. *British Medical Journal*, 321(1355), 1–4.

Weiskopf, C.S. (2005) Nurses' Experience of Caring for Inmate Patients. *Journal of Advanced Nursing*, 49(4), 336–343.

Wood, F. (2007) The Challenge of Providing Palliative Care to Terminally Ill Prison Inmates in the UK. *International Journal of Palliative Nursing*, 13(3), 131–134.

World Health Organisation (WHO) (2002) *National Cancer Control Programme: Policies and Management Guidelines* (2nd edn). Geneva: WHO.

Index